# (Re)designing the Continuum of Care for Older Adults

Farhana Ferdous • Emily Roberts
Editors

# (Re)designing the Continuum of Care for Older Adults

The Future of Long-Term Care Settings

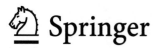 Springer

*Editors*
Farhana Ferdous
Department of Architecture
Howard University
Washington, DC, USA

Emily Roberts
Oklahoma State University
Stillwater, OK, USA

ISBN 978-3-031-20969-7        ISBN 978-3-031-20970-3    (eBook)
https://doi.org/10.1007/978-3-031-20970-3

This Springer imprint is published by the registered company Springer Nature Switzerland AG
The registered company address is: Gewerbestrasse 11, 6330 Cham, Switzerland

# Foreword

The title of this timely volume highlights the pressing need for re-examining and revisioning the current long-term care system. Kane and Kane[1] (p. 4) defined long-term care as "a set of health, personal care and social services delivered over a sustained period of time to persons who have lost or never acquired some degree of functional capacity." Although this definition captures the core mandate of the long-term care provision, especially in North America over the decades, upon closer examination, it also suggests where we may have missed the mark. By and large, the ethic of care and caring for health and personal care has been predominantly shaped by clinical and health-related quality of life outcomes, largely foregoing the complex and integrated reality of older adults in their psychological, social, cultural, and spiritual inclinations. The relational nature of caring with the potential of independence and interdependence has been generally relegated to a unidimensional and undifferentiated framing of care. We have come far in the movement promoting person-centered care or person-oriented care in the last several decades, but not far or fast enough to have a transformational and systemic change of culture in long-term care.

Long-term care in the nursing home context is currently going through a critical phase after the pandemic's effect on outbreaks in the care facilities and resulting high number of deaths of residents and staff. The sobering reality of the pandemic has raised the curtain that has kept the systemic gaps and fault lines in our long-term care system out of our collective sight for decades. Important to note that the challenges faced by residents, care staff, and administration in this time of crisis do not represent failure or shortcoming of any particular group of organizations, providers, or individuals, rather they are indicative of the limitations at the macro levels of social values and resulting structural mechanisms and culture of care to provide long-term care. Regrettably, it has taken an outbreak of COVID-19 proportions to make those challenges come to sharp focus in our collective consciousness. In this

---

[1] Kane, R. A., & Kane, R. L. (1987). *Long-term care: Principles, programs and policies.* New York, NY: Springer Publishing Company.

critical time to re-envision long-term care that may embrace a transformational change of the current system and culture, this edited volume is a timely contribution to shed light on the care innovations, challenges, and potentials in this care sector.

This volume offers an impressive collection of multidisciplinary contributions on diverse settings of long-term care, as well as on a myriad of topics spanning the continuum of long-term care, including gerotechnology, community-based care, diverse ethnicity of the residents, design for people with dementia, acute care, end-of-life care, adaptive reuse, impact of COVID-19, and continuing care retirement community (CCRC). It is worthwhile to note the overlap of the topics across setting types, such as the technology innovations and rehabilitation options in both care facilities and community. Several innovative projects and non-traditional options are part of this volume, such as the Rehabilitation and Architecture project (REARCH), Adult Family Care (AFC), adaptive reuse of closed malls, vertical CCRC, etc.

The readers of this volume will be challenged and rewarded with an in-depth understanding of distinct, yet complementary topics in long-term care that are relevant for contemporary times. Collectively, the chapters provide layers of insights on public policies, quality of care practices, and residents' quality of life, as impacted by the characteristics of the setting type, built environment, social contexts, and technological solutions. The diversity of topics covered in the volume is a testament to the complexity of what we know as long-term care; we can appreciate that making reforms in the current system is neither easy nor clear-cut. Nonetheless, the authors provide us a clear understanding of the challenges, highlight solutions, and shed light on pathways to move forward in a constructive way for improved care and support for older adults with disability who need support and care on an ongoing basis.

The continuum of long-term care that consists of community-based home care, institutional long-term care facilities, memory care, etc. is arguably here to stay for the foreseeable future. However, in the context of community-based care to foster aging-in-place, it is important to generate innovative solutions to unbundle the location-based care in more institutional settings and decentralize care and support in the community, e.g., community-based healthcare hubs. The community at large could also serve as a social ecosystem for interactions, activities, and support, which is a critical component in the older adults' functioning and quality of life. There is no one solution for the provision of long-term care, rather the settings and care levels need to recognize the diverse care and social needs of older adults in the community. Many older adults are "stuck in place" and would benefit in relocating to a congregate care setting, as many others with strong informal support networks, may thrive in their current communities with additional support.

Given the reality of the pandemic, it is important to share some reflections on the role of the physical environment of a care facility on infection prevention and control. Although it is too early to have substantial evidence on the built environmental impact on outbreak management or mitigation, based on emergent evidence, we can note the advantages of self-contained small homes (e.g., 12–16 bed households) with a clustered arrangement of rooms, activity, and dining areas—for more effective infection prevention and control, responsive management of residents with dementia, and care interactions. Smaller group size provides the option to compartmentalize residents who might be at greater risk of infection, as well as isolate residents who are infected. Separating or grouping residents on floors with more than 60 residents and rooms with 2–4 residents is highly challenging. In conjunction with physical isolation, dedicated staffing would need to be established for affected residents to minimize transmission of the virus in the facility through staff. A majority of the residents in care homes live with cognitive decline and may have difficulty adhering to social distancing from other residents. They may have higher levels of anxiety at a time of isolation along with the reduced number of planned activities. A smaller group size facilitated by a household setting can provide the much-needed hands-on or close-proximity care and support from staff at a time of an outbreak. Beyond the possible benefit of outbreak prevention and control, there is evidence on the positive influence of small homes or household model on increasing residents' social engagement levels, decreasing anxiety and aggression, supporting mobility, and reducing use of psychotropic medications.

This is a time to galvanize our collective will and commitment to make meaningful and sustainable reform in long-term care on policy and practices by re-envisioning the current care model. There is no better time to embrace innovative care approaches, increase financial resources to support policies and practices that prioritize residents' safety and quality of life, staff safety and work culture, investments in physical infrastructure, higher staffing ratios, consistent staffing models, and increased wages for care aides. We are at a crossroads for long-term care homes. Let's have an honest discussion on the question—how can we create a community of care that is authentic and honors our elders and their care partners (healthcare workers and families) in providing a safe environment without compromising dignity, values, and comfort? How do we unbundle long-term care from care facilities and bring it to community homes more effectively and sustainably? A coordinated national effort is needed to focus on ramping up promising efforts and generating innovative solutions. If we don't act to meaningfully change the related policies and practices in the foreseeable future, tomorrow may become the same as yesterday's news as we flip back to the past "normal" in a default mode of operation. This is the charge and challenge in the coming days.

The contributions in this volume do not make unrealistic claims or far-fetched promises, instead they offer useful insights into a host of salient topics in long-term care that need to be thoughtfully engaged with to advance our understanding of the challenges and potentials, and subsequently identify areas for impacting policy and practice. The need for providing long-term care to those of us who need that support is here to stay, regardless of the location of care. This is the time for a moral response on part of the policy-makers, care providers, healthcare professionals, and industry stakeholders to pay serious considerations to these ongoing and emergent issues and take necessary actions to create a more meaningful and effective generation of "long-term care" for our current and future older adults needing ongoing care.

Chair and Professor, Department of Gerontology          Habib Chaudhury
Simon Fraser University,
Vancouver, BC, Canada

# Preface

## Continuum of Care Environments in the Post-COVID-19 Era

The global population of adults 65 years of age and older will increase dramatically over the next several decades, presenting economic and social challenges requiring sustainable solutions. These health and socioeconomic challenges will have implications for individuals older than 65 years and their families and communities, requiring integrated solutions that should be addressed simultaneously through the lens of realistic and evidence-based goals. The future design of aging programs, environments, and technologies may then support intergenerational solidarity and include specific targets to reduce inequalities between women and men, multiple generations, older populations, and among different subgroups, with particular attention being paid to vulnerable populations who are marginalized. While there is a growing body of research relating to these factors, there is less focus on the continuum of long-term care settings on residents' health, functioning, and quality of life along with associated design strategies on several unexamined issues in the continuum of care.

*(Re)designing the Continuum of Care for Older Adults: The Future of Long-Term Care Settings* presents a collection of essays focusing on the role of the built environment in the continuum of long-term care by representing recent advances in theoretical understanding, methodological innovations, and empirical evidence. This edited volume offers contributions from notable researchers and scholars in environmental gerontology and healthcare architecture on new and emergent research that can effectively inform and reshape the planning and design of long-term care environments. With diverse topics in theory, substantive issues, and methods, the volume covers a range of innovative programming, environments, and technologies which can impact the changing needs and support for older adults and their families across the continuum of care.

Recently, almost all healthcare settings have been particularly hard-hit by the novel coronavirus (COVID-19) pandemic, which can be lethal to older adults with or without any underlying health conditions. The double societal hit of our aging community and infectious disease outbreaks like COVID-19 have raised great concerns for the future of care settings for older adults in need of long-term care. The Centers for Disease Control and Prevention (CDC) have reported that 8 out of 10 deaths in the USA have been in adults 65 years or older due to COVID-19 (CDC, 2020). The confined living arrangements in some care settings (i.e., sometimes 3 or 4 residents to a room), combined with understaffing and failure to comply with infection-control guidelines, have been associated with high infectious disease rates across the USA. In addition to the need for improved safety precautions for infection control, it is imperative that mental health and psychosocial support be concurrently delivered, calling attention to the urgent need for alternatives to traditional care settings.

The lessons we have learned through the COVID-19 health crisis about staffing shortages, turnover, and dangerously confining environments allow us to broaden the lens on new care environments that are designed to be inclusive, progressive, and convergent with the needs of an aging population. When considering the physical environment of care facilities, both the ambient environment and specific design features are considered as key elements that could influence the physiological and psychological health and well-being of its immediate users. This volume has four thematic sections which focus on (1) home and community-based care, (2) facility-based care, (3) memory and end-of-life care, and (4) evidence-based applied projects and next steps. This comprehensive view of the continuum of long-term care environments for older adults addresses the physical environment, design context, theoretical underpinnings, strengths and limitations of contemporary practice, and future care opportunities. Instead of taking one side of the above views, each subset of chapters will open up the grounds for critical discussions that are much needed in this design and research sector.

## Part I: Home and Community-Based Care

Social separation is a significant public health issue and is linked to vulnerability in negative mental health outcomes. This book section addresses this confluence of issues relating to home care and family caregiving. The physical and mental challenges of aging can impact how an older adult takes care of activities of daily living at home such as bathing, eating, and toileting, calling to attention the adjustments in the home that can create a supportive, safe, and engaging environment. These adjustments are not only important for the individual in need of support, but for family members who provide care and who may have problems with balance and frailty, and/or struggling mobility themselves. Adjustments in the home environment may also include technologies to aid in reducing social isolation, as COVID-19 has pushed many lives at home into isolation while reducing the availability of medical services.

In *Bridging the Digital Divide: Smart Aging-in-Place and the Future of Gerontology*, Rotem Arieli, Manuela E. Faulhaber, and Alex J. Bishop explore the impact of the emerging field of gerontechnology in aging-in-place for older adults who wish to remain in their home. They provide an overview of the literature related to older adults' use, access, barriers, and understanding of assistive smart technologies, emphasizing current gaps and future directions. In an aligned chapter entitled *How Environmentally Embedded In-Home Sensors Are Revolutionizing Independent Living and Family Caregiving: A Literature Review*, Dr. Kari Lane and Erin L. Robinson describe the influence that in-home sensors can play in enabling independence for care recipients and caregivers in the home. They argue embedded sensors can have an impact on the health of older adults and may assist older adults in living independently longer. They explore how older adults feel about accepting this technology in their homes and privacy issues are also discussed. This is followed by the chapter, *The Home as a Place for Rehabilitation After Stroke* by Marie Elf and Maya Kylén. Elf and Kylén use empirical research to describe the experiences of post-stroke individuals living at home. They address findings within the REARCH (Rehabilitation and Architecture) project, and the purpose was to explore environmental factors to fulfill person-centered rehabilitation. In the final chapter of Part I, Kelly Munly, Karen A. Roberto, and Katherine R. Allen explore the benefits of home-like settings for adult family care (AFC). They provide a brief history of AFC and present findings from a qualitative study that explored experiences of how they navigated their own personal circumstances.

## Part II: Facility-Based Care

This book section enumerates the unique issues and themes relating to physical and philosophical programmatic change in facility-based care occurring both in the USA and internationally. While the COVID-19 pandemic has been highlighted with images of older adults who are quarantined in closed long-term care settings, research prior to the pandemic highlights key frameworks relating to culture change and the small house model of care. These frameworks include shared goals, expectations, and consistency in leadership; frontline staff empowerment through the strength of teamwork; and the balance of choice, risk, and autonomy for residents in these settings. The physical environment has a direct impact on the social environment in these care settings, and while the actuality of "home" is a very personal distinction based on the history and past preferences of each individual, the shared themes in this section relate to the core elements of long-term care: the need for and the provision of care.

Leading off for Part II, Sheila L. Molony and Jude Rabig provide a background to theory of at-homeness in long-term care in *A Theory of Creating At-Homeness Across the Long-Term Care Continuum*. At-homeness is an experience of person-environment harmony that holds the potential for thriving in residential long-term care. The theory introduces the concept of *at-homeness* as a central construct to integrate theories of caring and thriving with key constructs related to deinstitutionalization, person-centered care, placemaking, and pattern language. In the following chapter, Alex J. Bishop and colleagues explore the potential of robotic health assistants in facility-based care in a chapter entitled *The Evolution and Rise of Robotic Health Assistants: The New Human-Machine Frontier of Geriatric Home Care.* The chapter identifies and conceptualizes functional elements necessary for successful adoption of robotic technology within geriatric healthcare environments. Maja Kevdzija then addresses the need to reconsider the design of rehabilitation clinics for stroke recovery in *Rehabilitation Clinics That Enhance Stroke Recovery: Rethinking the Same-for-All Design Approach.* The chapter aims to explore the possibilities for designing rehabilitation clinics that support patients' activity and well-being during recovery. Maja introduces a new perspective on the design of rehabilitation clinics to creating specifically designed environments for different rehabilitation goals. In the final chapter of Part II, Shreemouna Gurung and Habib Chaudhury address the importance of the individuality of preferences through person-centered care in resident mealtimes in the chapter entitled *Exploring the Role of the Built Environment in Person-Centered Care During Mealtimes in an Ethno-Specific Long-Term Care Home.* This chapter offers insights on how the built environment influences mealtime care practices in an ethno-specific care home that promotes person-centered care (PCC).

## Part III: Memory Care and End-of-Life Care

This book section addresses issues relating to memory care for individuals living with dementia. It is estimated that 5.4 million Americans have some form of dementia and these numbers are expected to rise in the coming decades, leading to an unprecedented demand for specialized programs, housing, and services. Historically a biomedical approach to dementia care has focused on symptoms, deficits, and emotionally charged metaphors about dementia that have influenced overall public perceptions. In response to these negative public perceptions, stakeholders in development, government agencies, and care administration have been moved to search for innovative options to create more autonomy and quality of life for individuals living with dementia in their care settings and communities. In addition, the values and norms of end-of-life care have been tested by COVID-19, yet environments to support choices for individuals at the end of life and their family members continue to advance. The final chapter in this section explores options for in-home services and facility-based settings at the end of life which are designed to provide comfort care as well as support for family members. Both nationally and internationally hospice and palliative care in hospital wards are being replaced by purpose-built care centers with multiple amenities such as family apartments, libraries, and centers for family gatherings.

Jeffrey Anderzhon starts off Part III with his broad chapter on the importance of design in memory care settings entitled *Designing for Dementia: An Approach That Works for Everyone.* This chapter discusses how dementia-specific environmental design has evolved, providing an appropriate stage for resident-centered care and for integrated programming that celebrates the individual. Kate de Medieros then applies similar reasoning in the exploration of the significance of how designed space can impact individuals living with dementia in the chapter *Communication and Environmental Positioning in Dementia Care Units: Dialogues Through Space and Place*. By presenting the illustrative case study, this chapter considers how staff and residents use conversational positioning to construct power relationships and identities. In the chapter entitled *Adaptive Reuse of Closed Malls for Dementia Programs and Services: Community Focus Group Feedback*, Emily Roberts and Heather Carlile Carter share community feedback on conceptual design for adaptive reuse of commercial spaces for dementia housing, programs, and services. This article describes the qualitative work by a Midwestern University research team and highlighted five principle themes relating to the barriers and benefits of adaptive reuse. Gesine Marquardt and Kathrin Bueter discuss the need for addressing how acute care facilities impact individuals with dementia in the chapter entitled *Extending the Continuum of Care for People with Dementia: Building Resilience*. The chapter transfers the evidence-based research findings into hospital design and elucidates ways to implement design criteria in acute care settings. The authors argue that dementia-friendly design criteria can help to build a continuum of care in hospital environments. In the final chapter of Part III, Sharmin Kader addresses design for end-of-life care settings in the chapter entitled *Designing the Post-Pandemic Hospice Environment: "The Last Place."* This chapter discusses eleven therapeutic goals of hospice care environment for dying experiences. The author argued that the physical settings of hospice along with the carefully designed organizational environment can contribute to the realization of desired therapeutic goals and have a positive effect on individuals at the end of life.

## Part IV: Evidence-Based Applied Projects and Next Steps

The evidence-based and applied projects section includes contributions presenting lessons learned to assist design professionals, educators, and policy-makers to develop care environments that are more effective in infection prevention, control, and social connectedness through evidence-based practices. This book section addresses the complex and multilayered impact of infectious disease outbreaks like COVID-19 on the trajectory of care for an aging population. By emphasizing different modes of applied design projects, the aim of this section is to bridge the gap between evidence-based research and practice-based design projects in the continuum of care settings. Significant discussion has come out of the COVID-19 pandemic throughout the healthcare industry and government agencies about necessary conversions of existing care settings, as well as the need for expanded quarantine and general patient care spaces in the time of a pandemic. Social isolation due to social distancing and quarantine is also impacting the mental and psychological well-being of older communities (Cudjoe & Kotwal, 2020). The design of spatial and physical environment of care facilities is an important aspect toward these steps, and the evidence-based applied projects section addresses these challenges by using the examples from practice-based design projects within long-term care environments. The chapters of this section show a diverse range of built and unbuilt project examples along with theoretical construct aligned within the global context of care environments.

Valerie Greer and Keith Diaz Moore lead off Part IV with the chapter entitled *Autonomy, Identity and Design in the COVID-19 Era*, describing the lessons learned across the continuum of care during the COVID-19 pandemic. They specifically examine independent housing and skilled care with a focus on how physical settings and technological systems can empower autonomy and identity in response to vulnerabilities exposed by the COVID-19 pandemic. In the chapter *Creating a Tailored Approach: The Transformation of Jewish Senior Life*, Emily Chmielewski and Melissa DeStout of Perkins Eastman architecture firm explore real-world outcomes of culture change in long-term care in a case study. They outline the design goals of both renovation and new construction and explain the process of redesigning the physical environment using research-based evidence to make more informed decisions. Upali Nanda and Grant Warner of HKS Architects share their research framework of enriched environments and illustrate the principles through a robust case study "The Vista at CC YOUNG" in the chapter entitled *Flexible and Enriched Environments for Senior Living and Aging-in-Place in Dense Urban Environments*. Similarly, Hui Cai, Caroline Coleman, and Dani Kolker share their case study in changing paradigms in *Envisioning Innovative Post-COVID Approaches Toward LTCF Design in Dense Urban Areas: Exploring an Evidence-Based Design Prototype*. They provide an extensive review and synthesis of the lessons learned from long-term care settings during and after the pandemic. Closing out this section, six colleagues of Gensler architecture firm address the next steps in approaching the care needs of an aging in the chapter entitled *Realizing the Future of Intergenerational Environments for Aging Through Design Research*. The Boomtown framework is an intergenerational community model that outlines recommendations and targeted interventions for physical and social architecture to promote longevity and make connection among its residents. In this chapter, Boomtown framework presents a conceptual model of intergenerational communities in which all people, regardless of generation or culture, can actively age in place.

*(Re)designing the Continuum of Care for Older Adults: The Future of Long-Term Care Settings* offers a framework of scholarship to provide a better understanding of advanced research and design of the built environment in specialized healthcare settings through a critical discussion of theoretical, methodological, and empirical evidence. More specifically, this volume presents a variety of the built environments in continuum of care through theoretical constructs and design features, as well as up-to-date empirical research findings in guiding new research and design. The key idea is to emphasize emergent, evidence-based design research and practice that can effectively inform and reshape the planning and design of long-term care environments in the future. By simultaneously focusing on theory and scholarship through in-depth essays and case studies, this book looks fundamentally toward the future. The volume can be used as a resource for all care administrators, healthcare design

professionals, and researchers in addressing design challenges and rethinking current/ contemporary issues in redesigning future care facilities.

Washington, DC, USA
Stillwater, OK, USA

Farhana Ferdous
Emily Roberts

# References

CDC. (2020). *Centers for disease control and prevention: COVID-19 and older adults.* Centers for Disease Control and Prevention. Retrieved 9 Nov 2020 from https://www.cdc.gov/coronavirus/2019-ncov/need-extra-precautions/older-adults.html

Cudjoe, T. K. M., & Kotwal, A. A. (2020, Jun). "Social distancing" amid a crisis in social isolation and loneliness. *Journal of the American Geriatrics Society, 68*(6), E27–E29. https://doi.org/10.1111/jgs.16527

Ferdous, F. (2021, Jan–Dec). Social distancing vs social interaction for older adults at long-term care facilities in the midst of the COVID-19 pandemic: A rapid review and synthesis of action plans. *Inquiry, 58*, 469580211044287. https://doi.org/10.1177/00469580211044287

# Contents

# About the Editors and Contributors

## Editors

**Farhana Ferdous, PhD**, is an assistant professor in the Department of Architecture at Howard University. She is an educator, designer, and scholar whose teaching and research career span the continents of South Asia, Australia, and North America. She continues to make symbiotic interconnections between design, practice, and research, especially one which is focused on health, design, and marginalized African American or aging population. Her inclusive teaching style and evidence-based pedagogical philosophy integrate diversity and communities of color by making symbiotic interconnections between two facets of architecture: environment and design. As an environmental gerontologist, Dr. Ferdous has published widely on urban and environmental design and environmental psychology for the elderly. Her co-edited volume *All-Inclusive Engagement in Architecture: Towards the Future of Social Change* published by Routledge (2021) is a groundbreaking critical discourse focusing on the impact of social engagement in architecture. Her scholarship has been supported by several research grants including from the American Association of University Women (AAUW) Fellowship (2013), Grantmakers in Aging (GIA) Fellowship (2013), Academy of Architecture for Health Foundation (2017), Toyota Individual Research Grant (2018), Graham Foundation Grant (2021), Alzheimer's Association Research Grant (2021), Innovations in Pedagogy/Teaching Fellowship (2021), and National Endowment for Humanities Fellowship (2022).

**Emily Roberts, PhD**, is an associate professor of Interior Design at Oklahoma State University and has a research focus in Environmental Gerontology, the study of the person-environment fit between older adults and the physical environment. She holds a PhD in Architectural Studies and a Master's degree in Gerontology from the University of Missouri-Columbia. She previously attained a Masters of Architecture from the University of New Mexico. As an Environmental Gerontologist, Dr. Roberts has studied the factors involved in aging in place, as well as evolving models of long-term care, particularly for older adults with dementia and their families. Dr. Roberts has conducted research in the United States, Europe, and Canada, focusing on government-funded community-based long-term care programs. She serves on the Editorial Board of the *Journal of Aging and Environment* and *Inquiry: The Journal of Health Care Organization, Provision and Financing* and serves as the Environmental Gerontology network chair for the Environmental Design Research Association.

## Contributors

**Katherine R. Allen** is Professor Emerita of Human Development and Family Science, Virginia Tech. She received the Ernest Burgess Award and the Alexis Walker Award, both given for lifetime achievement in scholarly contributions to family science from the National Council on Family Relations. She studies marginalization, vulnerability, reflexivity, and innovation over the family life course using feminist, intersectional, and qualitative approaches. Her recent work includes intergenerational family tensions around technology, lesbian mothers' experiences with relational dissolution and child loss, older women's family relationships when surviving gynecological cancer, and the interconnection among scholarship, pedagogy, and praxis using autoethnographic and critical approaches.

**Jeffrey Anderzhon, FIFA**, is an architect specializing in environments for the elderly and is Principal at Crepidoma Consulting, LLC. He holds a Bachelor of Architecture degree from Illinois Institute of Technology, is a past member of the Alumni Board of Directors, and received the 2008 Alumni Professional Achievement Award. He is a member of the College of Fellows, American Institute of Architects and co-author of the books *Design for Aging Post Occupancy Evaluations: Lessons Learned from Senior Living Environments* and *Design for Aging, International Case Studies of Building and Program* and has written numerous articles on environments for the elderly. He served as the 2006 Chair for the AIA Design for Aging Knowledge Community; 2007 and 2011 Jury Chair; 2009 juror for the International Association of Homes and Services for the Ageing Design Symposium; and juror for the Design for Future Aging, Student Competition, Yonsei University, Seoul, Korea, in 2006 and 2007.

**Rotem Arieli** is a PhD candidate in Human Development and Family Studies at Iowa State University. She has a Master of Science degree in Human Development and Family Studies from Iowa State University and a Bachelor of Science degree in Family Studies and Human Development from Kansas State University. Rotem has presented her research at state, national, and international conferences, receiving the 2021 Young Research Investigator Award at the International Centenarian Consortium. She recently co-authored a book chapter focused on environmental supports for centenarians (people aged 100+), and her current research focuses on the well-being and social health of older adults, with active interests in gerontechnology, social support, and exceptional longevity.

**Alex J. Bishop, PhD, FGSA**, is a professor in the Human Development and Family Science Department and the Bryan Close Professor of Adulthood and Aging in the

College of Education and Human Sciences at Oklahoma State University, Stillwater, Oklahoma. He is also a fellow member of the Gerontological Society of America. Dr. Bishop maintains an interest in examining well-being among old and very old adults who age in place. Of particular interest is understanding how socially assistive robotic technology can be used to passively and actively monitor the health and well-being of homebound older adults receiving home healthcare services. Dr. Bishop's work is focused on integrating technology-based applications, innovations, and education to further modernize the home healthcare industry and enhance the future of work in geriatric care.

**Kathrin Bueter** is a post-doctoral research associate at the Chair of Social and Health Care Buildings and Design in the Faculty of Architecture at Technische Universität Dresden, Germany. Her work focuses on designing architecture for persons living with dementia. Recent publications include a Construction and Design Manual on Dementia-friendly Hospital Buildings. In 2017, she completed a doctoral thesis at TU Dresden with a dissertation on "Dementia-friendly Acute Care Hospitals." She graduated from the University of Applied Sciences and Arts Hannover with a Master's degree in Interior Design in 2011, with a final thesis on designing dementia-friendly holiday accommodation.

**Hui Cai, PhD**, is Associate Professor and Chair at the Department of Architecture, and Associate Director of the Institute of Health and Wellness Design at the University of Kansas. Cai received her PhD degree from the Georgia Institute of Technology. Dr. Cai's research focuses on using evidence-based design approach to analyze the relationship between culture, human behavior, and the physical environment in healthcare settings and healthy communities. Cai disseminates her work extensively through numerous publications in academic journals. She has received several awards, including the International Academy Award for Best Research project, AIA-AAH/AAH Foundation Burgun Fellowship, 2021 HCD 10 Healthcare Design Educator, 2021 Foundation for Health Environments Research Grant, and the inaugural Wilbur H (Tib) Tusler, Jr. Health Design Research Prize. She serves on the Board of Directors for Environment Design and Research Association.

**Barbara W. Carlson, RN, PhD, FGSA**, is the Ziegler Endowed Chair in Nursing Science and Associate Dean for Research, Scholarship, and PhD Studies at the Fran and Earl Ziegler College of Nursing. Her research focuses on cerebral blood flow during sleep and cognitive decline in older adults. A national expert in biobehavioral science, her work involves the design and application of minimally invasive physiological sensors and wearable devices, signal processing and analysis, behavioral observation methods, neurocognitive testing, inflammatory/immune markers, epigenetics, and the integration of physiologic and behavioral measures. Her current randomized clinical trial examines impact of vaccines to boost innate immunity in nursing home residents.

**Heather Carlile Carter** completed her PhD in Human Environmental Sciences with an emphasis in Architectural Studies at the University of Missouri, Columbia. She has an active research program. Her interests include the impact of material culture on place meanings, older person residential care environments, sustainable environments, and interior design pedagogy. One of Dr. Carter's areas of focus is people's behavior within and attachment to their interior environments, particularly how older people transition out of the houses they live in for many years and what possessions they choose to keep to make place in their new environments. She is a professional member of the Interior Design Educators Council (IDEC), the American Society of Interior Design (ASID), and the International Interior Design Association (IIDA). She has National Interior Design Qualifications (NCIDQ) certification and is a US Green Building Council's Leadership in Energy and Environmental Design Accredited Professional (LEED AP).

**Habib Chaudhury, PhD**, is Professor in the Department of Gerontology, Simon Fraser University, Canada. He has extensive research experience in the field of environmental gerontology. He conducts research and consulting work in the following areas: physical environment for people with dementia in long-term care facilities, memories of home and personhood in dementia, community planning and urban design for active aging, and dementia-friendly communities. Projects have been funded by the Public Health Agency of Canada (PHAC), Canadian Institute of Health Research (CIHR), Social Science and Humanities Research Council (SSHRC), Canada Mortgage and Housing Corporation (CMHC), CapitalCare Foundation, and the Centre for Health Design. Published books include *Environments in an Aging Society: Autobiographical Perspectives in Environmental Gerontology* (*Annual Review of Gerontology and Geriatrics*, Vol 38, 2018; co-edited with F. Oswald), *Remembering Home: Rediscovering the Self in Dementia* (Johns Hopkins University Press, 2008), and *Home and Identity in Later Life: International Perspectives* (Springer Publishing Company, 2005; co-edited with G. Rowles). Dr. Chaudhury conducts research consulting with various national and international organizations in the areas of planning and design of senior housing and long-term care facilities. He is also affiliated with the Centre for Research on Personhood in Dementia at the University of British Columbia, Vancouver, and Alzheimer Catalonia, Barcelona, Spain. He serves as the Editor-in-Chief of the *Journal of Aging and Environment*

**Emily Chmielewski, EDAC**, is a founding member, senior associate, and director of Perkins Eastman's Design Research Department, an industry forerunner of practice-based environment-behavior research. She is an advocate for research in practice and helps create better-built environments by pushing the boundaries of professional knowledge and improving environmental design through design research. Emily's research primarily focuses on senior living and K-12 educational environments. Her studies have ranged from concise environmental audits that gather major lessons learned to more in-depth research that evaluates multiple aspects of a facility's physical environment and building occupants' satisfaction and use patterns.

**Caroline Coleman, Assoc. AIA, EDAC,** is a Project Coordinator in the Healthcare design group at The Beck Group in Dallas, Texas office. Coleman received her undergraduate degree in Architectural Studies and Master of Architecture degree at the University of Kansas. During her graduate education in Kansas, Coleman was selected to study at the Institute of Health and Wellness Design where she completed research exploring the impact of health on community resilience. In collaboration with Dani Kolker, Coleman developed a prototype continuous care retirement community as her final capstone project. Her project received honorable mention for the student work, Healthcare Environment Award.

**Tama Duffy Day, FACHE, FASID, FIIDA, LEED AP,** is a Principal, the Global Leader of the Senior Living Practice, and an advisor to the Health Sector at Gensler. A leader in the health industry for over four decades, she challenges conventional thinking and develops solutions to reimagine longevity in an age-inclusive world. Actively leading projects across the world, she is a frequent speaker at events and conferences such as Milken Institute's "Future of Health" Summit, the Agile Ageing Alliance "Societies Leaders Forum," Environments for Aging, and the Mayo Clinic "Transform." Her work has been published in *Forbes*, *Interior Design* magazine, *Fast Company,* and *The McMorrow Reports*. She is an active member of Women in Healthcare and is on the Washington, DC Mayor's Age-Friendly Task Force. She serves on the boards of the Capitol Hill Village and The CARITAS Project and on Advisory Boards for the Healthcare Facilities Symposium, Marymount University, and Medical Construction and *Design* Magazine. A frequent author and blogger, she has hosted and been a guest on numerous podcasts featured on the Gensler Design Exchange platform on topics ranging from Equity by Design and Psycho-Oncology, to Sound Health and Rethinking Patient-Centered Design. She is one of the few design professionals inducted as a fellow into the American College of Healthcare Executives.

**Kate de Medeiros, PhD,** is the O'Toole Professor of Gerontology in the Department of Sociology and Gerontology, a research fellow at the Scripps Gerontology Center, and an affiliate faculty member in the Women, Gender, and Sexuality Studies program at Miami University, Oxford, Ohio. Her dementia-related research includes work on living alone with dementia, risk and value in nursing homes, the meaning of place and friendships in long-term care, self and personhood, and the role of the participatory arts in improving quality of life. She co-developed (with C. Lyketsos) the Neuropsychiatric Inventory Clinician Rated assessment, a revised tool to measure behavioral changes in people with dementia. Her other age-related research has focused on narratives in later life, the meaning of suffering in old age, and agist language and practice. Her research has been funded by the National Institutes of Health and the Alzheimer's Association. She has authored or co-authored four books on aging, over 45 journal articles, and numerous book chapters. She is currently the editor of *Narrative Works*, a journal which includes narrative scholarship from a variety of disciplines.

**Melissa DeStout, AIA, LEED AP BD+C, CPHD,** is a senior associate and architect at Perkins Eastman, specializing in designing environments with senior living providers across the United States. Her work ranges from complex renovations to new construction across all levels of care. She frequently works with clients from early strategic and master planning efforts through to the completion of the work in a project management role. Melissa's passion for the well-being of the residents and staff occupying her designs as well as her love of nature have led her to focus her work in senior living on sustainable concepts, particularly biophilic design.

**Stella Donovan** is a Research Communications Strategist for the Gensler Research Institute. She translates research from teams around the world into engaging and actionable deliverables. She has received numerous editorial awards and prizes, including a recent Hermes Award for Gensler's Research Catalogue, Volume 3. Prior to Gensler, Stella worked as a book editor for social science publications.

**Marie Elf** is a Professor of Nursing at Dalarna University in the Department of Nursing. I have a position as program director for the nursing program. I am originally qualified as a nurse, have a PhD in architecture, and have since worked across several academic environments in nursing, architecture, and health services with a focus on architecture and its impact on the patient's health and well-being. Ever since I graduated in healthcare architecture, I have devoted myself to research to provide evidence on the built environment and its impact on the health and well-being of older people and patients with stroke. Today I combine my knowledge of nursing and architecture in my research. I lead several projects with a focus on care and rehabilitation at home for people with frail health. My research includes person-centered care, participation, and support for self-care – always with a question about how the environment looks like and is experienced: Is it promoting or hindering?

**Manuela E. Faulhaber** is a PhD student in Human-Computer Interaction at Iowa State University. She holds a Master of Science degree in Human-Computer Interaction as well as a Bachelor's degree in Psychology and Sociology, both from Iowa State University. Ella has presented research at over a dozen national and international conferences and co-authored a book chapter on Internet Gaming Disorder. She is a recipient of the Vera Whinery Memorial Scholarship, International Merit Scholarship, and Mary Zetta Lind Scholarship Award. Her research interests include user research, technology, and social media.

**Valerie Greer, AIA, LEED AP**, is an assistant professor in the School of Architecture and a faculty affiliate with the Center on Aging at the University of Utah. A licensed architect with experience working from design through construction on complex building types, Valerie teaches studios and seminars that investigate themes of social, environmental, and health impact. Her research focuses on design and health environments, resilient places for aging, and adaption to climate change. Valerie is currently a principal investigator on a research project that utilizes photovoice methods to investigate healthy aging in place during the COVID-19 pandemic.

**Shreemouna Gurung** is PhD candidate in the Department of Gerontology at Simon Fraser University, Vancouver, Canada. Her research is focused on person-centered care for ethnically diverse older adults in long-term care homes.

**Nadia Firdausya Jones, PhD**, is a senior data analyst at Oklahoma Department of Mental Health and Substance Abuse Services in Oklahoma City, Oklahoma. She received a doctoral degree in Human Development and Family Science from Oklahoma State University, Stillwater, Oklahoma. Dr. Firdausya Jones has contributed to various projects involving the development of socially assistive robotic devices and technology tools for geriatric and mental health care. Her research and professional interests focus on the interconnection between mental and physical health relative to the use of clinical interventions designed to passively and actively monitor physiological stress and cognitive functioning for improved mental health functioning wellness.

**Sharmin Kader, PhD, Assoc. AIA**, is an architectural designer, researcher, and educator with over a decade of experience. Her project areas focus on healthcare facilities, student living-learning environments, and senior living. She worked as a lead design researcher in architectural and engineering firms. Currently, she is working as a postdoctoral research scholar at Kent State University. She has developed expertise in the post-occupancy evaluation (POE) process, and she has developed the first-ever POE tool for hospice care environment, *Hospice Environmental Assessment Protocol* (HEAP). She has been the recipient of several awards and honors throughout her academic and professional career. Three of her practice-based research projects received the Certificate of Research Excellence. She served as a Chair of the Board of the Environment Design Research Association (EDRA) for two consecutive years. In 2019, she presented a webinar on the "end-of-life care environment" organized by the Academy of Architecture for Health of the American Institute of Architects (AIA AAH). She has presented her work at national and international venues and has served as a reviewer of many conferences, AIA Convention, HERD journal, and others.

**Maja Kevdzija, PhD, EDAC**, is an assistant professor in Healthcare Design at the Faculty of Architecture and Planning at TU Wien, Austria. She obtained her PhD in 2020 at the Faculty of Architecture at Technische Universität Dresden, Germany. Her research study on mobility-supporting rehabilitation clinics for stroke patients was awarded the Healthcare Environment Award 2020 in the Post-Graduate Student category, the 2021 European Healthcare Design Award in the Design Research category, and the 2021 EDRA Certificate of Research Excellence (CORE) with Merit

Status. In her research, she is exploring at how the built environment may support and enhance the recovery of stroke patients in rehabilitation settings.

**Dani Kolker, Assoc. AIA, EDAC, LEED AP BD+C**, is a Tradewell Fellow/ Medical Planner at EYP Architecture and Engineering. Kolker received her Master of Architecture degree from the University of Kansas. During her graduate studies at the University of Kansas Institute of Health and Wellness Design, Kolker focused her research on pediatric behavioral health design post-COVID-19. Kolker has received several recognitions including a St. Louis AIA scholarship and Healthcare Environment Award honorable mention in the student design work category in collaboration with Caroline Coleman.

**Maya Kylén, PhD**, in gerontology, is a researcher and teacher at Lund University. She belongs to the Applied Gerontology Research Group at the Institution of Health Sciences and has focused her research on the relationship between place, health, and well-being along the process of aging, as well as exploring attitudes to user involvement in research on aging and health. She is the principal investigator of a large project exploring the relationship between health and economic factors that incentivize or disincentivize relocation in older age. Since 2018, she is also working as a researcher at Dalarna University, School of Education, Health, and Social Studies. Together with Professor Marie Elf, they explore how factors in the built and social environment can support a person-centered rehabilitation process at home among people with stroke.

**Kari Lane, PhD, RN**, is an associate teaching professor at the University of Missouri's Sinclair School of Nursing. Dr. Lane completed her doctorate in Nursing and Aging at the University of Iowa. She was a 2008 NICGNE Archbold Scholar and a 2013 NHCGNE Claire M Fagin Fellow. Dr. Lane's expertise lies in gerontology, long-term care, and health sensors to monitor for chronic health changes. Dr. Lane also has a strong interest in hearing impairment in older adults and interventions to assist in communication. She teaches geriatrics and pathophysiology at the school of nursing.

**Laura Latham** is the design director at the Gensler Research Institute and is dedicated to visualizing and communicating research to inform the design of all aspects of life—how we live, work, play, and care. Laura has led Gensler's research focused on longevity and intergenerational community models. In Laura's previous role as a design director in Gensler's brand design practice, her work spanned many industries including hospitality, finance, travel, corporate and residential real estate, designing places, spaces, print, and digital communications that create rich user experiences.

**Gesine Marquardt** is an architect and has been a professor of Social and Health Care Buildings and Design in the Faculty of Architecture at Technische Universität Dresden, Germany, since 2015. In her academic and design work, she develops architectural concepts for the healthcare sector in a society impacted by demographic change. Her publications focus on the dissemination of knowledge about dementia-friendly architecture. From 2012 to 2017, she headed an Independent Junior Research Group funded by the German Research Association after her postdoctoral work at the Johns Hopkins Medical Institutions in the USA. Her 2007 dissertation on dementia-friendly architecture earned her several academic awards.

**Sheila L. Molony, PhD, APRN, GNP-BC, FGSA, FAAN**, is a professor of Nursing at Quinnipiac University. She is a fellow of the American Academy of Nursing and the Gerontological Society of America. Dr. Molony is currently engaged in an R21 study to develop new positive psychosocial outcome measures that are meaningful and useful for people living with dementia (individuals with a diagnosis and care partners). Dr. Molony's doctoral and postdoctoral work focused on the development and testing of a measure to quantify the experience of at-homeness and person-environment integration.

**Keith Diaz Moore, PhD, AIA**, is Dean of the College of Architecture and Planning at the University of Utah and has served as both interim Chief Sustainability Officer and interim Senior Vice President for Academic Affairs (iSVPAA). Dr. Diaz Moore is an international expert in the connection between culture, health, and place, particularly regarding design for people experiencing dementia with several books, over 40 refereed publications, and more than 100 presentations on the topic. Whether in his academic, professional, or community roles, he is an ardent proponent for the power of good design to promote health and social well-being.

**Kelly Munly** is an assistant professor in the Penn State Altoona Department of Human Development and Family Studies, with a research and teaching focus on adult development and aging; her doctoral degree in human development, as well as gerontology and future professoriate certificates, is from Virginia Tech. In academia, government contract settings, nonprofits, and direct care settings, she has studied and worked with a range of topics, including community-based long-term care and caregiving relationships, intersectionality, critical race theory, autoethnography, intergenerational programming, community-based public health intervention, and substance use disorder prevention and treatment across the lifespan.

**Upali Nanda, PhD**, is Principal and Global Director of Research for HKS, an international architectural firm where she spearheads and leads research projects globally. She also teaches as Associate Professor of Practice at the Taubman School of Architecture and Urban Planning at the University of Michigan and serves as the Executive Director for the nonprofit Center for Advanced Design Research and Education. Her award-winning research around health and well-being, neuroscience and architecture, sensthetics, point of decision design, enriched environments, and outcome-driven design has been widely published. She has won various research and innovation awards, including the 2015 HCD 10 Researcher Award and the 2018 Women in Architecture Innovator Award.

**Tim Pittman** is a Research Strategy and Communications Director for the Gensler Research Institute. He holds a Bachelor's degree in Visual and Environmental Studies from Harvard University and a Master's degree in City Design and Social Science from the London School of Economics. His core areas of expertise include survey design, data visualization, and the translation of research findings into actionable insights. His work has been featured in publications including the *Harvard Business Review*, *Corporate Real Estate Journal*, and *Fast Company*; and received numerous both design and editorial awards, including a recent Hermes Award for Gensler's Research Catalogue, Volume 3.

**Jude Rabig** is a nurse gerontologist whose practice, research, and writing focus on the small house model of residential long-term care. She served as the founding Executive Director of the Robert Wood Johnson National Green House® Project and led the initiative for five years. She then established Rabig Consulting to assist organizations in the USA and Canada to implement small house projects. She has served on task forces, including the University of Minnesota's National Advisory Group Study of State Nursing Home Regulations, the Specialty Subgroup for review of Residential Health Care Facilities Guidelines for Design and Construction of Health Care Facilities, and the Pioneer Network National Fire Protection Code Revision Task Force. She has been an Atlantic Philanthropies Hartford Foundation Practice Change Fellow and a Center for Medicare and Medicaid Innovation Advisor. She holds a PhD in gerontology from Union Institute and studied Social Entrepreneurship at the Stanford School of Business.

**Karen A. Roberto** is University Distinguished Professor; Executive Director of the Institute for Society, Culture, and Environment; and Senior Fellow at the Center for Gerontology at Virginia Tech. Her research includes studies of rural older women, dementia family caregiving, and elder abuse. Much of Dr. Roberto's research relies on community-based samples, combines quantitative and qualitative methodologies, and includes interviews with older adults, family members, and formal service providers. She is the recipient of the Gerontological Society of America Behavioral and Social Sciences Distinguished Mentorship Award and the Gary Andrews Visiting Fellow Award from the Australian Association for Gerontology.

**Erin L. Robinson** is an assistant professor at the University of Missouri School of Social Work and has expertise in public health social work and gerontology. Dr. Robinson's primary research focus is on older adult health, health communication, eldertechnology, and social support networks. She collaborates with an interdisciplinary research team from engineering, nursing, occupational therapy, and medicine to develop a state-of-the-art monitoring technology for older adults, which uses in-home sensors to detect early signs of illness and functional decline. A large part of Dr. Robinson's work is around developing a sensor-enhanced care coordination model for older adults.

**Weihua Sheng, PhD**, is a professor at the School of Electrical and Computer Engineering, Oklahoma State University (OSU), USA. He is the Director of the Laboratory for Advanced Sensing, Computation, and Control (ASCC Lab, http://ascc.okstate.edu) at OSU. Dr. Sheng received his PhD degree in Electrical and Computer Engineering from Michigan State University in May 2002. He obtained his MS and BS degrees in Electrical Engineering from Zhejiang University, China, in 1997 and 1994, respectively. Eight of his publications have won the best paper or best student paper awards in major international conferences. His current research interests include social robots, wearable computing, human-robot interaction, and intelligent transportation systems. His research has been supported by US National Science Foundation (NSF), Department of Defense (DoD), Oklahoma Transportation Center (OTC), etc. Dr. Sheng is a senior member of IEEE and is an Associate Editor for *IEEE Robotics and Automation Magazine*.

**Sofia Song** leads cities research at the Research Institute, where she leads a cross-disciplinary team that includes architects, planners, economists, and technologists, to generate new insights and knowledge that extend beyond a single building to communities, neighborhoods, and cities. She positions Gensler as a cities thought leader to influence change at the city scale. Prior to Gensler, she was a founder and head of research at a start-up that created a transparent marketplace for senior living in the USA. She was also the former head of research at proptech companies such as StreetEasy.com and Compass. Sofia has a background in economics and urban planning.

**Grant Warner, AIA, LEED AP**, is a principal at HKS. Grant is passionate about designing senior living environments where residents and their care-partners can thrive. He leads the early planning and design stages of projects, learning from clients and care partners to program and design the best environment for their unique needs. Grant values empathy, creativity, and innovation and infuses these values into the firm's projects. A board member of SAGE, an enthusiastic participant in The Sleepover Project, and speaker at numerous national conventions on aging, Grant is a devoted advocate for our elders, enjoys teaching others, and loves collaborating with each community to find ways design can help improve quality of life.

**Nicholas Watkins, PhD**, is Gensler's Health Sector Research Lead. His professional work focuses on the interactions between humans and their built environments that reflect excellence in design and contribute to well-being and productivity. His research findings on healthcare, workplace, arts + culture, and education settings can be found in several refereed publications and venues. He has served as an EDRA board member and chair, and his design research of workplace settings has impacted organizations' national and international guideline development. He was recognized as one of the top ten leaders in healthcare design with an HCD 10 honor during the award's inaugural year.

# Part I
# Home and Community-Based Care

# Bridging the Digital Divide: Smart Aging in Place and the Future of Gerontechnology

Rotem Arieli, Manuela E. Faulhaber, and Alex J. Bishop

## 1 Introduction

Research has established that there are barriers specific to older adults, known to possibly contribute to the *digital divide* of understanding and engaging with technologies (Neves & Vetere, 2019; Schlomann et al., 2020). As the number of older adults continues to climb (Greenwald et al., 2018; Mendel & Toch, 2019), effective technology integration remains important to address. Studies have linked the importance of information and communication technologies with improved satisfaction and well-being in later life (Bong et al., 2019; Schlomann et al., 2020). Improving information and communication technologies may help older adults to live independently for longer while positively influencing health and social connection (Czaja et al., 2018; Schulz et al., 2015; Schlomann et al., 2020).

Older adults may experience significant physical, cognitive, and environmental changes as they age which may create opportunities for interventions focused on mitigating losses and maintaining quality of life (Van Patten & Maye, 2020). This topic is important and relevant as older adults may not want to move from their

R. Arieli (✉)
Department of Human Development and Family Studies, Iowa State University, Ames, IA, USA
e-mail: rotem@iastate.edu

M. E. Faulhaber
Department of Human-Computer Interaction, Iowa State University, Ames, IA, USA
e-mail: manufa@iastate.edu

A. J. Bishop
Department of Human Development and Family Science, Oklahoma State University, Stillwater, OK, USA
e-mail: alex.bishop@okstate.edu

© The Author(s), under exclusive license to Springer Nature
Switzerland AG 2023
F. Ferdous, E. Roberts (eds.), *(Re)designing the Continuum of Care for Older Adults*, https://doi.org/10.1007/978-3-031-20970-3_1

homes, rather deciding to "age in place," or remain in their homes for as long as possible (Mois & Beer, 2020; O'Brien et al., 2020; Pino et al., 2015). Living at home may come with needing some assistance, which is often left to an informal caregiver, like a family member or other loved ones (O'Brien et al., 2020). Even if physical needs, such as help with activities of daily living (ADLs), are not needed, there are social needs to address (Alves-Oliveira et al., 2015). This chapter offers an overview of the current literature on topics in and around the field of gerontechnology with a focus on aging in place, finishing with potential future directions.

## 2   Social Robotics for Aging in Place

Although aging in place is preferred for the majority of older adults, there are important safety and social concerns to consider. Some examples include limited social interaction or isolation, safety concerns navigating home space, and lack of noticing important changes in health, hygiene, or nutrition (Mois & Beer, 2020). Older adults may need home modifications to continue aging in place, assuring that the home environment maximizes their health and safety (Pynoos et al., 2018). In addition, assistive technologies can help empower older adults to maintain autonomy while prioritizing safety in the home (Ghorayeb et al., 2021). As Mois and Beer (2020) address, smart home technology may allow for home environments to assist older adults in performing tasks and prolonging autonomy in the home, especially if age-related declines start to accumulate.

To capture an example of social technologies and robotics enhancing well-being components of independent living, we first introduce some smart home features from the 2012 movie titled *Robot & Frank* (Schreier, 2012). In the film, an older adult named Frank adamantly chooses to age in place, against suggestions from his children who prefer that he reside in a skilled nursing facility. In a kind of compromise, Frank's son buys him a socially assistive robot, and Frank despises it at first, not wanting nor trusting it (Schreier, 2012). Over time, the movie addresses two main components: (1) hesitation to accept socially assistive robots in the home, including issues like privacy, usability, autonomy, and resistance to accepting help, and (2) benefits of the socially assistive robot, including assistance with cleaning, medication reminders, medical health monitoring, nutrition improvement, and finding a wellness hobby, such as gardening as in the film. Overall, the film demonstrates an example—albeit an entertaining one—to present a glimpse into some important concepts covered in this chapter.

The field of smart aging in place and expanding social robotics for older adults are vast, especially as society advances toward a more digitally focused way of life. Maintaining and improving social connections through social technologies may benefit older adults' quality of life (Alves-Oliveira et al., 2015; Mois & Beer, 2020; Pu et al., 2019). Additionally, technology can play a vital role in enhancing quality of life and autonomy for individuals as they age (Schulz et al., 2015). Older adults experiencing physical limitations and/or disabilities may be unable to remain living at home, resulting in a potential move to an institutionalized setting; this could potentially obstruct independent lifestyles, in turn leading to worse mental and/or physical health, lower quality of life, and increased care costs (Wang et al., 2019). This demonstrates a potential gap for various smart technologies to fill.

One type of assistive technology for promoting aging in place includes robotic technology for assistive care. As Hung and authors (2019) explain, physically assistive robots (PARs) aim to help perform physical tasks like body lifting, and socially assistive robots (SARS) focus on supporting the social and psychological needs of older adults. In a meta-analysis on the effectiveness of social robots, Pu et al. (2019) identified the Personal Assistive RobOt (PARO) as the most popular among socially assistive animal-like robots in research with older adults. PARO appears as a baby harp seal with friendly features (Pu et al., 2019) and has been measured alongside several mental health outcomes (e.g., depression, loneliness, quality of life) among older adults (Chen et al., 2020), as well as with later-life cognitive functioning (Van Patten & Maye, 2020). Older adults may have felt particularly attached to or positively impacted by PARO due to the *humanizing* component of the companionship created with the seal (Van Patten & Maye, 2020). Although interacting with live animals can enhance older adults' well-being, the burdens of caring for live animals limit this option, so animal-type SARs may be a better fit (Pu et al., 2019). Animal-like SARs could be helpful in homes or therapy settings for older adults as they may provide the positive effects of live animals without added associated risks (Pu et al., 2019; Thodberg et al., 2016). Additional animalistic social robots examined in Pu et al.'s (2019) meta-analysis alongside PARO include AIBO the robotic dog, NAO the humanoid communication robot, two health-care-specific robots called iRobiQ and Cafero, and a humanoid communication robot with features of a young boy. SARs with friendly, humanizing features may allow older adults to feel a personal connection, which may enhance mental and emotional well-being (Chen et al., 2020; Van Patten & Maye, 2020).

As Pu et al. (2019) suggested, social robots may help with stress, loneliness, medication use, social interaction, and overall engagement for older adults. One recent study created a "conversation-based" medication management system for older adults, utilizing a companion health robot alongside a cloud-based application (Su et al., 2021). Utilizing verbal conversation, older adults can create medication reminders, and the robot can begin conversations to check medication adherence. The authors included a caregiver feature, digitally connecting a trusted caregiver with medication updates even if geographically distanced. The piloted project demonstrated high levels of satisfaction from participants (Su et al., 2021), presenting an example of integrating robots into different domains of older adults' lives.

Another recent study examined perspectives from 16 independently living older adults as they observed scenarios with three companion robots (i.e., a robotic dog, a moving toylike vehicle, and a speaking assistant; Coghlan et al., 2021). The participants identified three important considerations for robotic companions: (a) maintaining autonomy, (b) maintaining dignity, and (c) having concerns about the potential impact on one's abilities/skills. Alongside the future of utilizing social robots among independently living individuals, these considerations can help advise user-centered designs of future companionate robots (Coghlan et al., 2021). Future studies with larger sample sizes and randomized controlled trials are needed to improve knowledge regarding the benefits of SARs.

Identifying the benefits of social robotics and smart home technologies must be addressed alongside whether older adults will approve of and use these technologies within their homes. Mois and Beer (2020) posited how research has largely supported older adults' "positive attitudes toward robots into their home if the benefit of using the robot is clear" (p. 63). As the literature demonstrates, technology acceptance and use consist of multiple components (e.g., attitude, intention, behavioral integration, Mois & Beer, 2020), which we discuss in greater detail in a later section.

## 3   Technology Literacy and Health

Technologies aimed toward enhancing older adults' health and well-being continue to improve and expand. However, a continuous challenge remains in addressing technological literacy (e.g., skills, learning, and understanding). Lack of technology literacy is a public health issue, as substantial amounts of information are already being shared across digital platforms, including banking, travel, and important health systems (Azzopardi-Muscat & Sørensen, 2019). Improving older adults' technological literacy can enhance their experiences with existing technologies and potentially increase the likelihood of introducing new technologies (Pourrazavi et al., 2020).

Addressing issues surrounding digital literacy can help narrow the digital divide for older adults (Servon, 2008; Tsai et al., 2017) and may have important implications. Greater technological literacy allows for greater autonomy related to technology use among older adults (González et al., 2015), and low technological literacy may exclude older adults from engaging in the digital world (Ma et al., 2020). Increased digital literacy may allow older adults to more easily connect through social, learning, or other online platforms from a geographical distance. For example, older adults could engage in online community forums, such as the crafting website "Ravelry," which is an online community platform for sharing current and past creative projects such as knitting, crocheting, and more, but may act as a social connection platform for its members (Winge & Stalp, 2014). Another digital application platform potentially useful for older adults to engage with is "Duolingo," an app focused on learning foreign languages, which may relate to the maintenance of cognitive processes in later life (Payne & Stine-Morrow, 2017). Further, the current global COVID-19 pandemic demonstrated the increased importance of digital literacy among older adults, both in terms of social connection across digital platforms and in health literacy for telehealth and communication with care providers.

Health literacy refers to "an individual's ability to understand and utilize health information…to maintain health" (Kim & Oh, 2020, p. 2). Literature has linked poor or limited health literacy to poor health outcomes (Kim & Oh, 2020), and health literacy remains an important component of race/ethnicity and education disparities in self-rated health and certain preventative health behaviors among older adults (Bennett et al., 2009). Further, the COVID-19 pandemic widened the scope of utilizing telehealth as a means of health checks and communication between older adults and their health providers (Centers for Disease Control and Prevention [CDC], 2020). Even before the pandemic introduced the crucial need for physically distant care, the American Medical Association (2020) identified increased interest in utilizing digital health tools among both older adult patients and health care providers from 2016 to 2019. However, without addressing technology and health literacy, physically distanced health measures could be more difficult for older adults.

Telehealth connects older adults and their health care providers without requiring geographic proximity. For older adults who may decide to age in place in a rural setting, this could be especially useful. Access to health care services remains a challenge for older adults residing in rural areas, as they may be geographically limited in accessing health services (Chu et al., 2021). Additionally, telehealth as a health care tool has the potential to improve access and continuity of health care, as well as potentially improve health outcomes, lower associated costs, and reduce the frequency and burden of traveling to in-person office visits (Quinn et al., 2018).

Digital health monitoring is another avenue that can cause strain regarding health literacy. Various health monitoring devices are available, varying in type, cost, ease of use, and more. A systematic review focused on health monitoring technologies aimed toward independently living older adults (Peetoom et al., 2015) and identified five main monitoring types: "in-home passive infrared motion sensors…body-worn sensors… video monitoring…pressure sensors…and sound recognition" (p. 2). A seemingly cost-effective digital health monitoring device is a wearable device such as a commercial smartwatch (e.g., Fitbit, Jawbone). Wearable devices are good examples of inclusive and universal designs as they are attractive to people of all ages. This may increase acceptability and use among older adults as the wearables are not viewed as "only for older adults." Health monitoring wearable devices can include features such as "the wearer's gait, walking speed, posture, respiratory rate, blood oxygen, heart rate, blood pressure, energy expenditure, position, and other related parameters" (Lu et al., 2020, p. 4). Wearable activity trackers provide opportunities for older adults to improve their well-being via adjustments to their health and lifestyle behaviors (Shin et al., 2019). Additionally, wearable health monitoring allows for "continuous, non-invasive, non-intrusive, and seamless surveillance" of older adults' physical health and well-being (Majumder et al., 2017, p. 35), potentially increasing their years of successfully aging in place. As Majumder et al. (2017) posit, this monitoring can collect comprehensive, longitudinal health information which then informs health professionals and potentially contributes to the future of cost-effective remote health care. Further, depending on the health monitoring device, information collected can often be directly shared with health care providers if chosen. Wearable health monitoring may allow for earlier detection of potential health-related issues, in turn leading to earlier medical attention, diagnoses, and treatment (Majumder et al., 2017).

Mercer et al. (2016) examined the usability and acceptance of wearable activity trackers among adults aged 50 and older with chronic illnesses who had never used activity trackers. The authors suggested several potential improvements for older adults' wearables: (a) increasing the pairing ability of the tracker to both personal computers and more basic Android phones; (b) providing a paper version of the instructions explaining how to use the device and interpret the collected information; (c) enhancing the device's associated app, including contrasting fonts, colors, and sizing; (d) creating a waterproof design of the wearable to reduce accidental damage and encourage water-based activity, which may be more low-impact; and (e) including a comprehensive setup by a real person to assist with setting up the tracker. Mercer et al. (2016) suggested that future research consider establishing "best practices for designing wearables for older adult populations" (p. 12) to improve the widespread use and associated benefits of wearable health devices.

Improving technological literacy among older adults helps older adults' autonomy with potential implications for caregivers and/or loved ones. Lindeman et al. (2020) examined several technology-based supports for caregivers of older adults to ease their workload during day-to-day activities. For example, enhancing older adults' technological literacy allows for greater independence with finding digital activities online (e.g., e-reader/Kindle, digital games like solitaire, video chatting with family or friends, listening to music, etc.), without being dependent on another person to facilitate the article search or video call. This shift provides autonomy for the older adults who then navigate their digital environments, as well as potentially decreasing the burden experienced by caregivers/loved ones (Lindeman et al., 2020). Overall, increasing technological literacy among older adults has numerous opportunities for enhancing well-being and independence for older adults, caregivers, other loved ones, physicians, and health providers.

## 4 Interface Usability, Design, and Accessibility

With the increase of older adults and the continuous development of new technologies, it is important to question the usability and inclusivity of designs. Older adults' technology use is generally increasing, as is the desire or requirement for technology use, yet there is also a general decline in certain physical and mental health factors in late life (Li & Luximon, 2020). Thus, examining mechanisms that influence usability among various digital interfaces for older adult users is crucial. Implications for advancing the field are vast. During the worldwide COVID-19 pandemic, older adults were potentially more isolated from others as they were at a higher risk for critical health issues with COVID-19 (Banskota et al., 2020). This might have limited their available in-person assistance with daily tasks and technological queries. However, even in a normal, non-pandemic era, improving self-efficacy in using various technology interfaces could benefit older adults. As older adults feel more in control of their abilities to independently surf the web or connect with loved ones via virtual platforms, there can be fewer unpleasant emotions related to technology use.

Improving the interface design and usability of various technologies geared toward older populations could have several positive implications, such as interfaces working for individuals of varying ability levels. This issue is greater than age; there are issues of ability levels across the lifespan, so this remains vital to address. The lack of customizability for individuals with physical issues (e.g., poor vision) and the high cost must also be addressed. During the current pandemic, improved interface design and usability could have helped older adults since in-person assistance for technological issues may have been less accessible due to the nature of the airborne virus. The next section will review several perspectives surrounding design principles, inclusive design, accessibility, and usability among older adults.

A study by Li and Luximon (2020) examined interface usability and design within mobile phone technology, presenting challenges experienced by older adults by interface type, accompanied by several important design implications for future gerontechnology creators. The authors investigated usability challenges by testing two types of mobile phone interfaces: (1) "menu-oriented design" and (2) "content-oriented design" (p. 5). Participants were asked to use a smartphone to perform different tasks on separate applications, followed by in-depth user interviews. Example tasks included, "Initiate a voice conversation with Kayan" or "Create a new contact named 'Li, 123456' and initiate a dialogue with him" (p. 8). Usability results concluded that older adults had an easier time navigating content via *content*-oriented design patterns rather than through *menu*-oriented design patterns (Li & Luximon, 2020). Content-oriented design patterns include list views, card views, or galleries and grids. Menu-oriented designs, which older adults experienced difficulty with, include collapsible menu navigation panes which require recall memory to retain information and unclear icons like the "hamburger" menu (i.e., three or four horizontal parallel lines close together which signify the menu button). The researchers presented a comprehensive list of 12 specific user interface recommendations for future gerontechnology creators to consider. Some of these include (a) enhancing visual differences between touchable and untouchable buttons, (b) avoiding scrollable menus, (c) providing clear and tactile feedback, and (d), if using icons, keeping them simple and perhaps including text explanations (Li & Luximon, 2020). Addressing the layout of information in applications used by older adults may make a difference in the decisions to use or avoid certain applications.

Research by Rivero Jiménez et al. (2021) aimed to increase therapeutic adherence for older adults using technology. To test usability for this project, they developed the Assistant on Case and Health Office (ACHO), a voice assistant helping recall medical appointments and timely medication reminders. Utilizing a co-design team of ten researchers alongside real older adult users (aged 65 and older, without impairments, living rurally), they tested the prototype's usability. Participants were observed interacting with the voice assistant, and then they quantitatively measured usability with the System Usability Scale. Results demonstrated ACHO as a reliable tool for older adults' daily use in increasing therapeutic adherence and provided a good example for co-design collaboration among researchers and older adults to successfully design and test a beneficial tool.

Another example of a usability-focused study investigated an application for improving quality of life among older adults with dementia (Rai et al., 2020). The researchers developed a touchscreen application aimed at providing mental stimulation to older adults by utilizing touchscreen functionality. Focus groups and individual interviews were conducted, as well as a feasibility trial to test real-world applicability. While iterating through the first paper prototype versions, researchers learned about the usability expectations of older adults and their mental models. Most older adult participants had some experience using technology, and participants reported being enthusiastic about the app, seeing it as an opportunity to engage. This study included the principles of cognitive stimulation therapy (CST) and individual cognitive stimulation therapy (iCST) with the help of technology, which can show improvement in life quality (Rai et al., 2020). Overall, a strong collaboration utilizing academic researchers, software developers, and older adults was suggested to design usable interventions for older adults.

Another component of usability and inclusive design is in designing the actual hardware (e.g., smartphone, tablet, laptop, etc.). An older adult population may experience different challenges regarding inclusive design. Vaportzis et al. (2017) utilized focus groups to investigate how older adults felt about tablets, including their familiarity, barriers, and advantages to using them, as well as how they interacted with them and how tablet design could benefit ease of use and overall usability. Their focus groups included 18 older adults with no previous experience using tablets in a qualitative research study to examine their attitudes toward tablets, learning to use them, and new technology in general. Some of the barriers they reported about using a tablet included (a) reservations about the cost of the tablet itself, demonstrating monetary accessibility, (b) lack of instructions and/or guidance, (c) lack of knowledge and/or confidence, and (d) health-related barriers. Common concerns and disadvantages identified by the focus groups regarding technology use in general as well as specifically tablet use included (a) worries regarding complexity and the sheer amount of technology available, (b) feelings of inadequacy compared to younger generations, (c) feelings that "screens and machines" [p. 6] take away from social interactions and communication, and (d) worries regarding negative features on the tablets themselves (e.g., button confusion, tablet weight; Vaportzis et al., 2017). Further, the study found that exposing participants to the hardware itself increased participants' interest in future usage. This demonstrates the importance of addressing perceived barriers experienced by older adults in learning to use new technology. In addition, the study identified key tablet recommendations specifically toward older users, such as (a) increasing keyboard and button sizes; (b) adding clear indications for each button's use; (c) limiting tablet weight to no more than 500 g; (d) finding ideal tablet screen size, as small tablet screens may be too small for comfort but larger tablets are perhaps too large to comfortably keep with them; and (e) providing a hard-copy tablet instruction manual clearly explaining each function (e.g., holding the power button for a few seconds to power off the tablet; Vaportzis et al., 2017). This study demonstrated inclusive designs for older adults focused on interface usability and inclusivity in the hardware design.

If the field of gerontechnology is to advance, several mechanisms of interface usability and design must be addressed. For starters, full consideration of physical and mental health variability among older technology users must be given. In some cases, usability design shifts could include adjusting security questions: as Smith (2019) posited, "Questions like 'What was the make and model of your first car?' may be quite pertinent for a 20-or 30-something user, but difficult to remember or even entirely irrelevant for an 80-something member of the silent generation" (p. 7). Considering physical and/or mental changes associated with the aging process may aid older adults in their prolonged abilities to work with and utilize new technologies. In addition, practitioners in the field should try to understand the reasoning behind older adults' decisions of using a new application. Further, gerontechnology creators may need to consider fewer changes within an already used application, as it may be frustrating and confusing if an application or device updates often and has new, unfamiliar changes. For cognitive adaptation, the same type of testing and sensitivity should be addressed to maintain clear, straightforward, and simple navigation directions and processes in the presence of ongoing cognitive impairment.

There are several future directions presented regarding usability and interface design for older adults. For one, there is the adaptation for physical health. As Smith (2019) posited, physical health components "still need to be considered by designers and communicators; and interfaces and devices should be adequately user tested to account for the diversity of bodies that use them" (p. 4). Future directions should also consider greater expansion of the person-centered teams for the process of research and designing new technology. This could first include adopting a co-design relationship, wherein researchers design the technological product or system alongside older adults (Sumner et al., 2020). Future research should advance the knowledge by evaluating more current design interfaces for older adults, as well as including them in the entire design process. By addressing barriers, technology can be made more available to older adults. Lastly, the topic of usability is quite complex. We do not want to minimize the daily usability issues older adults encounter. Managing usability issues is not simple, and addressing them requires a substantial shift in how technology is typically designed. Going forward, a substantial shift in how technology is typically designed for usability is necessary, as Rivero Jiménez et al. (2021) and Rai et al. (2020) demonstrated by including researchers, software developers, and older users to create and test their applications.

## 5   Technology Acceptance, Use, and Privacy

Although gerontechnology has the potential to enhance older adults' quality of life (Halicka, 2019), we must first acknowledge the barriers restricting older adults from engaging with gerontechnology, such as technology acceptance, use, and privacy. For older adults to consider integrating new technologies into their lives and likely their homes, their concerns must be addressed. One such concern may be privacy related to new technologies, especially with applications' potential to collect immense amounts of sensitive information (Fournier et al., 2020). Additionally, technology acceptance may be more complicated for older adults, as it may include emotions like anxiety and self-efficacy related to technology (Jarvis et al., 2019). Research has noted barriers to adopting technologies like "a lack of awareness, access, skills, and experience...decreased confidence in ability to use the technology...and physical/cognitive declines" (Berkowsky et al., 2017, p. 2). For gerontechnology to enhance and augment the lives of older adults, barriers to technology acceptance and use must be dealt with.

Research has identified multiple complex barriers to technology acceptance and use. Peek et al. (2014) explained that ambivalent attitudes toward technology were held by many older adults: "on the one hand, they recognize that such technologies could support independent living...on the other hand, they do not feel that they personally need them" (p. 227). Further, Schulz et al. (2015) identified barriers regarding users' abilities, needs, and preferences lining up with the features of the technology at hand. We must also consider societal factors as potential barriers to technology use and acceptance, including social and health policies and the influence of one's environment(s).

Schulz et al. (2015) identified five core life domains at the center of technology development: "(a) physical and mental health; (b) mobility; (c) social connectedness; (d) safety; and (e) daily activities and leisure" (p. 726). Furthermore, the technology acceptance model (TAM; Davis, 1989) plays a role in technology usage and acceptance, as one of the most influential conceptual models in explaining older adult technology use. Specifically, older adults' "perceptions of ease of use" are vital as they can strongly influence technologies' perceived usefulness (Roberts et al., 2019, p. 2). One emerging technology is virtual reality (VR) research with older adults. Although VR research with older adults is limited (Roberts et al., 2019), studies seem to show VR may improve memory function (Optale et al., 2010), balance (Bisson et al., 2007; Kim et al., 2009), and strength and physical activity from movement games like Wii Fit (Liao et al., 2015).

A study by Roberts and authors (2019) assessed how VR simulation experiences influenced participants' perceived usefulness of the technology among 41 community-residing older adults. The researchers received several recommendations from participants on improving VR equipment for older users, resulting in six components: "body movement, hearing, vision/glasses, nausea from sensation of motion, undesirable to put on a headset, and worry about remembering how to use the equipment without assistance" (p. 6). Some participants had difficulty with their glasses under the goggles, while others had difficulty identifying where the sound was coming from or turning enough to see everything in the goggles. Some of the barriers concerning older adults using VR included (a) improving the technology itself (allowing for a fit over larger glasses or improving image quality), (b) more social interaction within the experience, and (c) some older adults may prefer other devices/technologies (e.g., may not want or need to view a movie through a headset when they have a television). Some benefits of VR among older adults included "a replacement for enjoyable activities (if limited by mobility)" and "good for retirement communities…watching movies…and keeping up with the times" (p. 7). Many participants expressed interest in engaging with VR again, especially if physical or mental mobility were to decline or if socially disconnected. Overall, the participants were impressed and enjoyed the VR experience, emphasizing the "great potential for… usefulness in the future" (Roberts et al., 2019, p. 8).

Another barrier to technology acceptance and use is privacy. Demiris et al. (2009) evaluated ten older adult participants' privacy experiences of being monitored via silhouette home monitoring while performing daily activity scenarios (i.e., eating a snack, or being visited in a test apartment). After the activity, participants were shown their videos and asked about initial reactions, thoughts about privacy, and personal willingness to install a monitoring technology in their homes. Results demonstrated that the majority of participants felt the silhouette did not violate their privacy as they were unrecognizable blobs. Notably, some participants mentioned that if such technology were installed in their homes, they would want the option to turn it off occasionally.

A similar study by McNeill et al. (2017) focused on understanding older adults' desired privacy protection via individual interviews with 20 participants. Identified themes included (a) self-protection from harm, (b) personal autonomy, (c) release from social expectations without fear of consequences, (d) control over disclosed information, (e) managing social image, (f) shared information impacting self-concept, and (g) withholding to protect others. The authors recommended that future designers establish privacy protection from the start and view older adults as active participants in their privacy/data decisions (McNeill et al., 2017).

Schomakers and Ziefle (2019) examined privacy concerns of older adults related to technologies for enabling successful aging in place via focus groups. They learned that most participants were concerned about lacking control and feeling they were subject to surveillance by technologies. Further, significant age differences suggested that older adults seemed more hesitant and careful toward aging in place technologies than younger adults (Schomakers & Ziefle, 2019). Jaschinski et al. (2020) mirrored this finding, providing evidence from a large-scale survey that older adults would prefer to age in place and lose some privacy, rather than having to age in an unfamiliar environment. This interesting finding illustrates the importance of aging in place among older adults, even as potential privacy compromises meant staying at home.

## 6  Conclusion and Future Directions

This chapter presented an overview of the current gerontechnology literature, focusing on where we are now, where the gaps are, and where to go from here. We covered issues among older adults' use, access to, and understanding of smart technologies focused on aging in place, including (a) social components of gerontechnology for aging in place, (b) technology and health literacy, (c) interface design and usability, and (d) technology use, privacy, and acceptance. By focusing on the gaps, barriers, and future potential for gerontechnology, this chapter may serve researchers and practitioners alike in expanding their knowledge and understanding of the benefits and challenges of gerontechnology as we look toward enabling successful aging in place. The rest of this chapter focuses on future directions for gerontechnology.

The research and gerontechnology design field should aim for greater inclusion of older adults within design teams. For example, co-design teams could be implemented, wherein researchers design the technological product or system together with older adults (Sumner et al., 2020). Co-design teams allow older adults to provide helpful ideas and suggestions as part of the target audience who will use the new technology (Sumner et al., 2020), which may increase their investment in the success of developing a consumable product for the masses. As Russo-Netzer and Littman-Ovadia (2019) stated, one crucial resource important in older adulthood is "being a part of something bigger than themselves" (p. 7), which a co-design team and collective purpose could provide. In addition to older adults, interdisciplinary collaboration teams could include "clinicians, social and behavioral scientists, and policy experts, but also include engineers, human factors specialists, computer scientists, designers, and informaticists" (Schulz et al., 2015, p. 731). More diverse perspectives may decrease shortsightedness in designing products with avoidable ability barriers.

In addition, future directions in gerontechnology must address privacy and security concerns clearly and upfront with older adults (Ray et al., 2019). Stating clear and understandable information regarding privacy and monitoring may help older adults feel less vulnerable to privacy threats and less likely to turn away from new technologies (Ray et al., 2019), especially when addressed alongside important factors like autonomy and ageism. Interestingly, a recent study by Ghorayeb et al. (2021) reported that older adults who lived with and utilized smart home monitoring technology over 8–12 months were less worried about privacy and trust over time, rather increasing their acceptance of smart technology in the home. Although limited in sample size (i.e., seven participants living with temporary smart home technology), the findings may have important implications regarding privacy concerns in theory vs. in practice over time. We have come a long way on issues of privacy and technology acceptance, but much more is needed as the gerontechnology field advances.

Future explorations should also explore how gerontechnology may relate to the interindividual differences of older adults. Alongside the age component, other factors contributing to the digital divide can include gender, education, income, and generational status (Pruchno, 2019). Expanding gerontechnology research from a more singular, homogenous view may allow for a broader understanding of technology use in later life across varied backgrounds and experiences. For example, future research can consider various older age groups (i.e., young-old vs. middle-old vs. oldest-old), cultures, spoken language preferences, physical and mental ability levels, health statuses, and many more individual characteristics to explore. Analyzing and improving technology ease of use, acceptance of new technologies, and addressing privacy and security concerns can help ease barriers for older adults. Potential benefits for improving the technology acceptance and use for older adults may include greater quality of life and well-being (Bong et al., 2019; Schulz et al., 2015; Sumner et al., 2020), benefiting individuals across the globe as we all continue to age.

Future gerontechnology studies should continue to explore how new technologies, such as VR, smart home surveillance, wearable trackers, medication adherence tools, and SARs, become a greater part of our changing world. Despite several concerns addressed in this chapter (e.g., privacy, usability, accessibility), we believe the potential for gerontechnology to enhance the lives of older individuals who age in place is vast. Whether it is the peace of mind for family members living afar, older adults having greater autonomy with their technology-related decisions, or simply staying socially connected during a worldwide pandemic, gerontechnology offers creative solutions that were never possible before.

As future technologies continue expanding, we must aim to address the diverse needs of individuals across the lifespan. This includes issues of accessibility, inclusivity, and differing ability levels, which may impact a greater proportion of the population in addition to older adults. Prioritizing inclusive design and utilizing the proposed recommendations may help address barriers experienced by individuals of any age. The topic of usability within technology applications is complex and requires a shift in mindset. It is important to include older adults as active participants in the process of crafting, ideating, and testing prototypes to create a useful and valuable piece of technology that can improve countless lives. The call to action is clear: a user-centered approach to expand current and future technology is necessary to create a technological future that is diverse and age-inclusive.

# References

Alves-Oliveira, P., Petisca, S., Correia, F., Maia, N., & Paiva, A. (2015). Social robots for older adults: Framework of activities for aging in place with robots. In A. Tapus, E. André, J.-C. Martin, F. Ferland, & M. Ammi (Eds.), *Social robotics* (pp. 11–20). Springer. https://doi.org/10.1007/978-3-319-25554-5_2

American Medical Association. (2020, Feb). *AMA digital health research: Physician's motivation and requirements for adopting digital health, adoption and attitudinal shifts from 2016 to 2019.* https://www.ama-assn.org/system/files/2020-02/ama-digital-health-study.pdf

Azzopardi-Muscat, N., & Sørensen, K. (2019). Towards an equitable digital public health era: Promoting equity through a health literacy perspective. *European Journal of Public Health, 29*(3), 13–17. https://doi.org/10.1093/eurpub/ckz166

Banskota, S., Healy, M., & Goldberg, E. M. (2020). 15 smartphone apps for older adults to use while in isolation during the COVID-19 pandemic. *Western Journal of Emergency Medicine, 21*(3), 514. https://doi.org/10.5811/westjem.2020.4.47372

Bennett, I. M., Chen, J., Soroui, J. S., & White, S. (2009). The contribution of health literacy to disparities in self-rated health status and preventive health behaviors in older adults. *The Annals of Family Medicine, 7*(3), 204. https://doi.org/10.1370/afm.940

Berkowsky, R. W., Sharit, J., & Czaja, S. J. (2017). Factors predicting decisions about technology adoption among older adults. *Innovation in Aging, 1*(3), igy002. https://doi.org/10.1093/geroni/igy002

Bisson, E., Contant, B., Sveistrup, H., & Lajoie, Y. (2007). Functional balance and dual-task reaction times in older adults are improved by virtual reality and biofeedback training. *CyberPsychology & Behavior, 10*(1), 16–23. https://doi.org/10.1089/cpb.2006.9997

Bong, W. K., Bergland, A., & Chen, W. (2019). Technology acceptance and quality of life among older people using a TUI application. *International Journal of Environmental Research and Public Health, 16*(23), 1–21. https://doi.org/10.3390/ijerph16234706

Centers for Disease Control and Prevention. (2020, June 10). *Using telehealth to expand access to essential health services during the COVID-19 pandemic.* https://www.cdc.gov/coronavirus/2019-ncov/hcp/telehealth.html

Chen, S.-C., Moyle, W., Jones, C., & Petsky, H. (2020). A social robot intervention on depression, loneliness, and quality of life for Taiwanese older adults in long-term care. *International Psychogeriatrics, 32*(8), 981–991. https://doi.org/10.1017/S1041610220000459

Chu, C., Cram, P., Pang, A., Stamenova, V., Tadrous, M., & Bhatia, R. S. (2021). Rural telemedicine use before and during the COVID-19 pandemic: Repeated cross-sectional study. *Journal of Medical Internet Research, 23*(4), 1–10. https://doi.org/10.2196/26960

Coghlan, S., Waycott, J., Lazar, A., & Neves, B. B. (2021). Dignity, autonomy, and style of company: Dimensions older adults consider for robot companions. *Proceedings of the ACM on Human-Computer Interaction, 5*, 1–25. https://doi.org/10.1145/3449178

Czaja, S. J., Boot, W. R., Charness, N., Rogers, W. A., & Sharit, J. (2018). Improving social support for older adults through technology: Findings from the PRISM randomized controlled trial. *The Gerontologist, 58*, 467–477. https://doi.org/10.1093/geront/gnw249

Davis, F. D. (1989). Perceived usefulness, perceived ease of use, and user acceptance of information technology. *MIS Quarterly, 13*(3), 319–340. https://doi.org/10.2307/249008

Demiris, G., Oliver, D. P., Giger, J., Skubic, M., & Rantz, M. (2009). Older adults' privacy considerations for vision based recognition methods of eldercare applications. *Technology and Health Care, 17*(1), 41–48. https://doi.org/10.3233/THC-2009-0530

Fournier, H., Kondratova, I., & Molyneaux, H. (2020). Designing digital technologies and safeguards for improving activities and well-being for aging in place. In C. Stephanidis, M. Antona, Q. Gao, & J. Zhou (Eds.), *HCI international 2020 – Late breaking papers: Universal access and inclusive design* (pp. 524–537). Springer. https://doi.org/10.1007/978-3-030-60149-2_40

Ghorayeb, A., Comber, R., & Gooberman-Hill, R. (2021). Older adults' perspectives of smart home technology: Are we developing the technology that older people want? *International Journal of Human-Computer Studies, 147*(102), 571. https://doi.org/10.1016/j.ijhcs.2020.102571

González, A., Ramírez, M. P., & Viadel, V. (2015). ICT learning by older adults and their attitudes toward computer use. *Current Gerontology and Geriatrics Research, 2015*(849), 308. https://doi.org/10.1155/2015%2F849308

Greenwald, P., Stern, M. E., Clark, S., & Sharma, R. (2018). Older adults and technology: In telehealth, they may not be who you think they are. *International Journal of Emergency Medicine, 11*(1), 2. https://doi.org/10.1186/s12245-017-0162-7

Halicka, K. (2019). Gerontechnology: The assessment of one selected technology improving the quality of life of older adults. *Engineering Management in Production and Services, 11*(2), 43–51. https://doi.org/10.2478/emj-2019-0010

Hung, L., Liu, C., Woldum, E., Au-Yeung, A., Berndt, A., Wallsworth, C., Horne, N., Gregorio, M., Mann, J., & Chaudhury, H. (2019). The benefits of and barriers to using a social robot PARO in care settings: A scoping review. *BMC Geriatrics, 19*(232). https://doi.org/10.1186/s12877-019-1244-6

Jarvis, M.-A., Sartorius, B., & Chipps, J. (2019). Technology acceptance of older persons living in residential care. *Information Development, 36*(2), 339–353. https://doi.org/10.1177/0266666919854164

Jaschinski, C., Ben Allouch, S., Peters, O., & van Dijk, J. (2020). The influence of privacy on the acceptance of technologies for assisted living. In Q. Gao & J. Zhou (Eds.), *Human aspects of*

*IT for the aged population: Healthy and active aging* (1st ed., pp. 463–473). Springer. https://doi.org/10.1007/978-3-030-50249-2_33

Kim, M. Y., & Oh, S. (2020). Nurses' perspectives on health education and health literacy of older patients. *International Journal of Environmental Research and Public Health, 17*(18), 6455. https://doi.org/10.3390/ijerph17186455

Kim, J. H., Jang, S. H., Kim, C. S., Jung, J. H., & You, J. H. (2009). Use of virtual reality to enhance balance and ambulation in chronic stroke: A double-blind, randomized controlled study. *American Journal of Physical Medicine and Rehabilitation, 88*(9), 693–701. https://doi.org/10.1097/phm.0b013e3181b33350

Li, Q., & Luximon, Y. (2020). Older adults' use of mobile devices: usability challenges while navigating various interfaces. *Behaviour & Information Technology, 39*(8), 837–861. https://doi.org/10.1080/0144929X.2019.1622786

Liao, Y. Y., Yang, Y. R., Wu, Y. R., & Wang, R. Y. (2015). Virtual reality-based Wii Fit training in improving muscle strength, sensory integration ability, and walking abilities in patients with Parkinson's Disease: A randomized controlled trial. *International Journal of Gerontology, 9*(4), 190–195. https://doi.org/10.1016/j.ijge.2014.06.007

Lindeman, D. A., Kim, K. K., Gladstone, C., & Apesoa-Varano, E. C. (2020). Technology and caregiving: Emerging interventions and directions for research. *The Gerontologist, 60*(supp_1), S41–S49. https://doi.org/10.1093/geront/gnz178

Lu, L., Zhang, J., Xie, Y., Gao, F., Xu, S., Wu, X., & Ye, Z. (2020). Wearable health devices in health care: Narrative systematic review. *JMIR mHealth and uHealth, 8*(11), e18907. https://doi.org/10.2196/18907

Ma, Q., Chan, A. H. S., & Teh, P.-L. (2020). Bridging the digital divide for older adults via observational training: Effects of model identity from a generational perspective. *Sustainability, 12*(11), 4555. https://doi.org/10.3390/su12114555

Majumder, S., Mondal, T., & Deen, M. J. (2017). Wearable sensors for remote health monitoring. *Sensors, 17*(1), 130. https://doi.org/10.3390/s17010130

McNeill, A., Briggs, P., Pywell, J., & Coventry, L. (2017). Functional privacy concerns of older adults about pervasive health-monitoring systems. In *Proceedings of the 10th international conference on pervasive technologies related to assistive environments* (pp. 96–102). https://doi.org/10.1145/3056540.3056559

Mendel, T., & Toch, E. (2019). My mom was getting this popup: Understanding motivations and processes in helping older relatives with mobile security and privacy. *Proceedings of the ACM on Interactive, Mobile, Wearable and Ubiquitous Technologies, 3*(4). https://doi.org/10.1145/3369821

Mercer, K., Giangregorio, L., Schneider, E., Chilana, P., Li, M., & Grindrod, K. (2016). Acceptance of commercially available wearable activity trackers among adults aged Over 50 and with chronic illness: A mixed-methods evaluation. *JMIR MHealth UHealth, 4*(1), e7. https://doi.org/10.2196/mhealth.4225

Mois, G., & Beer, J. M. (2020). Chapter 3: Robotics to support aging in place. In R. Pak, E. J. de Visser, & E. Rovira (Eds.), *Living with robots: Emerging issues on the psychological and social implications of robotics* (pp. 49–74). Academic Press. https://doi.org/10.1016/B978-0-12-815367-3.00003-7

Neves, B. B., & Vetere, F. (2019). *Ageing and digital technology* (1st ed.). Springer. https://doi.org/10.1007/978-981-13-3693-5

O'Brien, K., Liggett, A., Ramirez-Zohfeld, V., Sunkara, P., & Lindquist, L. A. (2020). Voice-controlled intelligent personal assistants to support aging in place. *Journal of the American Geriatrics Society, 68*(1), 176–179. https://doi.org/10.1111/jgs.16217

Optale, G., Urgesi, C., & Busato, V. (2010). Controlling memory impairment in elderly adults using virtual reality memory training: A randomized controlled pilot study. *Neurorehabilitation and Neural Repair, 24*(4), 348–357. https://doi.org/10.1177/1545968309353328

Payne, B. R., & Stine-Morrow, E. A. L. (2017). The effects of home-based cognitive training on verbal working memory and language comprehension in older adulthood. *Frontiers in Aging Neuroscience, 9*, 256. https://doi.org/10.3389/fnagi.2017.00256

Peek, S. T. M., Wouters, E. J. M., van Hoof, J., Luijkx, K. G., Boeije, H. R., & Vrijhoef, H. J. M. (2014). Factors influencing acceptance of technology for aging in place: A systematic review. *International Journal of Medical Informatics, 83*, 235–248. https://doi.org/10.1016/j.ijmedinf.2014.01.004

Peetoom, K. K. B., Lexis, M. A. S., Joore, M., Dirksen, C. D., & De Witte, L. P. (2015). Literature review on monitoring technologies and their outcomes in independently living elderly people. *Disability and Rehabilitation: Assistive Technology, 10*(4), 271–294. https://doi.org/10.310 9/17483107.2014.961179

Pino, M., Boulay, M., Jouen, F., & Rigaud, A.-S. (2015). "Are we ready for robots that take care for us?" Attitudes and opinions of older adults toward socially assistive robots. *Frontiers in Aging Neuroscience, 7*, 141. https://doi.org/10.3389/fnagi.2015.00141

Pourrazavi, S., Kouzekanani, K., Bazargan-Hejazi, S., Shaghaghi, A., Hashemiparast, M., Fathifar, Z., & Allahverdipour, H. (2020). Theory-based E-health literacy interventions in older adults: A systematic review. *Archives of Public Health, 78*(72). https://doi.org/10.1186/s13690-020-00455-6

Pruchno, R. (2019). Technology and aging: An evolving partnership. *The Gerontologist, 59*(1), 1–5. https://doi.org/10.1093/geront/gny153

Pu, L., Moyle, W., Jones, C., & Todorovic, M. (2019). The effectiveness of social robots for older adults: A systematic review and meta-analysis of randomized controlled studies. *The Gerontologist, 59*(1), e37–e51. https://doi.org/10.1093/geront/gny046

Pynoos, J., Steinman, B. A., & Nguyen, A. Q. D. (2018). Environmental assessment and modification as fall-prevention strategies for older adults. *Clinics in Geriatric Medicine, 26*(4), 633–644. https://doi.org/10.1016/j.cger.2010.07.001

Quinn, W. V., O'Brien, E., & Springan, G. (2018, May). *Using telehealth to improve home-based care for older adults and family caregivers*. AARP Public Policy Institute. https://www.aarp.org/content/dam/aarp/ppi/2018/05/using-telehealth-to-improve-home-based-care-for-older-adults-and-family-caregivers.pdf

Rai, H. K., Schneider, J., & Orrell, M. (2020). An individual cognitive stimulation therapy app for people with dementia: Development and usability study of thinkability. *JMIR Aging, 3*(2), e17105. https://doi.org/10.2196/17105

Ray, H., Wolf, F., Kuber, R., & Aviv, A. J. (2019). "Woe is me": Examining older adults' perceptions of privacy. In *Extended abstracts of the 2019 CHI conference on human factors in computing systems* (pp. 1–6). https://doi.org/10.1145/3290607.3312770

Rivero Jiménez, B., Conde Caballero, D., Jesús-Azabal, J., Luengo-Polo, J., Bonilla-Bermejo, J., & Mariano Juárez, L. (2021). Qualitative research in evaluation. An usability evaluation protocol for the Assistant on Care and Health Offline (ACHO). In J. García-Alonso & C. Fonseca (Eds.), *Gerontechnology III* (pp. 43–53). Springer. https://doi.org/10.1007/978-3-030-72567-9_5

Roberts, A. R., Schutter, B. D., Franks, K., & Radina, E. E. (2019). Older adults' experiences with audiovisual virtual reality: Perceived usefulness and other factors influencing technology acceptance. *Clinical Gerontologist, 42*(1), 27–33. https://doi.org/10.1080/07317115.2018.1442380

Russo-Netzer, P., & Littman-Ovadia, H. (2019). "Something to live for": Experiences, resources, and personal strengths in late adulthood. *Frontiers in Psychology, 10*, 1–14. https://doi.org/10.3389/fpsyg.2019.02452

Schlomann, A., Seifert, A., Zank, S., Woopen, C., & Rietz, C. (2020). Use of information and communication technology (ICT) devices among the oldest-old: Loneliness, anomie, and autonomy. *Innovation in Aging, 4*(2), igz050. https://doi.org/10.1093/geroni/igz050

Schomakers, E. M., & Ziefle, M. (2019). Privacy concerns and the acceptance of technologies for aging in place. In J. Zhou & G. Salvendy (Eds.), *Human aspects of IT for the aged population: Design for the elderly and technology acceptance* (1st ed., pp. 313–331). Springer. https://doi.org/10.1007/978-3-030-22012-9_23

Schreier, J. (Director). (2012). *Robot & Frank* [Film]. Samuel Goldwyn Films.

Schulz, R., Wahl, H.-W., Matthews, J. T., De Vito Dabbs, A., Beach, S. R., & Czaja, S. J. (2015). Advancing the aging and technology agenda in gerontology. *The Gerontologist, 55*(5), 724–734. https://doi.org/10.1093/geront/gnu071

Servon, L. J. (2008). *Bridging the digital divide: Technology, community and public policy.* Blackwell Publishing.

Shin, G., Jarrahi, M. H., Fei, Y., Karami, A., Gafinowitz, N., Byun, A., & Lu, X. (2019). Wearable activity trackers, accuracy, adoption, acceptance and health impact: A systematic literature review. *Journal of Biomedical Informatics, 93,* 103153. https://doi.org/10.1016/j. jbi.2019.103153

Smith, A. W. (2019). User experience design for older adults: Experience architecture and methodology for users aged 60+. In *SIGDOC 19: Proceedings of the 37th ACM International Conference on the Design of Communication, 17* (pp. 1–9. https://doi.org/10.1145/3328020.3353952

Su, Z., Liang, L., Do, H., Bishop, A., Carlson, B., & Sheng, W. (2021). Conversation-based medication management system for older adults using a companion robot and cloud. *IEEE Robotics and Automation Letters, 6*(2), 2698–2705. https://doi.org/10.1109/LRA.2021.3061996

Sumner, J., Chong, L. S., Bundele, A., & Lim, Y. W. (2020). Co-designing technology for aging in place: A systematic review. *The Gerontologist, 61*(7), e395–e409. https://doi.org/10.1093/ geront/gnaa064

Thodberg, K., Sørensen, L. U., Christensen, J. W., Poulsen, P. H., Houbak, B., Damgaard, V., Keseler, I., Edwards, D., & Videbech, P. B. (2016). Therapeutic effects of dog visits in nursing homes for the elderly. *Psychogeriatrics, 16*(5), 289–297. https://doi.org/10.1111/psyg.12159

Tsai, H. S., Shillair, R., & Cotten, S. R. (2017). Social support and "playing around": An examination of how older adults acquire digital literacy with tablet computers. *Journal of Applied Gerontology, 36*(1), 29–55. https://doi.org/10.1177/0733464815609440

Van Patten, R., & Maye, J. (2020). Assistive robots in the homes of aging adults. *International Psychogeriatrics, 32*(8), 905–907. https://doi.org/10.1017/S1041610220000800

Vaportzis, E., Clausen, M. G., & Gow, A. J. (2017). Older adults perceptions of technology and barriers to interacting with tablet computers: A focus group study. *Frontiers in Psychology, 8.* https://doi.org/10.3389/fpsyg.2017.01687

Wang, S., Bolling, K., Mao, W., Reichstadt, J., Jeste, D., Kim, H. C., & Nebeker, C. (2019). Technology to support aging in place: Older adults' perspectives. *Healthcare, 7*(2), 60. https:// doi.org/10.3390/healthcare7020060

Winge, T. M., & Stalp, M. C. (2014). Virtually crafting communities: An exploration of fiber and textile crafting online communities. *Textile Society of America Symposium Proceedings*, Paper 889. http://digitalcommons.unl.edu/tsaconf/889

# How Environmentally Embedded In-Home Sensors Are Revolutionizing Independent Living and Family Caregiving: A Literature Review

Kari Lane and Erin L. Robinson

## 1 Introduction

Aging in place is a term used to describe older adults' ability to live in their own homes, neighborhood, and/or community. While this is a goal for many older adults and their caregivers, older adults will need support both physically and mentally for them to be successful at aging in their own homes (Fänge et al., 2012). Various supports exist that can enable the aging population to remain in their homes safely, including home-based healthcare services, community resources, and transportation services, among others. In addition, over the last decade, advances have been made in embedded, in-home, sensor technology that facilitates healthy aging in place.

Sensors have been used in the healthcare industry to detect various human biological features, such as heart rate, respiratory rate, motion, time in bed, and falls. They are often small electronic devices that are programmed to detect specific biological, chemical, or physical processes and then transmit the data for algorithmic analysis and data prediction. Once the sensors collect data, the data is transmitted to a central location where computers use algorithms to interpret the data and then communicate those computer interpretations to healthcare staff. Ideally, the healthcare staff uses the data to determine trends and changes in health status, either acute changes or chronic changes. Healthcare providers can use data monitoring trends and changes in health status to help keep patients out of the hospital and remain living independently.

K. Lane (✉)
Sinclair School of Nursing, University of Missouri, Columbia, MO, USA
e-mail: laneka@missouri.edu

E. L. Robinson
School of Social Work, University of Missouri, Columbia, MO, USA

Some sensors work outside of the body (like a smartwatch or thermometer), some inside the body (like a pacemaker), and some are embedded in the environment. Body-worn sensors can provide location-based and geographic data for a person. However, several drawbacks exist, such as individuals forgetting to wear the sensor or losing the sensor (Reeder et al., 2013). Environmentally embedded sensors aim to maintain or improve the wellness of the aging adult automatically and unobtrusively. The sensors can detect changes in physiological or behavioral indicators to recognize changes in typical patterns that may indicate a corresponding health issue. Once the computer has provided some pattern recognition, the data is sent to either the patient, a designated family member, or a healthcare provider for further interpretation, follow-up, and referrals. The purpose of this chapter is to explore the ability of embedded sensors to monitor activity patterns, falls and fall risk, and chronic health issues. This literature review was conducted using CINHAL and PubMed databases using keywords embedded sensors, older adults, health outcomes, depression, mental health, diabetes, activity pattern recognition, falls, fall risk, driving, and chronic health conditions.

## 2   Embedded Activity Sensors

In a broad sense, activity monitoring can be used to determine changes in human behavior that may correlate with impending healthcare conditions. Kim et al. (2010) used activity pattern discovery with a probability model. The sensors used in this research were motion sensors embedded in different parts of a person's home (Kim et al., 2010). These sensors can detect simple activities such as ambulation or falls. However, researchers often want to identify more complex activities, such as taking medications, cleaning, bathing, wandering, or falling. The algorithms in this study for complex activities had poor prediction abilities (Dernbach et al., 2012).

Monitoring persons in multi-resident households or long-term care settings are more complex, and body-worn sensors require more extended time frames to set up. Sensors embedded in the environment work well; however, it is essential that these sensors can differentiate between residents. These authors used clustering methods on data from an embedded sensor tracking system to separate the activity of two residents with low error rates (Müller & Hein, 2019).

## 2.1   Embedded Sensors for Activity Pattern Recognition

Assistive technology is being used more frequently in healthcare situations to recognize activities such as taking medications or self-harm behaviors. One of the most frequently used assistive technology recognition behavior recognition activities is ambulation or step counting. Recognizing activity patterns has the potential to assist clinicians in determining if health changes have occurred over time. Automatic activity pattern recognition may provide an earlier indication of changes in a health condition. Many activity patterns are currently being investigated including ambulation, sleep, wandering, medication management, driving, mental health, and more.

### 2.1.1 Identifying Behaviors Related to Diabetes

Embedded activity sensors have been used to detect behaviors and prompt interventions for diabetic patients (Dernbach et al., 2012). Cook's team worked to use sensors to identify chewing and ambulation in diabetic patients. Their team was able to identify when participants were ambulating and when they were chewing food, allowing them to focus on specific behaviors that diabetic patients must deal with. Very complex behaviors were more difficult to differentiate. Chatterjee and colleagues used embedded in-home sensors to monitor patients with diabetes. They monitored activity within the home to predict blood sugar levels for the next day and provided their participants with motivational messaging to help improve activity within the home.

Several researchers have used self-management applications via smartphones to assist participants in self-managing their diabetes. The applications typically monitor activity, food intake, medication management, and foot care. Other applications provide appointment reminders and text messages on adherence to treatment plans. Researchers have found these types of feedback devices do assist in diabetes self-management.

Persons with diabetes that are at high risk for diabetic foot ulcers have the potential to decrease that risk when wearing a plantar pressure feedback insole system. The system included pressure detecting insoles and a smartwatch application. Participants in the control group had more high-pressure alerts than the intervention group, and significant differences were detected after 16 weeks of using the device. While specific events that triggered high-pressure alerts were likely different for each participant, commonly reported events included sitting, driving, and standing for prolonged periods. The research team noted that significantly fewer alerts were reported while participants were walking. This embedded sensor technology could have a huge impact on the incidence of diabetic foot ulcers by providing individualized biofeedback.

### 2.1.2 Identifying Behaviors Associated with Cognitive Impairment

Embedded sensors have been used to identify behaviors associated with mild cognitive impairment in older adults living in community settings. Tagged personal items tracked missed medications and monitored activity and sleep patterns. Mild cognitive impairment participants were less active, had more sleep interruptions, and forgot their medications more often than the group without mild cognitive impairment. In addition, over 80% of participants found the system acceptable (Rawtaer, 2020).

Persons with cognitive impairment can develop activity patterns that indicate a progression in their disease state. Sensors embedded in the environment can assist caregivers at home or healthcare providers outside of the home to determine disease progression. When activity patterns are relayed to caregivers, more accurate assessments of typical behavior at home can be determined which assists with assessing their cognitive status. Multiple researchers have found significant results using these methods.

### 2.1.3 Driving Patterns

Seelye et al. (2018) used unobtrusive passive sensors to monitor older adult driving patterns over 6 months. Participants with mild cognitive impairment drove fewer miles and spent less time on the highway per day than cognitively intact participants. In addition, drivers with mild cognitive impairment drove in similar patterns every day with fewer deviations from their typical driving pattern (Seelye, 2018). One research team examined an unobtrusive monitoring device placed in the vehicle. They wanted to see if they could determine differences between drivers with mild cognitive impairment and those without cognitive impairment. They found that they were able to assess driving with each drive the person undertook. They also found that those persons with mild cognitive impairment drove fewer miles and spent less time on the highway than their cognitively intact counterparts. In addition, their driving habits changed less frequently than cognitively intact participants. Technology in this area is still expanding and we will see further initiatives soon.

### 2.1.4 Mental Health

Typically, mental health behavior assessment is highly dependent on self-report. Embedded sensors have the potential to monitor these behaviors unobtrusively in a more objective manner. Mental health has been monitored with embedded sensors in terms of activity recognition, such as time spent in bed. Early detection of an acute exacerbation of mental illness is ideal in maintaining treatment. Mohiuddin et al. (2013) used embedded sensors to monitor changes in individual residents' activity patterns. When changes were noted, the system notified the resident, who then was able to take appropriate action. Amor (2011) used a similar system embedded in the environment to detect changes in activity patterns and alert residents of those changes with the intent to initiate early interventions to prevent acute exacerbations of bipolar disorder. Amor's team did note that the behavior activity patterns were quite different on weekdays versus weekend days (Amor, 2011). Schutz and colleagues (2021) examined several factors including late-life depression; while they were unable to detect changes in depression that were positive, they could detect worsening depression using their embedded sensors. Researchers found changes in depression were preceded by reduced exercise duration and the use of active applications. In both depression and anxiety groups, persons moved less in their home or left their home to a lesser extent than was typical.

## 2.2 Embedded Sensors for Fall Risk and Fall Detection

Over 1.6 million older adults are treated for falls and fall-related injuries in the hospital emergency departments every year. Injuries include fractures, head injuries, death, and loss of independence and quality of life. Ideally, clinicians would be able to accurately identify fall risk in their patients in real time to provide timely interventions to reduce actual falls (DeLaHoz & Labrador, 2014). Researchers have found that gait parameters decline when a resident is at higher risk for falls. These parameters are gait speed, stride length, stride width, and swing time variability (Taylor et al., 2013; Protas et al., 2005; Mari et al., 2014; Rantz et al., 2014).

Sensors embedded in the living environment have been used to provide estimates of typically completed assessments when in physician offices only once or twice a year. Sprint et al.' (2015) work estimated a Timed Up and Go (TUG) test. The TUG test is an ambulation test that estimates fall risk. The subject is asked to sit in a chair, and when told to go, stand up, walk to a line, turn, and walk back to the chair and sit down. The line is placed 3 m from the chair. The clinician measures the time in seconds to complete the task (Rolenz & Reneker, 2016). Sprint et al. (2015) explored various research teams that had attempted to estimate the TUG time using different embedded sensors. Multiple teams had examined this issue from various perspectives and sensor applications from embedded object sensors, smartphone technology, and Kinect technology (Stone, 2013; Mellone, 2011; Milosevic, 2013; Austin, 2011). Kinect technology is a component used in video games that senses motion. Kinect technology is produced by Microsoft. Kinect technology uses cameras, infrared projectors, and motion detectors to perform real-time gesture recognition, body detection, movement detection, and speech recognition.

Since Sprint et al.' (2015) review, several researchers have estimated TUG time using remote environmentally embedded sensors. Elledge (2017) used OmniVR motion sensors to examine the concordance between clinician-administered fall risk tests and the motion sensors. The OmniVR is a motion sensor tracking device that performs gait and flexibility assessments using a three-dimensional (3D) camera. Elledge found statistically significant correlations for both the TUG test and the sit-to-stand test. Data suggest that the OmniVR can be used to determine fall risk in an older adult's home, improving accessibility to fall risk assessments in a comfortable real-world setting (Elledge, 2017).

The Microsoft Kinect system has been used to detect fall risk in older adults' homes. These systems were used to measure gait speed, height of the individual walking, stride time, and stride length. They were eventually used to estimate TUG time. An average in-home gait speed for each resident was computed from all walks in their home over 7 days. Results indicate that the average in-home gait speed was a better predictor of the mobility level of participants. In addition, the average in-home gait speed can be measured continuously and unobtrusively (Stone, 2015).

In further work using the Microsoft Kinect system, gait parameter estimates were used to predict the odds and probability of a fall event based on changes in those gait parameters. The researchers found that a change in gait speed over time was significantly associated with a likelihood of a fall. The model estimated that a cumulative decrease in gait speed of 5.1 cm/s over 7 days of in-home gait speed was associated with an 86% probability that the resident would fall within the next 3 weeks compared to a 20% probability of participants with no change in gait speed (Phillips, 2018).

After the continued development of these sensors and commercialization, other researchers have pursued fall detection and early bed exits. Using an innovative depth sensor on two in-patient units, fall risk, probability of bed exit, and fall detection were evaluated. Found a 54% fall rate reduction. The comparison unit without the sensors had a 58% increase in fall rates. An unobtrusive fall detection sensor system can provide staff a heightened awareness of potential falls, allowing them to implement fall risk reduction interventions earlier (Potter, 2017).

Several researchers have examined the use of accelerometers to detect fall risk and falls with some of these studies that required step detection while others did not. However, many studies used treadmills or other artificial means of ambulation instead of ambulation in their natural environment (Riva, 2013; Taraldsen, 2011; Mico-Amigo, 2016).

Smart sock technology has been trialed in a hospital situation to prevent falls. The technology is called PUP® (Patient is UP) and uses a smart sock with sensors embedded into the sock material. Two studies were conducted, one clinical trial and one observational study. The clinical trial demonstrated a reduction in falls from 4 to 0 per 1000 patient days, while the observational study at a separate facility found falls were reduced from 4 to 1.3 per 1000 patient days. In all, patients spent 1694 and 2286 patient days wearing the socks (clinical trial and observational study, respectively). The PUP® smart sock technology may be a key new technology that has the potential to make a significant impact on fall rates.

An additional concern of healthcare providers is actual falls. Timely fall detection is essential to provide medical assistance. Embedded motion sensors, depth sensors, and smart carpets have been used to detect falls in home settings. Several researchers have used smart carpets to detect falls. Muheidat et al. (2016) measured the sensitivity and specificity of their smart carpet using simulated falls to be 81% and 98%, respectively. Accuracy was 96%. Researchers used sensors embedded in the carpet and machine learning to detect both gait and falls. In addition, the team used video to assist in training classifiers (Muheidat & Tyrer, 2016).

## 2.3   Embedded Sensors for Chronic Illness Detection

To monitor vital signs such as heart rate, respiratory rate, blood pressure, or oxygen saturation ($SpO_2$) in a traditional manner, a healthcare provider must interact with the resident using a device to measure these vitals. Many residents require some vital sign monitoring, and some require frequent essential sign monitoring due to underlying conditions. Residents find attaching the devices themselves troublesome to either connect or wear for an extended period. Indeed, the ideal resolution would be to monitor vital signs without having to encounter the patient. Sensors embedded in the environment pose several advantages: the resident does not have to handle any equipment, skin irritation is no longer an issue, and vitals can be measured without knowing when they are measured. When a resident does not know their vitals are being measured, the change of "white coat syndrome" (falsely elevated vitals) is reduced (Montoya, 2017).

Embedded sensors allow for remote monitoring of residents without the resident interacting with a device. Sensors available today include sensors to monitor such vital signs as heart rate, respiratory rate, SpO2, temperature, and blood sugar levels (Malasinghe et al., 2019). The goal of embedded sensors is to speed the recognition of illness and keep long-term care residents out of the hospital. Rantz et al. (2012) utilized automated data processing algorithms to alert clinicians that something has changed in the resident's vital signs (respiratory rate, heart rate, time in bed, bed restlessness, gait parameters, and fall risk). Clinicians then used trend analysis to visualize vital sign changes and used this data together with a nursing assessment to determine if the physician needed to be notified of the change. The embedded sensors have been shown to detect changes in health status earlier than nursing assessments which often indicate an impending change in underlying conditions (Rantz et al., 2012).

Detecting an illness before it manifests using biomarker levels and therapeutic medication delivery can decrease the severity of biomarker levels. This research explores the use of body-implanted devices to monitor biomarker levels and medication delivery. Implantable therapeutic drug management may be able to provide continuous and automatic diagnosis and treatment. Point-of-care treatment using implantable chips that interact with implanted drug devices can increase patients' compliance who require constant monitoring, as in chronic diseases. Implantable sensors can be expected to interface with the body's biochemistry providing instantaneous treatment interventions (Ngoepe et al., 2013).

Sensors embedded in clothing can assist older adults with chronic illnesses such as Parkinson's disease by helping with posture and movement. Morone et al. (2021) described the use of a posture shirt to assist persons with Parkinson's disease in their posture and gait. The shirt is called K1 Posture Keeper® (e-Keep, Dual Sanitaly, Turin, Italy). This commercially available shirt was developed to stabilize and correct trunk, curved back, or kyphosis among other issues commonly found in Parkinson's patients. The research team used a baropodometric assessment comparison with and without the K1 Posture Keeper®. Participants found the shirt to be comfortable and easy to wear and the weight load between feet (caused by asymmetry of patient's posture) decreased significantly by 17–10% immediately. At the 1-month measuring point, the change decreased to 12%.

Additionally, participants with neurological paralysis have an interest in assistive technology that has the potential to improve their function, health, and well-being. A garment tested by Bastien and colleagues (2021) was deemed acceptable. Participants and clinicians alike also wanted to ensure the process for obtaining the garments was easy and accessible (Table 1).

## 3   Living with Sensors and Privacy Implications

Older adults have been willing participants in many research studies using embedded sensors to detect changes in health conditions and monitor for health risks such as falls. Older adults are more likely to be accepting of embedded sensors rather than smartwatch or wearable sensors, especially those born before 1946. One study examined willingness to adopt embedded sensors. The sensors were believed to help keep participants healthy and maintain independence. The participants were willing to adopt the sensors and were later more motivated if a decline in functional status was determined.

One goal of embedded sensors is to minimize all privacy intrusions. The systems are designed to be private, with encrypted security features and confidential log-in credentials. Galambos and colleagues (2019) found that participants were also willing to share their health data with healthcare providers and designated family members although future research is needed to determine any issues with privacy breaches.

Because healthcare data contains information that some individuals may take advantage of ensuring the security of such data is a high priority. Whether data breaches are intentional or unintentional, organizations are held accountable or criminally liable based on several pieces of legislation meant to protect healthcare data. IT professionals need to be included in research development discussions to ensure privacy concerns are addressed adequately.

## 4   Conclusion

Preventing hospitalization in older adults is of high importance. Older adults typically have two to five chronic health conditions to manage. As these chronic conditions are exacerbated, older adults need more acute care and possibly hospitalization. During hospitalization, the older adult loses even more muscle strength and vital capacity, decreasing their functional ability and quality of life. Essential interventions to prevent hospitalization include actively facilitating early illness detection, ambulation, and socialization.

**Table 1**  Characteristics of included studies

| Article citation | Purpose | Variables | Results | Findings |
|---|---|---|---|---|
| Austin (2011) | To describe the longitudinal analysis of in-home gait velocity collected unobtrusively from passive infrared motion sensors | In-home gait velocity, gait density, gait evolution | Estimation of gait density at time X = $f(\theta_t) \approx f(\theta_t')$ fort, $t \in [a,b)$ Gait evolution $$h = \left(\frac{4\sigma^5}{3n}\right)^{1/5}$$ | Austin (2011) calculated an algorithm to estimate the evolution of gait velocity over time. Austin also demonstrated monitoring the evolution in gait velocity adverse outcomes in older adults |
| Baker et al. (2021) | Baker et al. (2021) tested a smart sock technology to determine if these smart socks helped to prevent falls in high-fall-risk patients admitted to the hospital | Patient days wearing socks, falls | Socks reduced falls from 4 to 0 per 1000 patient days ($p < 0.01$) | Baker et al. (2021) saw a significant reduction in falls rates in their clinical trial |
| Chatwin et al. (2021) | Chatwin et al. (2021) investigated if a smart insole causes a reduction in plantar pressure | Pressure points on plantar surface | Control group saw more high-pressure points than intervention groups ($p = .05$) | Continuous plantar pressure feedback via smart insole is effective in reducing pressure points and preventing ulceration |
| Dernbach et al. (2012) | Dernbach et al. (2012) used a smartphone application to recognize both simple and complex behaviors in patient homes | Behaviors | The algorithm for complex behaviors had poor predictive ability; however, the model was still able to differentiate between simple and complex behaviors | Both simple and more complex behaviors were able to be differentiated using this smartphone application |
| Elledge (2017) | The purpose of this study was to determine the concordance of fall risk scores as measured by a motion sensor, with clinician-rated fall risk | Fall risk scores Functional Reach, 10-foot Timed Get Up and Go, Sit-to-Stand | Intraclass correlations .85 and significant Correlations for functional reach and Sit-to-Stand were significant at .05 and Timed Get Up and Go was significant at .01 | High concordance was found between motion sensor and clinician ratings. The sensor ratings were more stable |

(continued)

**Table 1** (continued)

| Article citation | Purpose | Variables | Results | Findings |
|---|---|---|---|---|
| Phillips (2018) | The purpose was to predict falls using data from unobtrusive sensors installed in assisted living facility apartments | Falls, gait speed, stride length | Cumulative change in speed over time was significantly associated with the probability of a fall ($p < .0001$). The odds of a resident falling within 3 weeks after a cumulative decline of 2.54 cm/s over 7 days is 4.22 (95% confidence interval [CI] = [2.14, 8.30]) | Results demonstrated the feasibility of using environmentally embedded sensors to measure gait parameters. The sensor system used here holds promise for monitoring older adults in their homes |
| Mari et al. (2014) | The purpose of this study was to determine the pattern of antagonist muscles in ankle and knee joints during walking. The participants all had cerebellar ataxia | Antagonist muscle co-activation indexes in ankles and knees, gait parameters | Both knee and ankle muscle co-activation indexes were positively correlated with disease severity. Ankle muscle co-activation was positively correlated with stance and swing duration variability. Significant negative correlations were observed between the number of self-reported falls per year and knee muscle co-activation | Mari et al. (2014) believed that the changes noted in this study would be important for creating braces to assist patients with cerebellar ataxia |
| Mellone (2011) | The purpose of this study was to determine if accelerometers found in devices such as smartphones could approximate a Timed-Get-Up-and-Go Test | Gait parameters | Each variable whose limits of agreement were within acceptable range was significant for gait phase, mean cadence, and gait coordination | Mellone (2011) hypothesizes that smartphone devices with accelerometers could become useful in eHealth applications |

(continued)

**Table 1** (continued)

| Article citation | Purpose | Variables | Results | Findings |
|---|---|---|---|---|
| Mico-Amigo, (2016) | To evaluate the accuracy of an algorithm based on acceleration, to determine gait parameters in older adults | Step duration | Low-back accelerations on average $22.4 \pm 7.6$ ms ($4.0 \pm 1.3$ % of average step duration) Between heel, accelerations were on average $20.7 \pm 11.8$ ms ($3.7 \pm 1.9$ %) Between low-back accelerations and heel, accelerations were on average $27.8 \pm 15.1$ ms ($4.9 \pm 2.5$ %) | This study demonstrated that gait parameters can be obtained from accelerometers |
| Milosevic (2013) | The purpose of this study was to quantify the parameters extracted from a smartphone accelerometer and gyroscope to calculate a Timed-Get-Up-and-Go test | Multiple parameters of the Timed-Get-Up-and-Go test | Participants with Parkinson's Disease required significantly more time to complete each phase of the test and the entire test than the healthy control individuals | Using a device such as a smartphone is an affordable option to detect gait parameters for instant results and performance over time |
| Montoya (2017) | Evaluate the ground truth of an off-the-shelf camera to detect vital signs accurately | Vital signs | Patients needed to be stable and the location of the patient's face had to be known | The camera estimates show a strong positive association with reference signals when the patient is stable |

(continued)

**Table 1** (continued)

| Article citation | Purpose | Variables | Results | Findings |
|---|---|---|---|---|
| Morone et al. (2021) | This study aims at investigating the short- and medium-term effects of a shirt with appropriate tie-rods that allows to correct the posture of the trunk | Symmetry, forefoot load, forefoot load time, time spent wearing the shirt | The results showed a significant improvement in symmetry of loads ($p = 0.015$) and an enlargement of the foot contact surface ($p = 0.038$) was found. A significant correlation was found between the change in forefoot load and time spent daily in wearing the shirt ($R = 0.575$, $p = 0.008$), with an optimal value identified at 8 h per day | The use of a postural shirt in patients with PD symmetrized the postural load and enlarged the foot contact surface improving their balance |
| Muheidat et al. (2016) | This study explored a smart carpet to detect gait parameters and to detect falls | Gait parameters and actual falls | Smart carpet has the ability to detect falls with 96.2% accuracy and 81% sensitivity and 97.8% specificity | Detecting falls in real time has significant clinical implications such as getting help to persons who have fallen minutes or hours sooner |
| Potter (2017) | Potter (2017) evaluated sensor technology to identify fall risk, and potential for early bed exit of high-risk patients | Potential bed exits, fall rates, fall rates with injury | The evaluation unit had 14 falls, for a fall rate of 2.22 per 1000 patient days, which was a 54.1% reduction compared with the Phase 1 fall rate ($z = 2.20$; $p = 0.0297$). The comparison medicine unit had 30 falls, a fall rate of 4.69 per 1000 patient days (a 57.9% increase as compared with Phase 1). | A fall detection sensor system affords a level of surveillance that standard fall alert systems do not have |

(continued)

**Table 1** (continued)

| Article citation | Purpose | Variables | Results | Findings |
|---|---|---|---|---|
| Rantz et al. (2012) | Test the implementation of an automatic fall detection system with rewind features | Gait parameters, actual falls, rewind of depth sensor images | The system was tested using "stunt actors" who fell from various positions in the step-down unit. The false positive rate was less than one fall per day per room (92% sensitivity, 95% specificity; 11 false alarms per month per room) | This feasibility study indicates that using embedded sensors in a hospital step-down unit detects falls, fall risks, and facilitates quality improvement after falls. These measures can be accomplished unobtrusively while taking into account patient privacy |
| Rantz et al. (2012) | Evaluate automated sensor health alerts and care coordination interventions to manage chronic conditions | Gait parameters, hand grips, functional ambulation profile | Intervention participants showed significant improvements (as compared to the control group) for the SPPB gait speed score at quarter 3 ($p = 0.030$), left-hand grip at quarter 2 ($p = 0.02$), right-hand grip at quarter 4 ($p = 0.05$), and the functional ambulation profile of the GAITrite at quarter 2 ($p = 0.05$) | Technological methods such as these could be widely adopted in elder housing, long-term care settings, and private homes where elders want to remain independent as long as possible |
| Riva (2013) | Determine fall risk without measuring gait parameters | Harmonic ratio (HR), index of harmonicity (IH), multiscale entropy (MSE), and recurrence quantification analysis (RQA) of trunk accelerations | MSE and RQA were found to be positively associated with fall history | MSE and RQA could be useful tools when identifying patients at high risk for falls |

(continued)

**Table 1** (continued)

| Article citation | Purpose | Variables | Results | Findings |
|---|---|---|---|---|
| Rolenz and Reneker (2016) | Does mild cognitive impairment alter the validity of several fall risk detection measures? | Gait parameters | The sensitivity of the TUG was only 20% with a specificity of 94.6% and the sensitivity of the 8UG was 64% with a specificity of 75.7%. The TUG identified fallers at significantly different rates than the 8UG and the ABC ($p < 0.05$) | The 8UG is recommended as a more appropriate outcome measure for identifying fall risk in community-dwelling older adults |
| Rawtaer (2020) | The purpose of this cross-sectional study was to establish the feasibility and acceptability of older adults with mild cognitive impairment (MCI) utilizing sensors in their home | Forgetfulness, step count, time spent away from home, television use, sleep duration, and quality | MCI participants were less active than the controls and had more sleep interruptions per night. MCI participants had forgotten their medications more times per month compared to controls. The sensor system was acceptable to over 80% (40/49) of participants, with many requesting for permanent installation of the system | System was both feasible and acceptable for seniors with MCI to use |

Embedded sensors can predict early indicators of health pattern changes which may eventually warrant hospitalization. Nurses and healthcare providers can use these early warning indicators with their skilled assessments to determine if physicians need to be notified and interventions implemented to prevent further functional decline. This paper has reviewed several types of embedded sensors that can detect changes in activity patterns, fall risk, actual falls, and vital signs.

Add info about how sensors are used and interpreted.

Add future research needs.

# References

Amor, J. D. (2011). Detecting and monitoring behavioural change through personalised ambient monitoring. *The British Library.* https://ethos.bl.uk/orderdetails.do?uin=uk.bl.ethos.548236

Austin, D. H. (2011). Unobtrusive monitoring of the longitudinal evolution of in-home gait velocity data with applications to elder care. In *Engineering in medicine and biology society, EMBC, 2011 annual international conference of the IEEE* (pp. 6495–6498).

DeLaHoz, Y., & Labrador, M. A. (2014). Survey on fall detection and fall prevention using wearable and external sensors. *Sensors, 14*(10), 19806–19842. https://mdpi.com/1424-8220/14/10/19806

Dernbach, S., Das, B., Krishnan, N. C., Thomas, B. L., & Cook, D. J. (2012). Simple and complex activity recognition through smart phones. *IEEE Xplore.* https://ieeexplore.ieee.org/document/6258525

Elledge, J. (2017). Concordance of motion sensor and clinician-rated fall risk scores in older adults. *CIN: Computers, Informatics, Nursing, 35*(12), 624–629. https://doi.org/10.1097/CIN.0000000000000378

Fänge, A. M., Oswald, F., & Clemson, L. (2012). Aging in place in late life: Theory, methodology, and intervention. *Journal of Aging Research, 2012*, 547562–547562. https://hindawi.com/journals/jar/2012/547562

Kim, E., Helal, S., & Cook, D. J. (2010). Human activity recognition and pattern discovery. *IEEE Pervasive Computing, 9*(1), 48–53. https://ieeexplore.ieee.org/document/5370804

Malasinghe, L. P., Ramzan, N., & Dahal, K. (2019). Remote patient monitoring: A comprehensive study. *Journal of Ambient Intelligence and Humanized Computing, 10*(1), 57–76. https://link.springer.com/article/10.1007/s12652-017-0598-x

Mari, S., Serrao, M., Casali, C., Conte, C., Martino, G., Ranavolo, A., et al. (2014). Lower limb antagonist muscle co-activation and its relationship with gait parameters in cerebellar ataxia. *The Cerebellum, 13*(2), 226–236. https://link.springer.com/article/10.1007/s12311-013-0533-4

Mellone, S. T. (2011). Suitability of a smartphone accelerometer to instrument the Timed Up and Go test: A preliminary study. *Gait Posture*, S50–S51.

Mico-Amigo, M. K. (2016). A novel accelerometry-based algorithm for the detection of step durations over short episodes of gait in healthy elderly. *Journal of Neuroengineering and Rehabilitation, 13*(38). https://doi.org/10.1186/s12984-016-0145-6

Milosevic, M. J. (2013). Quantifying Timed-Up-and-Go test: A smartphone implementation. In *Body Sensor Networks (BSN), 2013 IEEE international conference* (pp. 1–6).

Mohiuddin, S., Brailsford, S. C., James, C. J., Amor, J. D., Blum, J., Crowe, J. A., et al. (2013). A multi-state model to improve the design of an automated system to monitor the activity patterns of patients with bipolar disorder. *Journal of the Operational Research Society, 64*(3), 372–383. http://wrap.warwick.ac.uk/47098

Montoya, M. C. (2017). *Non-contact vital sign monitoring in the clinic.* Doctoral Thesis. University of Oxford. https://ora.ox.ac.uk/objects/uuid:488287d9-edf0-44de-9f83-ef25ef79a2e4

Muheidat, F., & Tyrer, H. W. (2016). Can we make a carpet smart enough to detect falls. In *Annual international conference of the IEEE Engineering in Medicine & Biology Society (EMBC)* (pp. 5356–5359). https://ncbi.nlm.nih.gov/pubmed/28269470

Müller, S. M., & Hein, A. (2019). Tracking and separation of smart home residents through ambient activity sensors. *Proceedings, 31*(1), 29. https://mdpi.com/2504-3900/31/1/29

Ngoepe, M., Choonara, Y. E., Tyagi, C., Tomar, L. K., Toit, L. C., Kumar, P., et al. (2013). Integration of biosensors and drug delivery technologies for early detection and chronic management of illness. *Sensors, 13*(6), 7680–7713. https://mdpi.com/1424-8220/13/6/7680/pdf

Phillips, L. D. (2018). Using embedded sensors in independent living to predict gait changes and falls. *Western Journal of Nursing Research, 39*(1), 78–94. https://doi.org/10.1177/0193945916662027

Potter, P. A. (2017). Evaluation of sensor technology to detect fall risk and prevent falls in acute care. *The Joint Commission Journal on Quality and Patient Safety, 43*(8), 414–421. https://doi.org/10.1016/j.jcjq.2017.05.003

Protas, E. J., Mitchell, K., Williams, A. L., Qureshy, H., Caroline, K. S., & Lai, E. C. (2005). Gait and step training to reduce falls in Parkinson's disease. *NeuroRehabilitation, 20*(3), 183–190. https://content.iospress.com/articles/neurorehabilitation/nre00281

Rantz, M., Skubic, M., Koopman, R. J., Alexander, G. L., Phillips, L. J., Musterman, K., et al. (2012). Automated technology to speed recognition of signs of illness in older adults. *Journal of Gerontological Nursing, 38*(4), 18–23. https://ncbi.nlm.nih.gov/pubmed/22420519

Rantz, M., Banerjee, T., Cattoor, E., Scott, S. D., Skubic, M., & Popescu, M. (2014). Automated fall detection with quality improvement "rewind" to reduce falls in hospital rooms. *Journal of Gerontological Nursing, 40*(1), 13–17. https://ncbi.nlm.nih.gov/pmc/articles/pmc4183454

Rawtaer, I. M. (2020). Early detection of mild cognitive impairment with in-home sensors to monitor behavior patterns in community-dwelling senior citizens in Singapore: Cross-sectional feasibility study. *Journal of Medical Internet Research, 22*(5), 1–10. https://ink.library.smu.edu.sg/sis_research/5129

Reeder, B., Chung, J., Lazar, A., Joe, J., Demiris, G., & Thompson, H. J. (2013). Testing a theory-based mobility monitoring protocol using in-home sensors: A feasibility study. *Research in Gerontological Nursing, 6*(4), 253–263. https://healio.com/nursing/journals/rgn/2013-10-6-4/{beb518d7-73ce-499d-9b9d-e5274f3ff168}/testing-a-theory-based-mobility-monitoring-protocol-using-in-home-sensors-a-feasibility-study

Riva, F. T. (2013). Estimating fall risk with inertial sensors using gait stability measures that do not require step detection. *Gait and Posture, 38*(2), 170–174.

Rolenz, E., & Reneker, J. C. (2016). Validity of the 8-foot up and go, timed up and go, and activities-specific balance confidence scale in older adults with and without cognitive impairment. *Journal of Rehabilitation Research and Development, 53*(4), 511–518. https://ncbi.nlm.nih.gov/pubmed/27532337

Seelye, A. M. (2018). Passive assessment of routine driving with unobtrusive sensors: A new approach for identifying and monitoring functional level in normal aging and mild cognitive impairment. *Journal of Alzheimer's Disease, 59*(4), 1427–1437. https://doi.org/10.3233/JAD-170116

Sprint, G., Cook, D. J., & Weeks, D. L. (2015). Toward automating clinical assessments: A survey of the timed up and go. *IEEE Reviews in Biomedical Engineering, 8*, 64–77. https://ncbi.nlm.nih.gov/pubmed/25594979

Stone, E. S. (2013). Mapping Kinect-based in-home gait speed to TUG time: A methodology to facilitate clinical interpretation. In *2013 7th international conference on pervasive computing technologies for healthcare (PervasiveHealth)* (pp. 57–64).

Stone, E. S. (2015). Average in-home gait speed: Investigation of a new metric for mobility. *Gait and Posture, 41*, 57–62. https://doi.org/10.1016/j.gaitpost.2014.08.019

Taraldsen, K. C. (2011). Physical activity monitoring by use of accelerometer-based body-worn sensors in older adults: A systematic literature review of current knowledge and applications. *Maturitas, 71*(1), 13–19.

Taylor, M. E., Taylor, M. E., Delbaere, K., Delbaere, K., Mikolaizak, A. S., Lord, S. R., et al. (2013). Gait parameter risk factors for falls under simple and dual task conditions in cognitively impaired older people. *Gait & Posture, 37*(1), 126–130. https://ncbi.nlm.nih.gov/pubmed/22832468

# The Home as a Place for Rehabilitation After Stroke: Emerging Empirical Findings

Marie Elf and Maya Kylén

## 1 Introduction

There is now evidence that the physical environment affects human health and well-being (Ulrich et al., 2010). Studies from different disciplines have shown that the built environment in care can be a mediating factor for experiences of care, patients' recovery process, and how care can be performed (Annemans et al., 2018; Duff, 2011; Lipson-Smith et al., 2021; Stevens et al., 2019). The environment can be described as multidimensional and includes the physical or built environment (e.g., spaces and objects), social (e.g., accessibility and quality of relationships), and professional environmental dimensions (e.g., activities that reflect the person's interest and ability). The environment provides opportunities, resources, requirements, and limitations for human actions and activities (Taylor, 2017). For people with physical disabilities, for example, after a stroke, extensive qualitative research has shown that environmental factors affect daily participation at the individual and societal levels (Hammell et al., 2015; Nanninga et al., 2015). These findings are not surprising; compared to healthy peers, people living with disabilities are more vulnerable to limitations in their home and community environments. Thus, a deviation between the individual's functional level and the requirements and constraints in the environment can affect the person's ability to perform daily activities and participate in everyday life (Brunborg & Ytrehus, 2014; Singam, et al., 2015), which can lead to reduced health and quality of life (Wottrich et al., 2012). In studies of disability in

M. Elf (✉)
School of Health and Welfare, Dalarna University, Falun, Sweden
e-mail: mel@du.se

M. Kylén
School of Health and Welfare, Dalarna University, Falun, Sweden

Department of Health Sciences, Lund University, Lund, Sweden
e-mail: maya.kylen@med.lu.se

rehabilitation medicine, the International Classification of Functioning, Disability, and Health (ICF) is often used (World Health Organization, 2001). This model describes health and functioning from a biological, individual, and social perspective (Cieza et al., 2002). The ICF defines factors important for health in four components: "b" (body functions), "s" (body structures), "d" (activity and participation), and "e" (environmental factors). It allows for identifying individual needs beyond their diagnoses and can help clinicians identify functional goals and select treatments. Although the ICF emphasizes the importance of environmental and personal factors for health and disability, the spatial and social environment is often neglected in the rehabilitation literature (Cott et al., 2007; Jansma et al., 2010). This gap may reflect that the definition of the environment in the model is abstract and does not provide direct guidelines on important environmental components needed to support rehabilitation.

The environment has become even more critical to address when increased care and rehabilitation occur in citizens' immediate environment and home (European Commission, 2019; SOU, 2020:19). There is thus a challenge for people with long-term and complex conditions and their families, care staff, and society to integrate the environment into care and rehabilitation. First, the environment is part of an individual's identity that must be considered when supporting the person in the home. There is no successful way to turn the home into an institution or make changes to support those in need of rehabilitation without ensuring joint decision-making with the person in question. In addition, society and its built environment are not planned and designed for solutions that include care and rehabilitation in the home. Health care also needs to shift from the traditional medicine paradigm focusing on diseases and treatments to encompassing the person's and their environment's experiences of care and rehabilitation. Despite this, the factors in the environment that can facilitate and/or hinder a person-centered rehabilitation process, especially health and well-being for people with stroke, are largely unknown.

Research on rehabilitation and the environment has been conducted mainly in hospitals, such as stroke units (Rosbergen et al., 2017; Shannon et al., 2019; Nordin et al., 2021), and not at home. For example, previous studies have shown that hospital rehabilitation environments can affect the patient's activity, early mobilization, and teamwork within the care team (Anåker et al., 2017, 2019, 2020; Shannon et al., 2019; Nordin et al., 2021). Research has shown a general need for improvements in rehabilitation environments. Even rehabilitation hospitals can cause patients to feel bored and lonely and create a lack of independence and control (Kenah et al., 2018; Anåker et al., 2019). These shared experiences will affect recovery and prevent individuals from leading or engaging in their recovery in meaningful ways. Studies have shown that patient outcomes vary among rehabilitation facilities (Reistetter et al., 2015). This may be due at least in part to differences in the built environment (Lipson-Smith et al., 2021; Anåker et al., 2017). This suggests that the design of rehabilitation environments can directly impact recovery for people who have had a stroke and affect their function in the long term. Thus, optimizing rehabilitation environments can support the patient's recovery and help avoid long-term physical disabilities, increasing the individual's quality of life while reducing dependence on societal resources.

## 1.1    Stroke and the Recovery Process

People with stroke are a large and older group of patients who often have a long-lasting physical, cognitive, and emotional disability after stroke (Rethnam et al., 2020). The rehabilitation process can take months or even years, and disabilities can be profound and lead to many limitations of activity and participation (Bernhardt et al., 2017; Arntzen et al. 2015; Rosewilliam et al. 2011; Sumathipala et al., 2012), such as reduced quality of life, social isolation (Kulnik et al., 2019), and adverse events such as falls. For many, these limitations are likely to change the way people perceive and engage with their home environment and surroundings (nanna). The patient may experience minor obstacles in the home as challenging to deal with after a stroke. There may be stairs, cramped spaces, or materials that make it difficult to function in daily life.

Poststroke recovery has been reported as difficult for many persons and their families. They describe the support after hospital discharge as inadequate and not patient-centered (Lindblom et al., 2020). In addition, older patients have much worse access to the rehabilitation after a stroke, even though they suffer from severe disabilities (Bhalla et al., 2004). Although they receive advanced clinical care in an acute environment, their rehabilitation and social needs tend to be neglected.

## 1.2    The Rehabilitation Pathway

The rehabilitation organization is different within and between countries (Bernhardt et al., 2017) and can occur in inpatient and outpatient settings (Adeoye et al., 2019). However, in most countries, the trend is shorter in the hospital and continued care and rehabilitation at home. In general, rehabilitation and recovery include three phases: (1) acute (0 to 7 days), (2) subacute (up to 3 months), and (3) poststroke (> 6 months). Regardless of the pathway and organization, rehabilitation after a stroke has been described as complex and fragmented, resulting in patients and their relatives having difficulty finding adequate and consistent care.

Early supported discharge (ESD) is an evidence-based outpatient model for patients with mild to moderate disability after stroke (Fisher et al., 2020). ESD means that an interdisciplinary team and the patient begin to plan the rehabilitation at the hospital and continue the rehabilitation at the patient's home. The model has a positive impact on people with stroke, including reduced hospital stays. Patients and staff have reported more opportunities for flexibility and a greater understanding of the patient's individual needs (Hitch et al., 2020). Despite promising results, ESD is not fully implemented in many countries due to a lack of resources and already established traditional processes. There are no studies on the role of the environment in an ESD organization.

## 1.3  Care and Rehabilitation Move from Hospitals to People's Homes

The reform with more rehabilitation in the home environment is more than an organizational change and requires a different approach for the staff to meet the patient and their relatives. Care needs to support the patient in becoming more independent and making their own decisions about care and rehabilitation. Above all, the home environment must be considered and included in rehabilitation in a much more advanced way than today. Rehabilitation in the home is a complex task. The home environment varies and differs considerably from an institutional environment regarding safety. There are solutions such as layouts, furniture, and free surfaces that can be obstacles at the same time to facilitate rehabilitation because they take place in a natural environment. For staff, it is crucial to change roles from a one-way expert provider to sharing decisions with the patient, which is far from a standard today (Downey et al., 2021; Van der Heide et al., 2018). Staff should not transfer the traditional expert role from institutional care to the patient's home.

## 1.4  Person-Centered Care and the Environment

Traditionally, rehabilitation medicine has focused on functional recovery rather than supporting people to understand and live with their changed situation and new self.

Person-centered care (PCC) aims to tailor care to the needs of patients with long-term conditions (Downey et al., 2021). The approach values the person's experiences, beliefs, personality, identity, and integration of the physical environment (Fazio et al., 2018; WHO, 2001; McCormack & McCance, 2006).

Extensive research has shown that patient-centered organizations result in greater satisfaction with care, greater job satisfaction among care staff, increased quality and safety in the care, and a greater quality of life and patient well-being (Rathert et al., 2013). However, few study on what person-centered care means for rehabilitation in the home and how the environment can be integrated into this process (Marcheschi et al., 2018).

An essential element of PCC is shared decision-making (Weston, 2001), in which professionals and patients work together to make health-care choices (Légaré et al., 2013). Shared decisions about adaptations and the use of the home environment after a stroke are complicated to fulfill. It is not easy to turn a private home into a caring and rehabilitative place. Conflicts can arise around goals and actions between the health care and the person in the home. For example, health services may want to adapt the environment to make it safer, such as installing holders and ramps, while the person wants to keep the home the way they are used to. This can be problematic, as the home is part of the person's identity. A home is also often a place where several family members gather and is important for the family's well-being. At the same time, the home can also be associated with an opposite feeling, where security is replaced by insecurity, for example, when health is fragile through a reduction in physical or mental well-being and abilities (Roxberg et al., 2020). Security can also be challenged when the home is turned into a care facility, which is often the case for in-home care services when technical equipment is needed for care, treatment, and rehabilitation (Landers et al., 2016).

## 2 Rehabilitation and Architecture: REARCH

Based on the problems identified in the introduction, the Rehabilitation and Architecture (REARCH) project (Kylèn et al., 2019) was formed. REARCH is framed by theories and research methods from different scientific disciplines and aims to gain in-depth knowledge into persons poststroke and their needs when rehabilitated at home. The focus is on how the environment is considered and affects the rehabilitation process from the perspective of different stakeholders.

### 2.1 Overarching Aims, Methods, and Participants

As described in Fig. 1, REARCH adopts a mixed method design, and combining quantitative and qualitative data sources provides a better understanding of complex research problems than either method alone. Data have thus far been collected using self-report questionnaires, semistructured interviews, medical records, and focus groups. Data were collected from 34 patients in their homes 3 months after stroke onset. In addition, eight practitioners (e.g., occupational therapists, physiotherapists, nurses) participated in focus group discussions on two occasions. The perspectives and experiences of various stakeholders were analyzed using

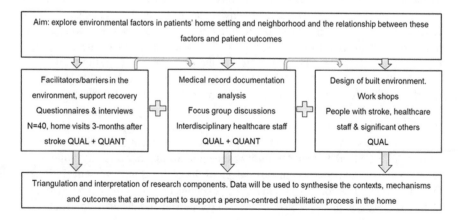

**Fig. 1** Methods flowchart

qualitative content analysis, and quantitative data were analyzed using descriptive statistics.

In addition, when the data were collected, the COVID-19 pandemic had its first outbreak. As a result, most of the clinical physical and rehabilitation medicine departments in Sweden and Europe had to stop their activities, at least for outpatients and patients being rehabilitated at home (Bersano et al., 2020). This was a unique situation, and a sample of patients interviewed in REARCH were thus invited to take part in follow-up interviews. These interviews were conducted by phone or video call.

## 2.2   Theoretical Underpinnings

To generate knowledge on the dynamic relationship between the person and the environment, REARCH is underpinned by several theories and frameworks that have guided the interpretation of data. These theories and models suggest that physical and experienced environmental aspects should be considered when creating person-centered stroke care and rehabilitation in the home. Moreover, providing high-quality science about environmental factors in the home is challenging for research and requires interdisciplinary knowledge and innovative research designs that are flexible and comprehensive.

To understand a person in relation to their environment, REARCH adopts a salutogenic understanding of health that emphasizes individual resources for promoting health (Antonovsky, 1987). According to this theory, the physical environment (e.g., home and neighborhood characteristics) and the various social processes and relationships in a home can be resources that contribute to health.

Another theory that explains how and why the environment is significant for health is the ecological theory of aging (ETA) (Lawton & Nahemow, 1973; Scheidt & Norris-Baker, 2003). ETA describes that a person's behavior results from the dynamic relationship between the individual's competence (e.g., cognitive, physical, and psychological skills) and the environment. When the demands from the environment are too high or too low in relation to a person's level of competence, this can result in negative consequences. For example, stairs in the home may require too much of a person with stroke, increase the risk of falling, and limit opportunities to move outside, which may lead to isolation and ill health. Hence, the lower the individual's competence, the more vulnerable they are to the demands of the environment (Lawton & Nahemow, 1973). ETA has primarily been used in REARCH to inform studies focusing on environmental factors and accessibility problems (Iwarsson et al., 2012). For example, the Housing Enabler instrument used to collect data defines accessibility as the relationship between the individual's functional capacity and the demands/design of the physical environment (Iwarsson & Ståhl, 2003). The concept is relative and explains how activity and participation restrictions arise in the relationship between the person and the environment.

However, it is not only the physical environment that is crucial for successful rehabilitation in the home. It is also important to understand place attachment and its significance for an individual's development. The physical environment is just space, while a home is a place filled with personal experiences, meaning, and social relationships, which over time transform a house (space) into a home (place) (Oswald et al., 2005). A person may experience the home differently than before the stroke. Emotional and cognitive ties to the home are closely related to well-being and identity. This is especially true for people with disabilities because familiarity with the home environment can maintain independence in everyday life (Nanninga et al., 2015). This means that when health-care practitioners step into a home and suggest or make changes, they must understand the concept of place attachment and listen to their needs and wishes. Therefore, the interviews with persons with stroke and focus group discussions with practitioners in REARCH included an exploration of place attachment in relation to rehabilitation practices and the possibilities and constraints of the built environment.

Another framework that has influenced REARCH is life-space mobility, which addresses the person's ability to move within their home environment and beyond (Fry & Keyes, 2010). People with stroke need to restore their previous identity and participate in activities outside the home environment (Lord et al., 2004), and any limitations are associated with worse perceived health (Leach et al., 2011). Research shows that people with stroke make fewer community trips than healthy adults in general (Robinson et al., 2011). Using life-space mobility has been possible to study persons' movement patterns in the home and neighborhood and thus reveal a person's daily life and possibilities for social participation after stroke. Life-space mobility also provides information on the degree of independence regarding assistance or mobility aids and the frequency of movements. Pain, difficulty walking, and depressive symptoms are negatively associated with life-space mobility (Rantakokko et al., 2019), which makes it even more important to be able to understand and consider physical environmental aspects beyond the home in rehabilitation after stroke.

## 3   Emerging Findings

### 3.1   Characteristics of the Rehabilitation at Home

Persons with stroke described rehabilitation at home to be dominated by the practitioner's perspective. Interventions focused mainly on functioning, such as impaired hand function, with limited home environment usage. In addition, activities primarily focused on the participants' self-care and indoor mobility and not on activities outside the home and possibilities to participate in society. The idea that practitioners follow what can be described as a generic approach to rehabilitation is an important but not a unique finding; many other studies have shown similar results. However, many opportunities and potential problems may be lost by not considering and using the environment in the rehabilitation process. Resources such as important persons in the community or the natural and/or built environment in the neighborhood are examples of resources that could be used to support the rehabilitation process. Likewise, home environment barriers can lead to reduced life-space and suboptimal rehabilitation outcomes, including worse perceived health and lower recovery after stroke and other long-term health conditions.

## 3.2  Shared Decision-Making

The persons with stroke were generally happy with the support they received. Yet, they experienced being informed rather than involved, meaning that the rehabilitation did not always correspond to their needs. As one participant expressed:

> We had no planning, I was advised … and received information from the start; I knew what was going on. Well, I cannot set any goals because I don't know what is needed. Because I cannot sit there and think, "Now I will do this and that to get well." I don't know; I just want to be as healthy as possible. (Male, age 65)

They obtained very brief information about their stroke and medications at the hospital. Very few described that they had taken part in a dialog about their health and environmental prerequisites at home primarily neglected. Thus, the practitioner's generic approach at the hospital ward was described as giving advice or providing information, which is not enough to reach the goal of shared decision-making. After hospital discharge, some persons with stroke experienced that they were more involved in planning their rehabilitation than at the hospital, which was also the view of the practitioners. The practitioners expressed in the focus group discussions that at home, they could pay more attention to what was important to the person and use those activities as an opportunity for the training, which also made the communication easier since the practitioner and the person with stroke were focusing on the same thing. This, in turn, was described as making it easier to involve the person in shared decisions about the rehabilitation:

> It is much easier, as we have said before; it is easier to get yourself focused on what is most important for the particular patient. (Quote from one of the focus group discussions)

However, few of the persons with stroke shared that they had experienced interventions based on their own goals. Some were even instructed to perform tasks or activities that they did not usually do or wanted to do in the future:

> No, I'm not using bus, but she who … the physiotherapist, says I have to test. (Male, age 46)

These contradictory findings in our material suggest that areas of health care can improve. If the goal of providing PCC is to be realized, practitioners must move away from a generic expert way of working and instead work together with patients and provide rehabilitation adapted to needs perceived and articulated by the person. From a patient perspective, this is a legal right that is especially important to adhere to in home and community care settings. For example, very few of the interviewed persons with stroke had housing adaptations, and many revealed that they had not been asked about their home environment before discharge from the hospital. Accessibility for those living with disabilities is a severe problem for individuals and society, yet health care continues to neglect the environment as a determinant for health and well-being. Thus, we argue that future care policy guidelines should incorporate the environment as a crucial part essential to providing PCC.

## 3.3   The Environment

The practitioners acknowledged that the environment contains much more than just the observable in the focus group discussions. They described the home as a social place imbued with meaning and intimately related to a person's identity, making it challenging, as they must carefully consider their needs and wishes:

> Yes, then you are inside… inside another person's home…so you cannot…of course you have to be a little careful when you start, before you know who it is you have to deal with, so to speak. (Quote from one of the focus group discussions)

The practitioners also expressed a huge contrast to the hospital, as the home offered many more opportunities. Even so, as the persons with stroke experienced that their home and neighborhood environments were hardly integrated into the rehabilitation, the opportunities the practitioners talked about seemed not always to be noticed or used. For example, some enjoyed gardening and longed to carry out activities outside the home, but such activities were hindered by barriers in the environment. Instead of overcoming these barriers with support from the practitioners, they were forced to put activities on pause. This is a concern because, following a stroke, patients expect that the home rehabilitation team will support them in managing cherished activities both inside and outside the home. In addition, the environment is important to consider from a safety perspective. The participants who reported one or more falls at home tended to live in homes with more accessibility problems. In addition, living in a home environment perceived to be supportive in everyday life was associated with living in a more accessible dwelling.

## 3.4   A Home Is a Social Place

A home is a place shared by many. For some, discharge from the hospital means to come home to a spouse; for others, it means to come home to a family with children still living there. Others come home alone. Nevertheless, in the context of home-based rehabilitation, regardless of the person's living situation, a home also becomes a workplace for practitioners delivering their services. In the focus group discussions, the practitioners acknowledged that family members could be a vital part of providing successful home rehabilitation. Still, they also shared that the relationship between them (the professionals and family members) could be complicated by, for example, different expectations of what the service should include or where it was delivered. Some family members felt too much responsibility on their shoulders and therefore wanted the rehabilitation to occur in a rehabilitation facility rather than at home:

> Many times, I think, you have to take that discussion with the relatives, because it is often they insist and want the patient to go (to the rehabilitation facility) because they feel that it is a too big responsibility forced on them. (Quote from one of the focus group discussions)

The practitioners also raised the shift in power that occurred when they entered a patient's home. At home, the patient was described as more empowered and had a stronger voice than the hospital, which the practitioners needed to respect and consider.

The fact that the person is integrated into a social context might explain the contradictory findings presented in the paragraphs above. Notwithstanding conflicting views, health care needs to adapt and find suitable solutions for addressing the challenges and possible integrated services where care and rehabilitation are provided at home rather than in institutions.

## 3.5   Adaptation to Life After Stroke in Light of the Coronavirus Pandemic

Following previously mentioned studies, we returned to the participants to learn how they lived with a complex health condition during a pandemic. The main finding was that they highlighted the importance of the physical and social environment in supporting their recovery. They expressed how the environment was a catalyst to mobilize their internal and external resources and thus enhance their possibility of engaging in meaningful activities. For example, places within and out of reach helped them manage the situation, exemplified by those living in apartment blocks in the city. Having a balcony supported a feeling of belonging despite the lack of social contact; seeing what was going on outside the street provided a sense of being part of everyday life in society. In addition, maintaining regular activities and structure in everyday life were also strategies they described, and this was eased by access to places outside of the home, such as nature and community places.

## 4   Conclusions

The lessons and the way forward show that there remains a lot to do to reshape the future of care settings in society for people with long-term conditions such as stroke. This is and will be an essential and complex task. In an ideal world, health and social care services should give patients great decision-making power and base their work on a holistic biopsychosocial model where the environment is taken into account, and the person's activity and participation in society is the goal of rehabilitation.

Society cannot achieve rehabilitation at home if a person is hindered from being at home due to limitations in the built environment. Therefore, we claim that the way forward must ensure that future efforts and guidelines capture the dynamics between people and the environment, which is not the case today. To inform such future policies and learn how to integrate the environment as a resource in the rehabilitation process, a first and important step is to listen to people who have experiences to share, a process that we have started in REARCH.

Moving care and rehabilitation to people's neighborhoods and homes is a global movement that society is not truly prepared for. We argue that researchers must use various methods and theoretical frameworks to inform clinical practice. In REARCH, we have observed that the environment in the home and the nearby surroundings have an impact on the person's capability to recover but are not fully integrated in the rehabilitation process. Based on our experience working with REARCH, we see a need to develop a new rehabilitation model that emphasize the environment and make use of what the individual has around them as part of the rehabilitation. This will add an important piece of the puzzle of how to improve the quality of life for people with stroke who are rehabilitated at home.

In addition, sustainable guidelines must be done together with those who will primarily be affected. To improve the current situation and promote the integration of the environment, researchers must use codesign methods and involve patients, caregivers, and multidisciplinary stroke teams to make changes that they know and have expertise in. This approach is crucial to meet the societal challenge described in this chapter. This will ensure that research best reflects people's different needs, preferences, and living environments.

**Acknowledgments** The authors thank the people with stroke and the professionals who participated in the REARCH study. We also wish to thank the Swedish stroke association for the contribution to this research.

# References

Adeoye, O., Nyström, K. V., Yavagal, D. R., Luciano, J., Nogueira, R. G., Zorowitz, R. D., et al. (2019). Recommendations for the establishment of stroke systems of care: A 2019 update: a policy statement from the American Stroke Association. *Stroke, 50*(7), 187–210. https://doi.org/10.1161/01.STR.0000158165.42884.4F

Antonovsky, A. (1987). *Unraveling the mystery of health: How people manage stress and stay well*. Jossey-bass.

Annemans, M., Van Audenhove, C., Vermolen, H., & Heylighen, A. (2018). The role of space in patients' experience of an emergency department: A qualitative study. *Journal of Emergency Nursing, 44*(2), 139–145. https://doi.org/10.1016/j.jen.2017.11.002

Anåker, A., von Koch, L., Sjöstrand, C., Bernhardt, J., & Elf, M. (2017). A comparative study of patients' activities and interactions in a stroke unit before and after reconstruction—The significance of the built environment. *PLoS One, 12*(7), e0177477. https://doi.org/10.1371/journal.pone.0177477

Anåker, A., von Koch, L., Heylighen, A., & Elf, M. (2019). "It's lonely": Patients' experiences of the physical environment at a newly built stroke unit. *HERD: Health Environments Research & Design Journal, 12*(3), 141–152. https://doi.org/10.1177/1937586718806696

Anåker, A., von Koch, L., Eriksson, G., Sjöstrand, C., & Elf, M. (2020). The physical environment and multi-professional teamwork in three newly built stroke units. *Disability and Rehabilitation*, 1–9. https://doi.org/10.1080/09638288.2020.1793008

Arntzen, C., Borg, T., & Hamran, T. (2015). Long-term recovery trajectory after stroke: An ongoing negotiation between body, participation and self. *Disability and Rehabilitation, 37*(18), 1626–1634. https://doi.org/10.3109/09638288.2014.972590

Bernhardt, J., Hayward, K. S., Kwakkel, G., Ward, N. S., Wolf, S. L., Borschmann, K., et al. (2017). Agreed definitions and a shared vision for new standards in stroke recovery research: The stroke recovery and rehabilitation roundtable taskforce. *International Journal of Stroke, 12*(5), 444–450. https://doi.org/10.1177/1747493017711816

Bersano, A., Kraemer, M., Touzé, E., Weber, R., Alamowitch, S., Sibon, I., & Pantoni, L. (2020). Stroke care during the COVID-19 pandemic: Experience from three large European countries. *European Journal of Neurology, 27*(9), 1794–1800. https://doi.org/10.1111/ene.14375

Bhalla, A., Grieve, R., Tilling, K., Rudd, A. G., & Wolfe, C. D. A. (2004). Older stroke patients in Europe: stroke care and determinants of outcome. *Age and Ageing, 33*(6), 618–624. https://doi.org/10.1093/ageing/afh219

Brunborg, B., & Ytrehus, S. (2014). Sense of well-being 10 years after stroke. *Journal of Clinical Nursing, 23*(7-8), 1055–1063. https://doi.org/10.1111/jocn.12324

Cieza, A., Brockow, T., Ewert, T., Amman, E., Kollerits, B., Chatterji, S., et al. (2002). Linking health-status measurements to the international classification of functioning, disability and health. *Journal of Rehabilitation Medicine, 34*(5), 205–210.

Cott, C. A., Wiles, R., & Devitt, R. (2007). Continuity, transition and participation: Preparing clients for life in the community post-stroke. *Disability and Rehabilitation, 29*(20-21), 1566–1574. https://doi.org/10.1080/09638280701618588

Downey, J., Bloxham, S., Jane, B., Layden, J. D., & Vaughan, S. (2021). Person-centered health promotion: Learning from 10 years of practice within long term conditions. *Healthcare, 9*(4), 439. https://doi.org/10.3390/healthcare9040439

Duff, C. (2011). Networks, resources and agencies: On the character and production of enabling places. *Health & Place, 17*(1), 149–156. https://doi.org/10.1016/j.healthplace.2010.09.012

European Commission State of Health in the EU: shift to prevention and primary care is the most important trend across countries. Press release; November 28th 2019. Retrieved December 19 from: https://ec.europa.eu/commission/presscorner/detail/en/IP_19_6336

Fazio, S., Pace, D., Flinner, J., & Kallmyer, B. (2018). The fundamentals of person-centered care for individuals with dementia. *The Gerontologist, 58*, 10–19. https://doi.org/10.1093/geront/gnx122

Fisher, R. J., Byrne, A., Chouliara, N., Lewis, S., Paley, L., Hoffman, A., et al. (2020). Effectiveness of stroke early supported discharge: Analysis from a national stroke Registry. *Circulation: Cardiovascular Quality and Outcomes, 13*(8), e006395. https://doi.org/10.1161/CIRCOUTCOMES.119.006395

Fry, P. S., & Keyes, C. L. M. (2010). *New frontiers in resilient aging: Life-strengths and well-being in late life*. Cambridge University Press.

Hammel, J., Magasi, S., Heinemann, A., Gray, D. B., Stark, S., Kisala, P., et al. (2015). Environmental barriers and supports to everyday participation: A qualitative insider perspective from people with disabilities. *Archives of Physical Medicine and Rehabilitation, 96*(4), 578–588. https://doi.org/10.1016/j.apmr.2014.12.008

Hitch, D., Leech, K., Neale, S., & Malcolm, A. (2020). Evaluating the implementation of an early supported discharge (ESD) program for stroke survivors: A mixed methods longitudinal case study. *PLoS One, 15*(6), e0235055. https://doi.org/10.1371/journal.pone.0235055

Iwarsson, S., Haak, M., & Slaug, B. (2012). Current developments of the Housing Enabler methodology. *British Journal of Occupational Therapy, 75*(11), 517–521. https://doi.org/10.427 6/030802212X13522194759978

Iwarsson, S., & Ståhl, A. (2003). Accessibility, usability and universal design—positioning and definition of concepts describing person-environment relationships. *Disability and Rehabilitation, 25*(2), 57–66. https://doi.org/10.1080/dre.25.2.57.66

Jansma, F. F., van Twillert, S., Postema, K., Sanderman, R., & Lettinga, A. T. (2010). Physical and rehabilitation medicine and self-management education: A comparative analysis of two approaches. *Journal of Rehabilitation Medicine, 42*(9), 808–814.

Kenah, K., Bernhardt, J., Cumming, T., Spratt, N., Luker, J., & Janssen, H. (2018). Boredom in patients with acquired brain injuries during inpatient rehabilitation: A scoping review. *Disability and Rehabilitation, 40*(22), 2713–2722. https://doi.org/10.1080/09638288.2017.1354232

Kulnik, S. T., Hollinshead, L., & Jones, F. (2019). "I'm still me–I'm still here!" Understanding the person's sense of self in the provision of self-management support for people with progressive neurological long-term conditions. *Disability and Rehabilitation, 41*(11), 1296–1306. https:// doi.org/10.1080/09638288.2018.1424953

Kylén, M., Von Koch, L., Pessah-Rasmussen, H., Marcheschi, E., Ytterberg, C., Heylighen, A., & Elf, M. (2019). The importance of the built environment in person-Centred rehabilitation at home: study protocol. *International Journal of Environmental Research and Public Health, 16*(13), 2409. https://doi.org/10.3390/ijerph16132409

Landers, S., Madigan, E., Leff, B., Rosati, R. J., McCann, B. A., Hornbake, R., et al. (2016). The future of home health care: a strategic framework for optimizing value. *Home Health Care Management & Practice, 28*(4), 262–278. https://doi.org/10.1177/1084822316666368

Lawton, M. P., & Nahemow, L. (1973). Ecology and the aging process. In C. Eisdorfer & M. P. Lawton (Eds.), *The psychology of adult development and aging* (pp. 619–674). https:// doi.org/10.1037/10044-020

Leach, M. J., Gall, S. L., Dewey, H. M., Macdonell, R. A., & Thrift, A. G. (2011). Factors associated with quality of life in 7-year survivors of stroke. *Journal of Neurology, Neurosurgery & Psychiatry, 82*(12), 1365–1371. https://doi.org/10.1136/jnnp.2010.234765

Lindblom, S., Flink, M., Sjöstrand, C., Laska, A. C., von Koch, L., & Ytterberg, C. (2020). Perceived Quality of Care Transitions between Hospital and the Home in People with Stroke. *Journal of the American Medical Directors Association, 21*(12), 1885–1892. https://doi. org/10.1016/j.jamda.2020.06.042

Légaré, F., & Witteman, H. O. (2013). Shared decision making: examining key elements and barriers to adoption into routine clinical practice. *Health Affairs, 32*(2), 276–284. https://doi. org/10.1377/hlthaff.2012.1078

Lipson-Smith, R., Pflaumer, L., Elf, M., Blaschke, S. M., Davis, A., White, M., et al. (2021). Built environments for inpatient stroke rehabilitation services and care: A systematic literature review. *BMJ Open, 11*(8), e050247.

Lord, S. E., McPherson, K., McNaughton, H. K., Rochester, L., & Weatherall, M. (2004). Community ambulation after stroke: How important and obtainable is it and what measures appear predictive? *Archives of Physical Medicine and Rehabilitation, 85*(2), 234–239. https:// doi.org/10.1016/j.apmr.2003.05.002

Marcheschi, E., Von Koch, L., Pessah-Rasmussen, H., & Elf, M. (2018). Home setting after stroke, facilitators and barriers: A systematic literature review. *Health & Social Care in the Community, 26*(4), 451–459. https://doi.org/10.1111/hsc.12518

McCormack, B., & McCance, T. V. (2006). Development of a framework for person-centred nursing. *Journal of Advanced Nursing, 56*(5), 472–479. https://doi. org/10.1111/j.1365-2648.2006.04042.x

Nanninga, C. S., Meijering, L., Schönherr, M. C., Postema, K., & Lettinga, A. T. (2015). Place attachment in stroke rehabilitation: a transdisciplinary encounter between cultural geography, environmental psychology and rehabilitation medicine. *Disability and Rehabilitation, 37*(13), 1125–1134. https://doi.org/10.3109/09638288.2014.955136

Nordin, S., Swall, A., Anåker, A., von Koch, L., & Elf, M. (2021). Does the physical environment matter? A qualitative study of healthcare professionals' experiences of newly built stroke units. *International Journal of Qualitative Studies on Health and Well-Being, 16*(1), 1917880. https://doi.org/10.1080/17482631.2021.1917880

Oswald, F., & Wahl, H. W. (2005). *Dimensions of the meaning of home in later life. Home and identity in late life: International perspectives* (pp. 21–45).

Rantakokko, M., Iwarsson, S., Slaug, B., & Nilsson, M. H. (2019). Life-space mobility in Parkinson's disease: Associations with motor and non-motor symptoms. *The Journals of Gerontology: Series A, 74*(4), 507–512. https://doi.org/10.1093/gerona/gly074

Rathert, C., Wyrwich, M. D., & Boren, S. A. (2013). Patient-centered care and outcomes: A systematic review of the literature. *Medical Care Research and Review, 70*(4), 351–379. https://doi.org/10.1177/1077558712465774

Reistetter, T. A., Kuo, Y. F., Karmarkar, A. M., Eschbach, K., Teppala, S., Freeman, J. L., & Ottenbacher, K. J. (2015). Geographic and facility variation in inpatient stroke rehabilitation: multilevel analysis of functional status. *Archives of Physical Medicine and Rehabilitation, 96*(7), 1248–1254. https://doi.org/10.1016/j.apmr.2015.02.020

Rethnam, V., Bernhardt, J., Johns, H., Hayward, K. S., Collier, J. M., Ellery, F., et al. (2020). Look closer: The multidimensional patterns of post-stroke burden behind the modified Rankin scale. *International Journal of Stroke*, 1747493020951941. https://doi.org/10.1177/1747493020951941

Robinson, C. A., Shumway-Cook, A., Ciol, M. A., & Kartin, D. (2011). Participation in community walking following stroke: Subjective versus objective measures and the impact of personal factors. *Physical Therapy, 91*(12), 1865–1876. https://doi.org/10.2522/ptj.20100216

Rosbergen, I. C., Grimley, R. S., Hayward, K. S., Walker, K. C., Rowley, D., Campbell, A. M., et al. (2017). Embedding an enriched environment in an acute stroke unit increases activity in people with stroke: A controlled before–after pilot study. *Clinical Rehabilitation, 31*(11), 1516–1528. https://doi.org/10.1177/0269215517705181

Rosewilliam, S., Roskell, C. A., & Pandyan, A. D. (2011). A systematic review and synthesis of the quantitative and qualitative evidence behind patient-centred goal setting in stroke rehabilitation. *Clinical Rehabilitation, 25*(6), 501–514.

Roxberg, Å., Tryselius, K., Gren, M., Lindahl, B., Werkander Harstäde, C., Silverglow, A., et al. (2020). Space and place for health and care. *International Journal of Qualitative Studies on Health and Well-Being, 15*(sup1), 1750263. https://doi.org/10.1080/17482631.2020.1750263

Scheidt, R. J., & Norris-Baker, C. (2003). The general ecological model revisited: Evolution, current status, and continuing challenges. *Annual Review of Gerontology and Geriatrics, 23*, 34–58. https://doi.org/10.1177/0269215510394467

Stevens, R., Petermans, A., & Vanrie, J. (2019). Design for human flourishing: A novel design approach for a more 'humane' architecture. *The Design Journal, 22*(4), 391–412. https://doi.org/10.1080/14606925.2019.1612574

Singam, A., Ytterberg, C., Tham, K., & von Koch, L. (2015). Participation in complex and social everyday activities six years after stroke: predictors for return to pre-stroke level. *PLoS One, 10*(12), e0144344. https://doi.org/10.1371/journal.pone.0144344

Shannon, M. M., Elf, M., Churilov, L., Olver, J., Pert, A., & Bernhardt, J. (2019). Can the physical environment itself influence neurological patient activity? *Disability and Rehabilitation, 41*(10), 1177–1189. https://doi.org/10.1080/09638288.2017.1423520

SOU 2020:19. *God och nära vård - En reform för ett hållbart hälso- och sjukvårdssystem*. Retrieved December 19 from: https://www.regeringen.se/rattsliga-dokument/statens-offentliga-utredningar/2020/04/sou-202019/

Sumathipala, K., Radcliffe, E., Sadler, E., Wolfe, C. D., & McKevitt, C. (2012). Identifying the long-term needs of stroke survivors using the International Classification of Functioning, Disability and Health. *Chronic Illness, 8*(1), 31–44. https://doi.org/10.1177/1742395311423848

Taylor, R. R. (2017). *Kielhofner's model of human occupation: theory and application*. Wolters Kluwer.

Ulrich, R. S., Berry, L. L., Quan, X., & Parish, J. T. (2010). A conceptual framework for the domain of evidence-based design. *HERD: Health Environments Research & Design Journal, 4*(1), 95–114. https://doi.org/10.1177/193758671000400107

Van der Heide, I., Snoeijs, S., Quattrini, S., Struckmann, V., Hujala, A., Schellevis, F., & Rijken, M. (2018). Patient-centeredness of integrated care programs for people with multimorbidity. Results from the European ICARE4EU project. *Health Policy, 122*(1), 36–43. https://doi.org/10.1016/j.healthpol.2017.10.005

Weston, W. W. (2001). Informed and shared decision-making: The crux of patient-centered care. *CMAJ: Canadian Medical Association Journal, 165*(4), 438–439.

Wottrich, A. W., Åström, K., & Löfgren, M. (2012). On parallel tracks: newly home from hospital—People with stroke describe their expectations. *Disability and Rehabilitation, 34*(14), 1218–1224. https://doi.org/10.3109/09638288.2011.640381

World Health Organization. (2001). *International classification of functioning, disability and health: ICF*. World Health Organization. https://apps.who.int/iris/handle/10665/42407

# Adult Family Care: A Homelike Environment for Community-Based Care

Kelly Munly, Karen A. Roberto, and Katherine R. Allen

A notable need for long-term care (LTC) services and housing has accompanied the aging of the population, both domestically and globally. Care and housing needs range from more independent models to more intensive supports for individuals facing cognitive and physical decline (Reeves et al., 2018; Wacker & Roberto, 2019). This need for housing includes the 61 million individuals in communities aging with and into disabilities (National Council on Disability, 2010; Okoro et al., 2018). The Americans with Disabilities Act (ADA) describes a person with a disability as an individual who either has or is seen as having a mental or physical impairment that significantly limits life activities (U.S. Equal Employment Opportunity Commission, n.d.).

Long-term care housing options for persons aging with and into disability include both large and small settings (Wacker & Roberto, 2019). Large settings include privately and publicly funded institutional care, such as nursing homes and assisted living facilities. A transition away from institutional care during the past 20 years has been driven by federal policy to curtail the cost of delivering institutional care, which tends to be approximately twice the cost of community-based care (Bagenstos, 2020; Integrity, Inc., 2019). In addition, both researchers and providers assert the value and importance of person-centered care that is often more easily provided in

K. Munly (✉)
Department of Human Development and Family Studies, Penn State Altoona,
Altoona, PA, USA
e-mail: kam6832@psu.edu

K. A. Roberto
Center for Gerontology and Institute for Society, Culture and Environment, Virginia Tech,
Blacksburg, VA, USA

K. R. Allen
Department of Human Development and Family Science, Virginia Tech,
Blacksburg, VA, USA

© The Author(s), under exclusive license to Springer Nature
Switzerland AG 2023
F. Ferdous, E. Roberts (eds.), *(Re)designing the Continuum of Care for Older Adults*, https://doi.org/10.1007/978-3-031-20970-3_4

53

smaller community-based, supportive housing, with the caveat that the definition of and research on person-centered approaches in LTC are still evolving (AARP Public Policy Institute, 2009; Li & Porock, 2014; Mollica et al., 2009; Mollica & Ujvari, 2020). Located within existing neighborhoods, these homelike settings provide greater opportunities for resident choice and integration with the community.

One such community-based housing option is adult family care (AFC; Mollica & Ujvari, 2020). Operating under a social care model in contrast to the medical model of nursing homes, AFC facilities (formerly known as adult foster care) are small residential care homes that typically provide support services, supervision, personal care, and, in some states, comprehensive medical care. Individuals generally reside in AFC homes because they do not have family who can take care of them or because their family is unable or unwilling to provide daily care (Wacker & Roberto, 2019). As gatekeepers to services and community engagement for AFC residents, AFC providers are uniquely situated between policy-informed regulations and the outcomes experienced by their residents (Munly et al., 2018).

The chapter begins with a brief overview of the history and national scope of AFC. Next is a description of the experiences of 26 AFC providers in North Carolina. The purpose of this qualitative study was to understand how providers navigated personal circumstances (e.g., work-family balance or the need to take care of older biological family members) and systemic conditions (e.g., insufficient Medicaid funding to provide for all of a resident's needs) to provide a homelike care context for their residents. The chapter concludes with a discussion of the study findings and recommendations for future AFC research and practice.

# 1 History and National Scope of AFC

AFC is not a new form of LTC in the United States. In colonial times, impoverished individuals with mental illness, as well as other impoverished children and adults, were sometimes placed with families in private homes but funded with public money. This practice stopped near the end of the 1600s with the inception of almshouses or charitable housing for impoverished individuals (McCoin, 1983; Morrissey, 1967). In the mid-1800s, US leaders began to encourage foster care as a form of care for individuals with mental illness (McCoin, 1983). In the 1950s, many psychiatrists began to applaud AFC as a solution for care for individuals with mental illness (McCoin, 1983). Research and general information on AFC dwindled, however, until the 1970s, when a greater emphasis on community placement of individuals with mental illness emerged (McCoin, 1983). AFC also began to be considered in the 1970s as a housing and care solution for frail older adults and for individuals with intellectual disabilities who were beginning to reenter the community from prior institutionalization (Birenbaum & Re, 1979; McCoin, 1983; Sherman & Newman, 1977). Furthermore, with the Supreme Court 1999 Olmstead Decision mandating that community-based care be made available to all individuals as an alternative to institutional care, there was renewed interest in AFC as a community-based option for care (National Council on Disability, 2004).

AFC encompasses many diverse care structures including adult board facilities, adult family care homes, boarding homes, board-and-care homes, community care homes, personal care homes, residential care homes, and shelter care facilities (McCoin, 1983). Definitions of these living environments often differ across and within states. For example, board-and-care homes are privately or publicly funded that typically have less than 12 adults not biologically related to the home manager. Services provided in board-and-care facilities often include a room, meals, house-keeping, and general protective oversight. This type of care has also historically provided end-of-life care to individuals, including persons of low income (Carder et al., 2006). Driven by different regulatory policies across states, board-and-care facilities are defined and licensed as assisted living in some states but as adult foster care in others (Carder et al., 2006; Morgan et al., 1993).

In 2009, in response to the variation in names and characteristics of care settings under the umbrella of adult foster care, AARP developed a consensus definition of AFC: care settings that provide residents who have physical and intellectual dis-abilities with a homelike and family-like environment with opportunity for 24-h care and community integration (AARP Public Policy Institute, 2009). Depending on types of funding available (e.g., Medicaid funding for adults experiencing pov-erty, with or without disability, or auxiliary grants for frail older adults), the person-alized nature and lower cost of AFC are appealing alternatives to institutional care for adults who are dependent due to an intellectual or physical disability or age-related frailty (AARP Public Policy Institute, 2009; Mollica et al., 2009; Mollica & Ujvari, 2020).

Most of what is understood about the current state of AFC across the nation is informed by AARP data gathered in 1996 and updated in 2009 and most recently in 2020 (AARP Public Policy Institute, 2009; Folkemer et al., 1996; Mollica et al., 2009; Mollica & Ujvari, 2020). Data sources included interviews with AFC provid-ers, community informants, and state officials. In December 2008, 64,189 residents across 30 states were being served by 18,901 AFC facilities (AARP Public Policy Institute, 2009; Mollica et al., 2009). There are now "38 states [that] include AFC among the array of LTSS [Long Term Services and Supports] residential care options available" and 18 states that "license AFC under assisted living regulations" (Mollica & Ujvari, 2020, p. 1).

AFC varies significantly across states, in terms of the name of the service (e.g., adult family care homes, adult foster care, domiciliary care), numbers of residents served within an AFC facility, regulations, and financing. In most states, there can be no more than five residents served per AFC home, though some states allow more (e.g., North Carolina allows six). Some states provide AFC licenses to provid-ers, and other states provide certifications. Some states regulate AFC through exist-ing assisted living conventions, and state regulations also include standards for Medicaid participation. AFC providers administrate and sometimes own the home in which care is provided; the home can be the provider's own residence but can also be corporately owned. Regardless of the AFC structure, providers are primary managers of their residences and the responsible party for their residents' well-being (Mollica et al., 2009).

AFC providers have a "willingness and ability" to provide service to individuals who are generally underserved "with high levels of need" and who, due to these significant needs, may not have other supportive care options (AARP Public Policy Institute, 2009, p. 2). As well as providing a service to an underserved group (i.e., adults with disabilities), AFC saves states money (AARP Public Policy Institute, 2009; Mollica et al., 2009). AFC does not have the overhead and extensive operating costs of larger facilities. Medicaid-funded residents usually pay for their room and board expenses with their Supplemental Security Income benefit, and Medicaid pays for some health and additional care services needed. However, the financial burden may be taken from the state and transferred to the AFC provider, as the provider must carefully balance a budget inclusive of home repair, cleaning services, additional respite service, and recreational activities for the residents. Therefore, depending on the funding mechanisms utilized by AFC agencies in each state, providers may only break even financially speaking.

## 2 North Carolina AFC Study Methods

Motivation for the study came from the first author's professional experience as an AFC respite worker and the limited information available about AFC providers (and residents) in the scholarly literature (Carder et al., 2006; Sherman & Newman, 1988). With a foundational understanding of AFC across the nation, North Carolina was selected as the study site because of its resistance to the Olmstead mandate. It was hypothesized that understanding providers' perspectives on and experiences of AFC as community-based care would shed light on issues of state policy implementation and the subsequent impacts on care contexts and care receivers.

### 2.1 Sample

Recruitment letters explaining the study were mailed to 84 providers in 4 racially diverse and centrally located counties in North Carolina that included both metropolitan and less populated areas (for details, see Munly et al., 2018). Providers were then contacted by telephone to invite them to participate in the study. To be eligible for the study, providers needed to be caring for two to six residents. Fifty-eight providers did not respond to telephone messages or indicated they were too busy or not interested in participating. The 26 AFC providers who participated in the study completed semi-structured, in-depth, telephone interviews in 2013–2014. Twenty-three providers identified as Black or African American women, two as Black or African American men, and one as a White male. Comprehensive demographics of the sample are provided in Table 1.

**Table 1** Select provider demographics

| Participants | Gender | Age | Race | Care work years | AFC years | Number of current AFC homes | Resident number by house (H) |
|---|---|---|---|---|---|---|---|
| Alex | M | 63 | Black | 25 | 25 | 2 | H1 = 6 |
| | | | | | | | H2 = 6 |
| Bernice | F | 58 | Black | 8 | 8 | 1 | H1 = 6 |
| Cadi | F | 41 | Black | 27 (since age 14) | 27 | 3 | H1 = 6 |
| | | | | | | | H2 = 6 |
| | | | | | | | H3 = 6 |
| Dan | M | 57 | White | 20 | 3 | 1 | H1 = 6 |
| Elon | F | 45 | Black | 15 | 8 months | 1 | H1 = 3 |
| Francis | F | 43 | Black | 8 | 3 | 1 | H1 = 4 |
| Gayle | F | 30 | Black | 2 | 1.5 | 1 | H1 = 3 |
| Helen | F | 62 | Black | 8 | 8 | 1 | H1 = 5 |
| Irene | F | 49 | Black | 20+ | 3 | 2 | H1 = 6 |
| | | | | | | | H2 = 6 |
| Joelle | F | 42 | Black | 5 | 5 | 2 | H1 = 6 |
| | | | | | | | H2 = 6 |
| Ken | M | 53 | Black | 28 | 16 | 1 | H1 = 6 |
| Leah | F | 37 | Black | 8 | 8 | 4 | H1 = 6 |
| | | | | | | | H2 = 6 |
| | | | | | | | H3 = 6 |
| | | | | | | | H4 = 2 |
| Miriam | F | 67 | Black | 45 | 18 | 1 | H1 = 1 |
| Nicole | F | 61 | Black | 3 | 3 | 1 | H1 = 5 |
| Olivia | F | 50 | Black | 5 | 5 | 1 | H1 = 2 |
| Patrice | F | 47 | Black | 16 | 16 | 1 | H1 = 5 |
| Qadira | F | 36 | Black | 17 | 3 | 3 | H1 = 4 |
| | | | | | | | H2 = 3 |
| | | | | | | | H3 = 1 |
| Rhonda | F | 69 | Black | 40+ | 31 | 1 | H1 = 4 |
| Shelli | F | 55 | Black | 18 | 14 | 1 | H1 = 6 |
| Tanya | F | ~55 | Black | 24 | 5 | 1 | H1 = 6 |
| Uniyah | F | 48 | Black | 25 | 3.5 months | 2 | H1 = 4 |
| | | | | | | | H2 = 6 |
| Veronica | F | 65 | Black | 7 | 7 | 1 | H1 = 4 |
| Wilma | F | 40 | Black | 20 | 4 | 1 | H1 = 6 |
| Xaveree | F | 53 | Black | 30 | 2 | 1 | H1 = 3 |
| Yolanda | F | 44 | Black | 17 | 17 | 2 | H1 = 3 |
| | | | | | | | H2 = 4 |

(continued)

**Table 1** (continued)

| Participants | Gender | Age | Race | Care work years | AFC years | Number of current AFC homes | Resident number by house (H) |
|---|---|---|---|---|---|---|---|
| Zada | F | 65 | Black | 13 | 13 | 6 | H1 = 6 |
| | | | | | | | H2 = 6 |
| | | | | | | | H3 = 6 |
| | | | | | | | H4 = 6 |
| | | | | | | | H5 = 6 |
| | | | | | | | H6 = 6 |

## 2.2 Procedures and Analysis

Interview questions relevant to the current analysis included the following: (a) Tell me about your experience of becoming an AFC provider. (b) Tell me about the general process of being matched with residents in your home. (c) What is your experience of family in your AFC home? (d) Tell me about professional supports that you find most helpful [in creating the home]. Least helpful? (e) How would you describe the way(s) in which you show "care" in your AFC environment? How do your residents show "care" to each other? How do they show "care" toward you? (f) Give me an example of how a resident exercised choice [in the home].

The constant comparative method of constructivist grounded theory (Charmaz, 2014) was used to analyze the data (for details about the process, see Munly et al., 2021). An integrative theoretical framework informed by theories of power (Foucault, 1977), care (Fisher & Tronto, 1990; Noddings, 2010; Tronto, 1998), and intersectionality (Allen & Henderson, 2022; Crenshaw, 1991; Few-Demo, 2014) informed analysis of the unpublished data and interpretation of the study findings presented in this chapter.

## 3 Results

Data analysis revealed how providers leveraged their power to support a sense of home. More specifically, the study findings shed light on four themes: (a) the AFC providers' motivations to create a home, (b) their skillful applications of a broad skill base to create a homelike setting, (c) the nature of provider practices supporting family-like relational ties and resident empowerment, and (d) community support for providers. See Table 2 for example quotes illustrative of the emergent themes.

**Table 2** Thematic findings: how AFC providers leveraged their power to support a sense of home

| Theme | Example |
|---|---|
| Motivations to create a home | *Cadi*: Actually, my mother … used to be a social worker for homes in the area … and she decided to open a facility for herself, and that's how … I got started at a young age. I love it, I love it. I mean, I love people … we have all ages and it's just like one big family and I love it.<br>*Francis*: I owned a group home before, and I've had a group home probably for about 3 years. And [I] was looking to get another business in the same industry … and ran across someone that was looking to sell her family care home. What keeps me going in the role is probably the compassion that I have for helping people. It's really rewarding to have someone come in and … to teach them independent living skills and get them to a point where they're able to be self-sufficient or live on their own. |
| Applications of broad skill base to create a homelike setting | *Rhonda*: You … give them the care they need. The food … their clothes, and I even have to, [if] they don't get enough money … buy their medicines.<br>*Xaveree*: I've been a nurse educator. I've worked in hospitals … providing medical surgical care, nursing care to patients, and I've done home care. My Master's is in healthcare management [and] administration. |
| Support of family-like relational ties (between and with residents) and resident empowerment | *Uniyah*: When they want something and can't remember where it is the other will get up and take them. I mean they are very attentive to each other. It's like being in the same situation and relating.<br>*Helen*: She buys her dirt, and she comes back, she plants her tomatoes, she harvests them, then she cuts down the stalks and cultivates her little land with her little shovel and what have you. *Very* active, very active. Um, she has her own little ole' refrigerator to make her salads and does her own little thing in her room. Very independent! |
| Community support for providers | *Shelli*: I've found cancer research of America to be really supportive…. The lady that I had that had cancer…She had brain, breast, and lung, and they were very supportive of her, and they treated her well. And when I would bring her for the visit, they were really kind.<br>*Yolanda*: Yes, we get training through an organization for free actually. There are some people that come out and do trainings with us on different procedures or different health problems or dealing with bipolar or dealing with whatever areas that these residents might have …. And we have to have data administration [training] also. |

## 3.1 Motivations to Create an AFC Home

The providers had diverse motivations to become AFC providers, including a penchant for caring for others, a need to care for their own biological family, and a desire or need to start a new business. In preparation for or in support of their role, providers brought diverse and varied certifications, representing healthcare, social work, caregiving, and business arenas.

Olivia was a provider whose community care orientation motivated her to start an AFC home (a motivation reflected by 20 of the providers), so that she would have the opportunity to apply this quality in a professional context:

I worked in a nursing home for years. And I've just always been compassionate. I've always dealt with the elderly, even at church or any social.... Actually, I wanted to go to school to be a nurse, but always … something came up, maybe finances or something like that, so I couldn't do it. And, one day I just decided "Hey, I'm going to do this. You know, I'm going to. This is what I want to do."

Three providers were motivated to create an AFC home because of care needs with their biological family members. For example, Alex started his AFC home to provide care for his parents and grandparents:

[T]he main purpose the business was opened was to provide care for immediate family members … because we had a situation in our family where we had family members that were … they were beginning to get up in age … and consequently as a result of that … my father felt like it would be … a great idea that if we opened a family care [so] that we could provide healthcare for our aging parents and grandparents. So, it was not opened as a means of income, a profiting income. It was open more in a sense to provide a service for family members.

Other providers ($n = 3$) described that they simply needed employment and that opening an AFC home was a practical move for them, particularly if they were able to bring some caregiving or business-related expertise to the new venture. For example, Wilma shared, "I've been in the mental health field for maybe 20 years. My husband was about to lose his job; we needed to open a business and that was something I was familiar with."

Nearly half of providers ($n = 11$) emphasized the business motivation for opening an AFC home, and they did not hesitate to share that they required separation between their personal and professional lives in doing so, even if also motivated by care. For example, Nicole expressed care for the residents in her home and the quality of life she and her husband facilitated for them through their business, but she emphasized that she saw it as a business, with her own home as a refuge: "Oh, good heavens, yeah! I don't live there. It's a total business for us. We live probably about 20 min away. So yeah, we come home, that's our refuge." Similarly, although Elon and her young daughter lived with her residents much of the time, she described taking weekends away to their actual home to support their family life, also noting, however, that her home was "right around the corner" from the AFC home:

I am a very family-oriented person and … so I do take maybe like every other weekend off to make sure that we – in my immediate family – we are spending quality time together and doing family things....We go back to our home which is right around the corner and kind of bring some normalcy back into our lives...balance out the two.

### 3.2   Adept Applications of a Broad Skill Base

The providers had a broad skill base that allowed them to negotiate personal circumstances and systemic conditions present in the AFC system in order to support their residents and the sustainability of their homes. The academic degrees that they earned informed their expertise as individuals who supervised all aspects of the home, from contractual paperwork to caregiving practice. For example, Leah brought a foundation of business education to her work, with undergraduate degrees in Accounting and Business Administration, supplemented by a Master's degree in Social Work. Other providers, such as Zada, brought a combination of prior professional experience that translated to the housing and business aspects of AFC work, along with a passion for making a difference in conditions for older adults' residents:

> I used to do real estate, what is called fix and flip. I made them look like they were very, very expensive homes because I wanted to give them the experience of having that feel of a home that was beyond their usual experience of having a rental property. So this man saw that, and he asked me if I had ever thought about family care, and I said, "No; what is that?" He said, "Well let me take you to a house." He took me to a family care home, and the home was very nice, and there were elderly people there ... there were two men sitting at the counter eating frank and beans. And the frank and beans appeared to have been cold, and they were just kind of piled up on the plate. My heart just dropped, and I said ... I can't save everybody, but those who will come into my home, I can care for them and make their lives better.

Other providers, such as Qadira, thrived due to their ability to jump into tasks and learn new skills and relevant knowledge quickly:

> [The home owner] said to me, "did you ever go take that test?" I said "yeah." He literally took the keys off of his key ring for his mom's house. He said, "go open that house next door." That's what I did. I started slowly learning, I wrote my rules, regulations, and I opened it up, kind of just like that, and it went from there, and once we got that one up, it turned a profit .... He was like wow ... and then he actually has a small cul-de-sac full of houses that he built. He pulled the key chain off another house and said, "hey open that one too."

## 3.3   Supporting Family-Like Relational Ties and Resident Empowerment

The skills providers brought to their AFC roles revealed much about the diverse kinds of contributions to thriving, homelike AFC settings, which include provider recognition of personal, family, and business investment; and a vision of what it takes to create a home. Providers demonstrated ongoing practice supporting strong relational, family-like ties, as well as empowering and protective practices with residents that could also be likened to practices in a supportive family and home.

All of the providers interviewed took great care, in some way, to sustain a comfortable and safe homelike context, which required consistent monitoring and discernment with intake processes. For example, Gayle discussed the standard North Carolina FL2 form that providers used as part of their screening process, as well as her perception of the "core group" that subsequent residents needed to fit. The FL2 form is North Carolina's LTC services prior approval form and solicits resident information categories including identification, admitting diagnoses, resident health information, and medication details (North Carolina Medicaid, 2018). Gayle stated, "We receive the FL2 and see if they're a good fit for our core group, which are ...

three males. They get along pretty well, and we don't want to disturb them." Alex, who had started his home for his family members, eventually began to take in individuals outside of his biological family. Consequently, like other providers, he began to put effort into making careful resident matches for the sake of maintaining a sense of home. For example, he required physical and psychological history forms to be completed to help him understand potential residents' conditions before their placement.

Patrice, who despite her caution did take in a resident with serious mental illness, talked about how there are residents that do not fit into the family care home paradigm: "And sometimes you want to meet with the clients also, just to get a feel, because you have to find a good fit, because some people are really very mentally ill and should not even be in a family care home or should be like maybe in a hospital." Similarly, Zada framed her matching process as one that considered both the potential residents, but also the realistic capacity of her staff, and thus the soundness of her AFC homes:

> I visit all of those people who will potentially come into my home and in my mind, I see them as "Would they fit into the home? In which home would they be most comfortable? And how could I serve them?" I think about my staff and myself: "Could I comfortably take care of this person? Would I want to be awake all night long while this person is walking the floor or tearing up furniture or running?" So I select people who I think would be compatible to the other people as well as to my staff.

Nearly all providers ($n = 23$) also contributed to a family-like sense of home and relational ties in their AFC contexts by overcoming a sense of authority in their care relationships and facilitating opportunities for or allowing naturally occurring reciprocity between residents or between residents and themselves and other care staff. For example, Bernice described how her residents have tended to look out for each other's needs:

> Yeah, they share with each other whatever … if they see one don't have it, [they will] give to the other one. Like if one don't have deodorant and they've got two or three, they give the other one. Whatever they have, they'll pretty much share it with each other.

Miriam described a similar kind of ongoing reciprocity in affectionate exchange, but between herself and her resident, empowering her resident by allowing herself (Miriam) to be cared for by her resident. Miriam's description of how her resident gifted her a meal at McDonald's indicated she was aware of the value of reciprocity present in this experience:

> Sometimes she treats me to something to eat if we go to McDonalds. [She says] "I'll pay for it," you know, that kind of thing. I let her do it. It's part of being in the community and caring about other people.

Positive interactions fostering a sense of homelike and family-like relational ties also took the form of facilitated social opportunities and interpersonal sharing. For example, Veronica described a prayer group that was facilitated at her home through a partnership with a resident's biological family member:

During that time, [a resident's] daughter started sort of a prayer group, and we'd get into what was called a circle of prayer, and all the ladies would pray and they could pray for different things –we weren't converting anybody to any religion, just praying together.

Five of the 26 providers lived in the AFC homes, and out of the 21 others who went to their own homes after work, a few lived near their AFC residences. Regardless of whether they lived in the AFC home or not, 18 providers considered their AFC residents to be like extended family. Only two providers felt strongly about creating an interpersonal boundary between their own lives and those of their residents, suggesting that they did not perceive residents as family. Furthermore, six providers acknowledged the complexities of differentiating their home from the AFC context and respecting that the residents had their own home in which they and their staff members were merely guests. For example, Dan explained positive and even empowering aspects of the boundary between staff and the residents of the AFC home where he served as an administrator. He described how an intentional separation between staff and residents empowered residents to feel that the facility was their home, not the staff's home. He clearly stated that the AFC facility was "not my house" and that the staff was also trained and supported to honor this separation:

Well, I'm definitely not a family member .... And I don't live there, I don't work there. I spend time there, but I am definitely the administrator. I'm not told to be a family member so to speak. And I think, you know, the household team ... when they're there working on their shift, they're there working on their shift. They're a member of the household, but ... they don't feel like ... their boundaries are when they clock in and when they clock out.

Olivia also saw herself as an outsider to the AFC home where she worked, and in this way, she respected the context as the home belonging to the residents:

So it has all the rules and regs that we have to follow by doctor's orders and things of that nature. It's not, you know ... to me when I think of a foster care home, I'm thinking you know ... they get x amount of dollars per month from the state or something like that, and it's like a *foster care* home. That's what *I* had envisioned, but the family care home ... the setting is just like they're at home, but I'm the one that has to follow all the rules and regulations. [Laughter]

Ten providers also felt that creating the home and a supportive, healthy family life entailed staying close to rules and regulations to best support resident safety and well-being. Following the rules seemed to be a priority, even in light of offering opportunities for choice. For example, Ken felt he might overstep rules and regulations (e.g., medication compliance or a physician's order) if he did not intervene in resident decisions. He described feeling compelled to intervene for the sake of his residents' well-being while trying to allow as much choice as possible with that as a priority:

Everyone loves certain things, and most times you tend to love the things that aren't good for you as far as your dietary needs. But we try to let them make appropriate choices as far as what they would buy – say when we're out to eat or whatever – what they would order. I try to give them as much liberty as possible with doing that. But then if it's something that I know that is not appropriate for their health, then I have to remind them, "You know that you're not supposed to be having this because of your high blood pressure or because of your cholesterol" or whatever.

## 3.4   Community Support for Providers

Over half of providers ($n = 14$) spoke positively about the community supports available to them. However, these positive narratives also revealed difficulties and how providers worked hard to support their residents in a system that is not always supportive or equitable. For example, Irene discussed frustrations with state-level supports but thrived professionally from a grassroots care provider network, which even inspired her to start a business to have the infrastructure to support other providers in similar situations:

> I have mentors that are in the business that were my proctors when I came into the business that I rely on, I call on. Because … the state is ever-changing …. We don't have the support that we need from the state unfortunately. They'll change law or change a rule and, you know, give you a month's worth of training that nobody could fit in because they are in different parts of the state. And if you can't … accommodate the schedule, then you just miss out! So, it is important to collaborate with other owners of facilities and have a network …. I'm finding there are a lot of providers who are aging out, who have been in the business 20 plus years, they're 62 now, they can retire, they're burnt out, tired [that] the state keeps changing. So, I'm starting a management company … we come in and help manage their home instead of letting them just lose it or give up their license or just throw it away because there's still a need.

Twenty-two providers spoke to the value of training opportunities that were provided that prepared them for the complex combinations of conditions experienced by their residents. For example, Joelle described the value of a dementia training that was provided to her, her siblings, and her parents who worked as a family to provide care for their residents. Similarly, Tanya described valuable county-level trainings that supported her understanding of her residents' health matters, stating "The county has these people that come in and train us for schizophrenia, dementia, bipolar [disorder] … they offer those trainings for us. They're very helpful."

## 4   Discussion

Study findings suggest that AFC providers worked hard to do what they needed to do to create a homelike environment for their residents, whether that meant being careful in matriculating new residents, whether that involved living in the home or living separately (and thus clearly defining the residents' home), and whether that meant providing choices and opportunities or applying policy to protect a resident's health and well-being. The providers' ability to overcome their own sense of authority in the caregiver-care recipient relationship allowed an opportunity for providers to be supported by the care context itself, which results in greater sustainability of their care efforts and AFC home. The ways in which providers navigated personal circumstances and systemic conditions to create a home for their AFC residents may be translated to additional LTC contexts (e.g., nursing homes, assisted living facilities) through the application of person-centered practices and community-based relational values (Arxer, 2019; Gilster et al., 2018; Murphy, 2019).

Providers effectively leveraged their power positions as authority figures in the AFC home and as liaisons with state regulatory agencies and supportive community resources. They used this power to bring maximum opportunity and benefit to residents, including a sense of being at home. As found in previous analyses (Munly et al., 2018), they leveraged their abilities and resources as they invested their expertise, time, and relationships to support the residents' experiences, even in the face of limited personal time and space and sometimes scarce resources. The AFC providers described diverse motivations for adopting their career choice, but in the end, all demonstrated adept applications of their broad skill base, whether related to caregiving or business operations. Their proficiency in both their practice of supporting family-like relational ties and resident empowerment contributed to a sense of home for the residents.

Although this study began to fill the gap in the knowledge about AFC, findings raise additional questions that need to be addressed. Further research is warranted to understand if the providers' perceptions of disconnect with state agencies and the dependence on grassroots networking are results of inadequacies on the level of state understanding and implementation of AFC as community-based care (National Council on Disability, 2003). It is also possible that agencies need to be more in contact with providers who have unique and specific insights from doing the actual day-to-day work.

Future research also needs to consider variability by state context. In the current paper, providers' experiences were presented from the state context of North Carolina. In North Carolina, providers were in direct contact and negotiation with government agencies, whereas in other states, like Virginia, there is the possibility of working under a nonprofit or private umbrella agency. Such an agency can provide an infrastructural buffer for government agency requirements and provide additional training supports and guidance to providers. However, an umbrella agency could also serve to limit individual providers in their independent efforts to facilitate optimal care climates. In addition to examining different state contexts, a full picture of the nature and contribution of AFC practice requires interviews with additional AFC stakeholders, such as Department of Social Services employees, AFC home support staff, AFC home residents, and residents' biological families.

Finally, to our knowledge, no published research focuses on how AFC providers and residents fared during the COVID-19 pandemic. Such an understanding will shed light on whether staff reports of "fear," "helplessness," "sadness," "grief," "anger," and "frustration" were uniquely experienced in skilled nursing facilities or in more homelike settings such as AFC as well (Freidus & Shenk, 2020). The long-term outcomes of COVID-19 on the health and well-being of AFC residents and providers also warrant attention. Research on this matter will be forthcoming for some time. For example, Prophater et al. (2021) looked at outcomes related to technology intervention across adult care communities during the pandemic, with AFC homes only 2% of the sample of 300, suggesting a need to look at AFC contexts in a greater depth. Researchers have been critical of policies responding to COVID-19 that keep households separate (including informal or professionally driven care contexts), which ignore the value of interdependence that is of great importance in disability and aging contexts, exacerbating conditions for those who are already isolated and inconsiderate of the networking needs of those on a smaller budget (Gulland, 2020).

## 5   Implications for Practice

As is the case with qualitative research, the findings from this study are not meant to be generalized but to create a foundation of understanding about AFC providers for informing future exploration of this form of care. Across AFC homes in North Carolina, providers demonstrated an investment in strong partnership with their residents, facilitating relational give and take among residents and between residents and the provider. In the current study, this presence of relational give and take was a marked quality of AFC setting success. Thus, the first implication of this research is the importance of states to go beyond training providers on good management practices (Reinardy & Kane, 1999; Sherman & Newman, 1979) to educating providers on the value of residents themselves for their contribution to the success of AFC settings. Educating providers on the value of residents as key contributors to the AFC context may require practice simulations and contemplative, reflexive exercises to try to understand the perspectives and positions of potential residents (Munly et al., 2016).

Furthermore, the profession of AFC providers demands that individuals be able to devote themselves fully to the role. Consequently, the second implication of this research is that providers, in the current system, should be trained to prepare for this level of professional immersion and dedication. Some providers were able to manage professional demands by integrating their biological family members into the experience, benefitting themselves and the residents. Such practices provide insight into promising practices that could be used to support sustainability in the AFC provider role.

A third implication of the current study is that regulatory agencies need to formally recognize and commend the massive administrative and care work that AFC providers are accomplishing. They must work to find ways to facilitate additional mechanisms of support for the providers, which may include advocating for increases in Medicaid funding so that providers are not funding residents' needs out of their own pockets. The quality of AFC as a community-integrated LTC option, fulfilling the requirements of the Olmstead Decision, will also remain optimal if quality providers are maintained; there is a danger of this not being the case if their professional demands are not adequately compensated. One possibility may be to support the roles of AFC providers through more focused efforts of existing supportive and regulatory agency staff. For example, the role of caseworkers has been described as essential for child foster care (CFC) provider connection with agencies, biological families, services, and resources (Dorsey et al., 2012). Similarly, caseworkers with a capacity to be more in contact with dedicated AFC providers and the realities of AFC homes could be a key point of state intervention to maximize agency connection with and understanding of AFC provider experiences and resident needs, consequently improving state care practices at large.

Finally, states and the public (e.g., families of potential and current residents, individuals residing in the same communities as the AFC homes, taxpayers potentially contributing to the funding of mechanisms of support) need to gain insights into how much providers are investing into their residents and AFC homes. This understanding will help the public and governments at local, state, and national levels to support providers in their strengths while also finding ways to augment that support so that they are not taking on relational and fiscal losses as part of their profession.

# References

AARP Public Policy Institute. (2009). *AARP public policy institute in brief (178). Building adult foster care: What states can do.* Author.

Allen, K. R., & Henderson, A. C. (2022). *Family theories today: A critical intersectional approach* (2nd ed.).

Arxer, S. L. (2019). Conclusion: A re-evaluation of institutionalized healthcare. In S. L. Arxer & J. W. Murphy (Eds.), *Community-based health interventions in an institutional context* (pp. 179–184). Springer. https://doi.org/10.1007/978-3-030-24654-9_13

Bagenstos, S. R. (2020). Take choice seriously in Olmstead jurisprudence. *Journal of Legal Medicine, 40*(1), 5–25. https://doi.org/10.1080/01947648.2020.1731320

Birenbaum, A., & Re, M. A. (1979). Resettling mentally retarded adults in the community. *American Journal of Mental Deficiency, 83,* 323–329.

Carder, P. C., Morgan, L. A., & Eckert, J. K. (2006). Small board-and-care homes in the age of assisted living. *Generations, 29,* 24–31.

Charmaz, K. (2014). *Constructing grounded theory* (2nd ed.).

Crenshaw, K. (1991). Mapping the margins: Intersectionality, identity politics, and violence against women of color. *Stanford Law Review, 43,* 1241–1299. https://doi.org/10.2307/1229039

Dorsey, S., Kerns, S. E. U., Trupin, E. W., Conover, K. L., & Berliner, L. (2012). Child welfare caseworkers as service brokers for youth in foster care: Findings from project focus. *Child Maltreatment, 17,* 22–31. https://doi.org/10.1177/1077559511429593

Few-Demo, A. L. (2014). Intersectionality as the "new" critical approach in feminist family studies: Evolving racial/ethnic feminisms and critical race theories. *Journal of Family Theory & Review, 6*(2), 169–183. https://doi.org/10.1111/jftr.12039

Fisher, B., & Tronto, J. (1990). Towards a feminist theory of care. In E. Abel & M. K. Nelson (Eds.), *Circles of care* (pp. 35–62). State University of New York.

Folkemer, D., Jensen, A., Lipson, L., Stauffer, M., & Fox-Grage, W. (1996). *Adult foster care for the elderly: A review of state regulatory and funding strategies.* AARP Public Policy Institute.

Foucault, M. (1977). *Discipline and punish.* Tavistock.

Freidus, A., & Shenk, D. (2020). "It spread like a wildfire": Analyzing affect in the narratives of nursing home staff during a COVID-19 outbreak. *Anthropology & Aging, 41*(2), 199–206. https://doi.org/10.5195/aa.2020.312

Gilster, S. D., Boltz, M., & Dalessandro, J. L. (2018). Long-term care workforce issues: Practice principles for quality dementia care. *The Gerontologist, 58*(Issue suppl_1), S103–S113. https://doi.org/10.1093/geront/gnx174

Gulland, J. (2020). Households, bubbles and hugging grandparents: Caring and lockdown rules during COVID-19. *Feminist Legal Studies, 28*(3), 329–339. https://doi.org/10.1007/s10691-020-09445-z

Integrity, Inc. (2019). *Three major benefits of community-based services vs. institutional care*. Integrity, Inc. https://www.integrityinc.org/3-major-benefits-of-community-based-services-vs-institutional-care/

Li, J., & Porock, D. (2014). Resident outcomes of person-centered care in long-term care: A narrative review of international research. *International Journal of Nursing Studies, 51*(10), 1395–1415. https://doi.org/10.1016/j.ijnurstu.2014.04.003

McCoin, J. (1983). *Adult foster homes: Their managers and residents*. Human Sciences.

Mollica, R., & Ujvari, K. (2020). *Adult family care: A viable alternative to nursing homes*. AARP Public Policy Institute. https://doi.org/10.26419/ppi.00128.001

Mollica, R., Simms-Kastelein, K., Cheek, M., Baldwin, C., Farnham, J., Reinhard, S., & Accius, J. (2009). *AARP Public Policy Institute research report. Building adult foster care: What states can do*. AARP Public Policy Institute. http://assets.aarp.org/rgcenter/ppi/ltc/2009_13_building_adult_foster_care.pdf

Morgan, L. A., Eckert, J. K., & Lyon, S. M. (1993). Social marginality: The case of small board and care homes. *Journal of Aging Studies, 7*, 383–394. https://doi.org/10.1016/0890-4065(93)90006-6

Morrissey, J. R. (1967). *The case of family care for the mentally ill*. Behavioral Publications.

Munly, K., Tilley-Lubbs, G., & Sheusi, C. (2016). Henry and Sneaky: Finding resolution to my ontological question about service. In G. A. Tilley-Lubbs & S. B. Calva (Eds.), *Re-telling our stories: Critical autoethnographic narratives* (pp. 105–122). Sense.

Munly, K., Roberto, K. A., & Allen, K. R. (2018). Understanding resilience of adult foster care providers. In B. Resnick, L. P. Gwyther, & K. A. Roberto (Eds.), *Resilience in aging: Concepts, research, and outcomes* (2nd ed., pp. 367–383). Springer.

Munly, K., Allen, K. R., & Roberto, K. A. (2021). Experiences of black women adult foster care providers for aging adults: Negotiating power and care. *Journal of Women & Aging, 34*, 692. https://doi.org/10.1080/08952841.2021.1919487

Murphy, J. W. (2019). A community-based organization. In S. L. Arxer & J. W. Murphy (Eds.), *Community-based health interventions in an institutional context* (pp. 11–21). Springer. https://doi.org/10.1007/978-3-030-24654-9_2

National Council on Disability. (2003). *OLMSTEAD: Reclaiming institutional lives* (abridged version). National Council on Disability. http://www.ncd.gov

National Council on Disability. (2004). *Consumer-directed health care: How well does it work?* National Council on Disability. http://www.ncd.gov

National Council on Disability. (2010). *The state of housing in America in the 21st century: A disability perspective*. National Council on Disability. http://www.ncd/gov/policy/housing

Noddings, N. (2010). *The maternal factor: Two paths to morality*. University of California Press.

North Carolina Medicaid. (2018). *Adult care home FL2 form*. https://files.nc.gov/ncdma/Adult-Care-Home-FL2-Form%2D%2DNC-Medicaid-372-124%2D%2D9.2018.pdf

Okoro, C. A., Hollis, N. D., Cyrus, A. C., & Griffin-Blake, S. (2018). Prevalence of disabilities and health care access by disability status and type among adults—United States, 2016. *Morbidity and Mortality Weekly Report, 67*(32), 882–887. https://www.cdc.gov/mmwr/volumes/67/wr/mm6732a3.htm?s_cid=mm6732a3_w#suggestedcitation

Prophater, L. E., Fazio, S., Nguyen, L. T., Hueluer, G., Peterson, L. J., Sherwin, K., Shatzer, J., Branham, M., Kavalec, A., O'Hern, K., Stoglin, K., Tate, R., & Hyer, K. (2021). Alzheimer's association project VITAL: A Florida statewide initiative using technology to impact social isolation and well-being. *Frontiers in Public Health, 9*, 720180. https://doi.org/10.3389/fpubh.2021.720180

Reeves, D., Pye, S., Ashcroft, D. M., Clegg, A., Kontopantelis, E., Blakeman, T., & Van Mawijk, H. (2018). The challenge of ageing populations and patient frailty: Can primary care adapt? *British Medical Journal, 362*, 1–7. https://doi.org/10.1136/bmj.k3349

Reinardy, J., & Kane, R. A. (1999). Choosing an adult foster home or a nursing home: Residents' perceptions about decision making and control. *Social Work, 44*, 571–585. https://doi.org/10.1093/sw/44.6.571

Sherman, S. R., & Newman, E. S. (1977). Foster-family care for the elderly in New York state. *The Gerontologist, 17*, 513–520. https://doi.org/10.1093/geront/17.6.513

Sherman, S. R., & Newman, E. S. (1979). Role of the caseworker in adult foster care. *Social Work, 24*, 324–328.

Sherman, S. R., & Newman, E. S. (1988). *Foster families for adults: A community alternative in long-term care.* Columbia University Press.

Tronto, J. C. (1998). An ethic of care. *Generations, 22*, 15–20.

U.S. Equal Employment Opportunity Commission. (n.d.). *Americans with disabilities act: Questions and answers.* https://www.eeoc.gov/laws/guidance/ada-questions-and-answers

Wacker, R. R., & Roberto, K. A. (2019). *Community resources for older adults: Programs and services in an era of change* (5th ed.). Sage.

# Part II
# Facility-Based Care

# A Theory of Creating *At-Homeness* Across the Long-Term Care Continuum

Sheila L. Molony and Jude Rabig

## 1 Introduction

> Architecture is basically a container of something. I hope they will enjoy not so much the teacup, but the tea. – Yoshio Taniguchi

Taniguchi is expressing his desire to create museum spaces where patrons will enjoy the experiences of engagement with art. Using this analogy, the "tea" of long-term care (LTC) design is *at-homeness*.

The crisis of COVID-19 in residential LTC settings, including nursing homes and assisted living facilities, has highlighted challenges in environmental design, staffing, training, and leadership (Zimmerman et al., 2021). It has also sensitized the public to the importance of connection, belonging, and feeling at home in the context of illness or disability. Predating COVID, the last 10 years have included critical shifts in thinking about LTC. These shifts include reimagining the older adult from a passive disabled person to be paternalistically "cared for" to an empowered individual able to express their own needs and preferences. There has also been a shift to a broadened concept of health, from a strictly physical deficit-based care model to a more holistic strength-based model of biopsychosocial, spiritual health. Together, these shifts are the basis of person-centered and person-directed care, which require reimagining the architectural and operational practices in LTC.

S. L. Molony (✉)
School of Nursing, Quinnipiac University, Hamden, CT, USA
e-mail: Sheila.molony@quinnipiac.edu

J. Rabig
Rabig Consulting LLC, Niskayuna, NY, USA
e-mail: juderabig@gmail.com

© The Author(s), under exclusive license to Springer Nature Switzerland AG 2023
F. Ferdous, E. Roberts (eds.), *(Re)designing the Continuum of Care for Older Adults*, https://doi.org/10.1007/978-3-031-20970-3_5

The founders of the Pioneer Network illuminated the critical role of the built environment in supporting or hindering person-centered care (Zimmerman et al., 2014). Subsequent efforts to deinstitutionalize the built environment have resulted in innovative models of residential LTC such as the Eden Alternative, the Green House Model, and related small house model dwellings. This chapter proposes a theory to guide ongoing efforts to enhance meaningful dwelling in meaningful environments.

The theory introduces the concept of *at-homeness* as a central construct to integrate theories of caring and thriving with key constructs related to deinstitutionalization, person-centered care, placemaking, and pattern language. *At-homeness* speaks to the need for a strong interdependence of the two components of creating a dwelling, both the built environment and the experiences that transpire in that place. The current theory is informed by a wealth of scholarship focused on meaningful environments (Rowles & Bernard, 2012). Three prerequisites are needed to generate the quantity and quality of person-environment integration necessary to potentiate thriving. These three prerequisites include:

- A built environment that enhances situational possibilities for experiences of home (referred to here as caring physical environments).
- Policies, practices, and individualized plans of care based on deep knowledge of meaningful experiences of home as defined by the resident (referred to here as a caring intentions).
- Day-to-day concrete actions that integrate the physical, social, and human environment by bringing the caring plan alive in practice (referred to here as caring actions).

The chapter will first review and define key concepts, models, and theories underpinning this work, synthesize these constructs, provide examples and resources for theory application, and offer future directions for research, policy, and practice.

## 2 Key Concepts and Models

Table 1 defines several key constructs that inform the Theory of Caring Environments. These concepts are shaped by decades of scholarship in environmental psychology, environmental gerontology, and social science and are grounded in Merleau-Ponty's (1962) philosophy of phenomenology that identifies subjective meaning in the context of the situation and arcs of possibility shaped by lived experience (Molony et al., 2007).

**Table 1** Conceptual definitions

| Concept | Definition |
|---|---|
| At-homeness | A situational lived experience of personal power, refuge, meaningful relationships, and self-reconciliation |
| Caring | Identifying what is most important to the individual in the context of their situation and acting upon that information to intentionally foster positive experiences |
| Deinstitutionalization | A process of removing organizational characteristics that obstruct mastery, goal setting, personal habits, and rhythms of daily life |
| Pattern language | The way that design and physical structures make an environment nurturing for human beings by being responsive to meanings and human relationships |
| Person-centered care | Values and preferences of individuals are elicited and, once expressed, guide all aspects of holistic health care |
| Thriving | Harmony between the personal, social, and built/natural environment |

## 2.1 Deinstitutionalization

Our elderly are left with a controlled and supervised institutional existence, a medically designed answer to unfixable problems, a life designed to be safe but empty of anything they care about. Atul Gawande (2014)

The nursing home is conceptualized as a location where clinical care is provided to frail older adults. Historically, it has been architecturally and operationally designed in the image and likeness of a hospital and meets the definition of a total institution characterized by Erving Goffman (1990). Traditional nursing homes house large numbers of individuals separated from the larger community. Residents bathe, eat, sleep, and socialize based on the facility-determined schedules with few choices left for individuals. Staff control and direct life, and residents are afforded little agency in determining care. As a result, they have diminished privacy, and they have a space to live in, but little opportunity to create a place.

Lieberman et al. (1968) examined 15 years of evidence regarding the psychological effects of institutionalization on older adults. They identified reduced capacity for independent thought and action, depressive mood, and low self-esteem. The individual's relationship with the environment becomes increasingly fractured as these various stresses are experienced. Carboni described homelessness as "a lived painful experience that brings about deep existential despair for the individual" (Carboni, 1990, p.33). As a result of her research, she posed the provocative question:

A pressing issue is whether nursing homes should exist at all if the consequence of being institutionalized is to be homeless, and if to be homeless is to lack meaning in life and to suffer intolerable pain, then can we justify providing and promoting this negative experience for the vulnerable and chronically ill elderly individual? Solutions to this dilemma might be found in the exploration and development of alternative settings in an attempt to move away from the total institution of the typical nursing home. (Carboni, 1990, p.36)

Many scholars have presented theories of positive aging and quality of life, with no definitive conclusion; however, most include that mastery over one's existence, goal setting, and proactive adaptation are necessary to achieve life satisfaction. The psychological effects of the institution create genuine obstructions to achieving positive outcomes. Thus, removing the institution from the LTC equation is fundamental and necessary to support the potential to achieve positive aging and thriving.

In 1997, a grassroots group of nursing home pioneers met to achieve radical change in LTC environments and organizational systems. This "culture change" movement known as the Pioneer Movement was deeply concerned with deinstitutionalizing and individualizing nursing home care (Miller et al., 2016). In addition to promoting resident-directed care (residents exercise choice and control over their own care), core components of culture change include close relationships between residents, family members, staff, and community, operational structures that empower staff to respond to resident needs and desires, collaborative and decentralized decision-making, systematic continuous quality improvement, and living environments designed to be a home rather than an institution (Miller et al., 2010; Zimmerman et al., 2016). In addition, the Pioneer Network recognized the critical role of the physical environment in fostering or constraining deinstitutionalization.

In 2003, the Green House Project® provided the first intentional attempt in the USA to deinstitutionalize the nursing home beginning with the design process (Kane et al., 2007). The physical design, architecture, leadership structure, staffing model, and approaches to care were radically redesigned to achieve the principles of culture change (Rabig et al., 2006). Based on European care home models, it envisioned creating a physical and experiential home for eight to ten people who required a nursing home level of care. In addition, it was planned to be a place to optimize the aging experience. Eagerness for change and early successful outcomes of the model staff, resident, and family satisfaction, as well as financial viability, led to the replication of the Green House® and related (generic) small house model of care in nursing homes and assisted living environments (Lum et al., 2008; Molony et al., 2011; Reinhard & Hado, 2021; Sharkey et al., 2011).

## 2.2 Pattern Language

Much of the initial design of the Green House was guided by the patterns found in *A Pattern Language: Towns, Buildings, Construction* by Christopher Alexander (Alexander et al., 1977). According to the text, a pattern is how physical design responds to meaning and human relationships. For example, in a keynote speech at the 1996 Conference on Object-Oriented Programming, Systems, Languages, and Applications (Alexander, 1996), Alexander explained it this way:

The idea that materialized in the published pattern language was, first of all, of course, intended just to get a handle on some of the physical structures that make the environment nurturing for human beings…People have asked me what kind of a process was involved in creating the architectural pattern language? One of the things we looked for was a profound impact on human life. We were able to judge patterns, and tried to judge them, according to the extent that when present in the environment, we were confident that they really do make people more whole in themselves.

It is worth noting here that this quote highlights the crucial role of the built environment in potentiating experiences of ongoing meaning-making and self-reconciliation inherent in *at-homeness*. Alexander developed 253 patterns. Each pattern describes a design problem and solutions that can be repeatedly used without ever doing it the same way. Many of Alexander's patterns were incorporated in the Green House® architecture, including Positive Outdoor Space, Common Areas at The Heart, Farmhouse Kitchens, A Room of One's Own, Sequence of Sitting Spaces, Bathing Room, Communal Eating, The Sunny Place, and others. As the original small house model has been replicated, new designs have maintained some of these critical elements and eliminated others that potentially contribute to or diminish human benefit. Some clearly reflect, and others blur the patterns of home compared to the patterns of an institution. Pattern language presents architecture and design in a distinctly abstract way. Salingaros (2000) describes this connection:

Pattern languages were revealed as the "taproot" of all architecture, from which design draws its life by virtue of satisfying human needs. This is true even if one disagrees with one or more of Alexander's patterns. Our results imply that design styles which cut themselves off from this source of life are condemned to remain forever sterile.

Future designers would benefit from reviewing and incorporating more patterns to support thriving.

## 2.3 Person-Centered Care

An expert panel convened by The Scan Foundation defined person-centered care (American Geriatrics Society, 2016, p.16):

Person-centered care means that individuals' values and preferences are elicited and once expressed, guide all aspects of their health care, supporting their realistic health and life goals. Person-centered care is achieved through a dynamic relationship among individuals, others who are important to them, and all relevant providers. This collaboration informs decision-making to the extent that the individual desires.

Person-centered LTC extends beyond traditional notions of medically defined health care and includes social, psychological, spiritual, and holistic health. Key concepts of person-centered care include forming and maintaining dynamic relationships with the person and significant others and building on that collaborative relationship to honor values, preferences, and life goals.

## 2.4 At-Homeness

*At-homeness* is the pre-reflective experience of feeling at home in the world. It is most often experienced within a particular place or space. One of the earliest references to the term *at-homeness* is in Seamon's publication, *A Geography of the Lifeworld (Routledge Revivals): Movement, Rest and Encounter* (1979). Seamon focused on the experience of rest and "being comfortable in and familiar with the everyday world in which one lives" (p. 70). Home is shared through rituals, traditions, and symbolic meanings. Home provides a space where we need not be constantly vigilant and can withdraw to return to ourselves (Bollnow, 1961). Phenomenological narratives describe it as a place where we have cherished possessions "pregnant with the meaning from which they emerged" (Baldurrson, 2002). At home, "we are looked for, named and important in someone else's world" (Norris, 1990).

The concept of *at-homeness* in this theory is derived from a meta-synthesis of 22 qualitative studies (Molony, 2010). The meta-synthesis describes home as both an existential place of situated human experience and an ongoing process to redefine and reshape the self in the context of changing health, function, environments, and lived experiences. Experiences of home are typified by experiences that have personal significance to the individual in the context of their history, self-concept, and social and physical world. These experiences center around four key sub-concepts: personal power, refuge, relationships, and self-reconciliation. *Personal power* consists of autonomy, choice, control, mastery, and contribution. *Refuge* is defined as holistic safety that includes emotional, social, spatial, and spiritual safety in the context of threats to self or wholeness. *Relationships* include cherished bonds with individuals, groups, pets, possessions, places, cultures, ideas, and values. *Self-reconciliation* means defining and redefining the self in the context of one's personal history, present situation, and anticipated future, connecting with one's strengths, integrating new identities into one's self-narrative, and opening a space for growth and possibility. *At-homeness* is created and recreated on an ongoing basis through *a personal process of engaging with the current place and situation*, integrating the past, shaping the present, and looking forward to the future.

The process of creating and maintaining *at-homeness* after a residential transition to LTC is particularly challenging due to the often involuntary nature of the move and the often co-occurring losses in health, function, and social interactions. Qualitative research describes three processes used to re-establish *at-homeness* during transition: closing one door and opening another, nesting, and moving the "meaning of me" forward (Molony, 2010). Closing one door and opening another means intentionally letting go of one's previous residence or situation and making up one's mind to move forward. Nesting is a process of placemaking by personalizing, investing time and work into the new environment, and/or creating shared experiences and engaging with others in new social relationships. Finally, moving the "meaning of me" forward requires a future orientation and may include sharing stories, sharing dreams, planning experiences to look forward to, engaging in creative endeavors that foster a sense of self, or connecting with culture, food, music, nature, the arts, or spiritual experiences that foster a sense of connection to something larger than oneself.

# 3 Theories

## 3.1 Caring Theories

Caring is a process of identifying what is most important to the individual in the context of their past and present situation, hopes, and dreams and then acting upon that information to intentionally foster positive experiences. Three nurse scholars offer theories of caring that inform this work; Benner and Wrubel (1989) identify caring as central to practice and is demonstrated by learning what matters to the individual. To gain empathy and understanding of what matters, one can listen, observe behavior, question, and reflect. Only by identifying what shows up as significant for the other person can one truly identify and act upon situational possibilities. What matters to an individual changes as the context changes, and it is therefore critical to realize that caring is dynamic and not limited to a one-time assessment or static care plan.

In the middle-range Theory of Caring, Swanson (1991) identifies caring processes including *knowing, being with, enabling, and maintaining belief. Knowing* means being open to another's reality, assessing capabilities and needs, being sensitive to nonverbal cues, attending to the other, engaging and sharing the genuine self, and learning what matters. *Being with* means being authentically present, being involved, and demonstrating warmth, love, compassion, expressive caring, and reciprocal sharing of expressive caring and feelings. *Enabling* means empowering, informing, explaining, validating, supporting, enhancing coping, generating alternatives, problem-solving, and removing all barriers to self-efficacy. *Maintaining belief* in the whole person is expressed by affirming experience, helping the person find meaning, offering realistic optimism, instilling hope, going above and beyond, and going the distance. Swanson also wrote that caring includes *doing for* others, activities that they are unable to do for themselves in a manner that optimizes or amplifies the person's abilities and contributions.

## 3.2 Theory of Thriving

Failure to thrive (FTT) has been identified as a life-threatening alienation between person and environment, typified by social isolation and withdrawal, physical and cognitive decline, depression, and weight loss. This description echoes many of the themes in Carboni's (1990) description of existential homelessness. *Thriving* is the antithesis of FTT and is defined by Haight et al. (2002) as harmony between personal, social, and built/natural environment recognized by indicators of social relatedness, giving of self, finding meaning, positive physical and cognitive function, positive affective state, and consistent weight. According to Haight et al., "… the variety of humans who enter in and out of the person's environment at different phases of life, can either manipulate the environment and person to contribute to optimum growth or interfere with the environment to hinder thriving and growth (p. 16)."

## 4  Synthesis: The Theory of Caring Environments

While exquisite experiences of *at-homeness* may occur organically and serendipitously, this theory is intended to guide *intentional action* to create and shape small, discrete person-environment experiences that enhance the likelihood of thriving in residential LTC environments. The theory hypothesizes that:

1. Caring environments: Built environments that incorporate a *pattern language* to foster humanistic social and experiential environments facilitate *nesting and self-reconciliation* (fundamental processes of *at-homeness*) to promote thriving.
2. Caring intention: Documents that guide and codify actions (policies, care plans) potentiate person-centeredness to the extent that they incorporate key elements of *caring* and *at-homeness*. If supported by adequate resources and put into action, these policies and plans potentiate *thriving*. These policies and plans are grounded in realistic optimism and informed by deep knowing of individual preferences, values, and needs. These policies and plans are created in collaboration with the person and their important others. They explicitly include ways to empower the individual and remove barriers to self-efficacy. They include careful consideration of ways to enhance personal power, refuge, significant relationships, and self-reconciliation. Throughout the transition process, they include strong support for closing one door and opening another, nesting and amending the self-narrative in a way that integrates the current situation into "meaning of me" and opens possibilities for projection into the future.
3. Caring actions: Offering as many discrete, individually meaningful experiences of *at-homeness* as possible and avoiding constraints that damage person-place relationships will enable situational *thriving*. This is accomplished through everyday concrete actions that bring caring plans and policies to fruition.

Carers can shape and change an experience by enhancing individual strengths and abilities, decreasing environmental constraints, or both. Examples may include designing and building spaces that remove disempowering barriers to wheelchair mobility, providing cognitive-behavioral therapy to remove disempowering thoughts that fuel depression, and using planned activities to call forth and celebrate the

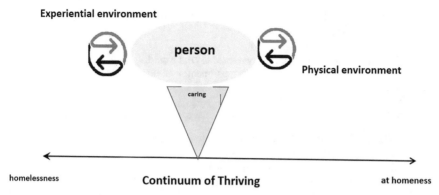

The community dwelling person who is transitioning from their existing home to a long-term care institution is travelling on a continuum of thriving. They are journeying between the psychosocial and emotional state of at-homeness where thriving is maximized, and a failure to thrive characterized by decline and despair. They are supported in the journey by carers who shape and influence the mutually interactive physical and experiential environments. Knowledge and implementation of caring practices which positively shape these forces will enhance and encourage movement towards at-homeness and maximize thriving.

**Fig. 1** Model of caring environments

creative self in persons living with dementia. Each carer has a role in enlarging the possibilities for person-environment integration and *at-homeness*. A diagram of the Theory of Caring Environments is illustrated in Fig. 1.

# 5 Application in Practice

## 5.1 Caring Environment

The built environment of the small house model nursing home provides one example of a caring environment. The bedroom and bathroom designs offer function-enhancing features; private rooms and "entry by doorbell" promote refuge, and closets, bathroom design, climate controls, and hallways intentionally facilitate independence in dressing, transferring, grooming, bathing, walking, and achieving personal comfort. Barrier-free access to outdoor courtyards and gardens, windows to inviting spaces, and welcoming shared spaces promote relationships with people and/or the natural world. The redesigned small house care model fosters empowerment and person-centered care. Whether or not the small house model is adopted, the use of pattern language in design guides the process toward wholeness and self-reconciliation. Questions in Table 2 highlighted in red indicate some preliminary data-gathering to inform design decisions.

**Table 2**  Questions to illuminate individual meanings and experiences of at-homeness

**EMPOWERING- Do What I Want**
- How would you finish this sentence?
  - •If I could do one thing that I really wanted to do, I would....
  - •If I could do as I pleased in my room/apartment, I would...
  - •If I were the boss in this place, I would...
  - •I wish I had the freedom to....
  - •I wish I had more choice about...

**EMPOWERING – Mastery, Meeting Needs, Feeling Useful**
- What helps the day go smoother for you?
- What helps you to take care of yourself and your needs?
- What helps you to feel a sense of accomplishment?
  - How would you finish these sentences?
    - o  I wish I could contribute to…
    - o  I wish I could take part in... (or play a role in)
    - o  I wish I could do… for others.
- What helps you to be your best or do your best?
- What would make you feel more comfortable in this space?
- What would help you to really know this place and get around better?
- What routines or rituals are important to you?

**REFUGE:**
- How would you finish this sentence?
- I feel safe when....
- I would feel safer if...
- I wish I had more privacy for...
- When I need time to heal or recuperate, or I just want to relax and feel better, I like to…
- Think about a moment when you felt really comfortable where were you? What were you doing?
- Think of a time when you felt at peace. Where were you? What were you doing?
- Do have any favorite smells? sounds? sights? tastes? textures/sensations?
- How important is it to you to journey or leave and return?

**RELATIONSHIP**
- Are there any things/objects/possessions that are important to you?
- Do you feel attached to particular…?
  - •Views or vistas or landscapes or nature?
  - •Ideas or stories?
  - •People or animals?
  - •Places/spaces?
  - •Cultures or ideas?
- How would you complete these sentences?
  - •I feel attached to....
  - •I feel needed by.... or I feel needed when ...
  - •...is just like family to me....
  - •...is my friend...
- What makes you feel like you are really part of a group?

**Table 5.2**  (continued)

**SELF-RECONCILIATION**

- How would you complete these sentences?
    - •If you REALLY want to know who I am as a person...you should know...
    - •I look forward to....
    - •I lose track of time when I....
    - •I experience joy and pleasure when...
- If I wanted you to tell "your story," what would some of the main points be? What would be insome of the chapters?
- What makes you feel connected with your past?
- What do you like to reminisce about?
- Can you tell me about an experience when you got over a rough time in your life? What helped you to get through it?

**INTEGRATION**

- Tell me about a place where you really felt like you were part of the place, or the place was partof you.
- Tell me about a place where you really "fit" or "belonged." Share your thoughts about thatplace. Can you describe it for me?
    - What do you feel? What do you see or hear or taste or smell? What are you doing? Are there other people or animals around?
- Tell me about another favorite place or space. Can you describe itfor me?
- Tell me about an experience where you have felt truly "at home" in the world. Describe that experience.
- Have you ever moved into a new place that didn't feel quite like home at first, but it felt more like home over time? Tell me about that.
- Are there little, "everyday" experiences that make you feel comforted and at home?

    Areas in red are suggested questions for architects and designers to incorporate in project planning interviews

## 5.2  Caring Intentions

The process of deinstitutionalization extends beyond the built environment. Feelings about a place are intimately connected with the experiences in that space. This supports the thinking that while the buildings are being constructed, the traditional staff role must be deconstructed – or in Lewin's theory of change framework – unfrozen and then exposed to new frameworks that support positive experiences for people and their supportive helpers (Lewin, 1951). For example, the small house model implementation team explores with the people who work in the houses the intentional shifts they will need to make in their previously learned institutional work behaviors, including developing an awareness of ageist stereotypes and the traditional system's focus on brokenness. Additionally, developing policies and practices that support collaborative partnership with the resident is essential.

Some examples of caring policies include resident involvement in decisions regarding the house where they live and policies on choice and care planning, which consistently and formally include the resident's voice and those who are important to the resident. Introducing and practicing these shifts constitute Lewin's moving phase of the change, ideally happening before the transition to the new building.

Refreezing or making the permanent changes involves post-occupancy work and may take an extended period. The process requires action accompanied by observation and good coaching until there is strong evidence that these "new" practices are routinely practiced. Educating, observing, coaching, and supporting are vital caring processes. They are consistent with culture change principles of continuous quality improvement and may be guided by systematic assessment of the degree to which *at-homeness* is identified and supported.

Using an assessment tool that intentionally seeks out individual meanings associated with the sub-concepts of *at-homeness* will provide a template for the caring plan. The caring plan identifies situational opportunities to enhance at-homeness and mitigate alienating, spirit-numbing experiences that may lead to a failure to thrive. A sample assessment guide (Table 2) and caring plan guideline (Table 3) were developed by the first author and pilot tested in a small feasibility study that demonstrated acceptability by nursing home residents and illuminated potential actionable person-centered approaches. Traditional care plans are oriented around medical categories, symptoms, behaviors, and diagnoses. Skillful medical care, symptom management, and risk mitigation remain essential using a caring framework, since pain, illness exacerbation, and excess disability disrupt refuge and relationships and foster disempowerment.

## 5.3    Caring Actions

An important component of *enabling at-homeness* is activating and engaging the other person in expressing their views, making choices, speaking up, and taking action to engage with the environment. The caring environment enables personal power by building knowledge and confidence in the person's ability to express their needs and wishes. As a result, an empowered person is involved in fulfilling their own needs and goals. This incorporates citizenship, choice, and co-production (Cottam & Leadbeater, 2004; Coulter, 2002) and emphasizes the quality of the relationships between flexible professionals and activated, empowered care recipients, representing a radical shift in power distribution and requiring a new mindset. Caring actions include recognizing behavior as a form of communication for persons with dementia (Kolanowski et al., 2021).

Caring actions before, during, and after transition to the nursing home are critical to the process of closing one door and opening another. The degree to which a person can feel at home in a residential LTC setting is dependent upon their previous experiences, needs, and expectations, the degree of choice in the move, individual

**Table 3** Guidelines for creating a dynamic caring plan

| |
|---|
| *Note*: Actions may include planning small experiences, training others in caring processes that optimize dignity, purchasing new technology, designing or redesigning the physical environment, and increasing the intensity of skillful health care. The prioritization of actions depends upon valuing and maintaining belief in a holistic well-being, and honoring "what matters" to the individual. |
| *Domain: Empowerment* is the power to do something, decide something, choose something, or refuse something. Spaces, places, social interactions, and experiences that provide opportunities for choice, control, success, mastery, and the chance to contribute and feel useful are empowering. |
| **What actions can be taken to *enable/empower* the person to:** |
| Enhance self-confidence in ability to speak up and advocate for their own needs and desires |
| Set a personally meaningful goal |
| Achieve a personally meaningful goal [Note: Small sub-goals may be needed] |
| Engage in routines/activities are familiar and/or preferred (e.g., help person feel "like themselves") |
| Participate in self-care |
| Care for loved others |
| Experience a sense of achievement and/or contribution |
| **What actions can be taken to *prevent* disempowering experiences that foster helplessness or feelings of uselessness** [e.g., use of infantilizing speech, unnecessary wheelchair or diaper use, discouraging self-care illness exacerbations]? |
| *Domain*: A *refuge* is a place to rest, heal, and recharge in times of duress. It is also a space of protection against threat, discomfort, intrusion, or harm. A refuge is characterized by comfort and contrast from the outside world where harsher conditions or rules may apply. In addition, returning to a welcoming, familiar, comfortable place is felt more keenly after traveling to a less familiar or hospitable situation. Therefore, journeying and returning reinforce refuge. Refuge includes personally meaningful boundaries that are respected and protected to keep out threats to physical, psychological, social, spiritual, or material well-being. However, boundaries that are perceived as confinement threaten selfhood and empowerment and are not considered refuge. |
| **What actions can be taken to improve the experience of *refuge*?** |
| Enhancing possibilities for relaxation, easing of vigilance, freedom from "rules" |
| Increasing familiarity and comfort of space |
| Providing opportunities to leave and return |
| Enhancing navigability and wayfinding |
| Fostering emotional safety |
| Promoting social safety |
| Protecting material safety (and safety for possessions/valuables) |
| Nurturing spiritual or existential safety |
| Safeguarding bodily or sensory safety (freedom from pain) |
| **What actions can be taken to *prevent* intrusions/experiences that threaten *refuge*** [e.g., placing a lock upon the door, trading a hospital-type bed for a comfortable bed or chair for person's home, identifying rules or practices that give perception of imprisonment)? |

(continued)

**Table 3** (continued)

| |
|---|
| *Domain: Meaningful relationship* connotes connectedness to cherished people, things, places, and/or ideas. This may include connection to family, neighborhood, culture, other individuals, or groups who are "like family," pets, personal possessions, symbols, values, or cherished places/ spaces. Salient positive relationships foster a feeling of belonging. Cherished possessions often serve as touchstones to favorite people, places, and experiences of the past, transporting the person like a portal to holistic experiences of the narrative self. The relationship to place involves mutuality. Investing time, energy, and decision-making into the environment as part of placemaking reaps a return of meaning, identity, and belongingness and strengthens relationship to place. |

**What actions can be taken to facilitate sense of belonging, connection, or *relationship* with?**

| |
|---|
| Significant others (family, friends, staff, peers, community, culture, group, pets) |
| Cherished possessions |
| Space/place |
| Nature |
| Important ideals or symbols |
| Higher power |

**What actions can be taken to *prevent* constraints on meaningful relationships** [e.g., lack of space for socialization, noisy, echoing environments, or tight spaces that do not permit easy interaction]?

| |
|---|
| *Domain: Self-reconciliation* is an ongoing process of self-recognition and integration of past, present, and future perceptions of self. Self-reconciliation is an ongoing reworking of "who am I" in the current place, body, relationship, or situation. Experiences such as illness, injury, functional decline, social disruption, or residential relocation pose challenges to the continuity of one's self-narrative and self-recognition. Memory loss related to advancing dementia may disrupt self-recognition and narrative continuity that may result in a lostness or frantic search for a familiar "home" experienced in the distant past. Connecting to self through arts, aromas, sensory experiences, or felt compassion and love may provide a bridge back to a more coherent present. |

**What actions can be taken to enhance one's sense of feeling like themselves or *self-reconciliation*?**

| |
|---|
| Routines or rituals of personal importance |
| Telling one's story or therapeutic reminiscence |
| Reconnecting with one's strengths |
| Aesthetic experiences |
| Familiar objects, photos, or music |
| Time for rest and recovery |
| Opportunities to experience being valued or loved |

**What actions can be taken to prevent loss of feeling like oneself** [e.g., loss of routines, loss of possessions, loss of coherence, illness, or medical concerns taking priority over "normal" life]?

engagement throughout the transition process, decision-making related to possessions, and personalization of the new environment (Cutchin, 2012).

Molony et al. (2011) followed 25 nursing home residents who were given a choice to stay in a traditional model nursing home or relocate to a new small house model facility. The nine residents who chose to remain in the traditional nursing home had adapted to the environment and achieved a sufficient level of person-environment integration to demonstrate a statistically significant difference in baseline *at-homeness* from those who elected to move. The remaining 16 residents had low levels of pre-move *at-homeness*. However, this group demonstrated a statistically significant increase in at-homeness 6 months after the move. The study also found a relationship between *at-homeness* and indicators of thriving, including a positive relationship between *at-homeness* and higher functional ability, and an inverse relationship between *at-homeness* and depressive symptoms.

A qualitative study by Cater et al. (2021) found that 62.8% of residents in adult foster homes in Oregon felt that their residence felt like home, compared to 48.9% of assisted living/residential care (AL/RC) dwellers and 30% of nursing home dwellers. Design decisions in the built and organizational environment (e.g., having a private room) played a significant role in the experience of home and often shaped the resident's ability to experience other key mediators of at-homeness: autonomy and social connectedness. Several other studies have highlighted the role of design in either enhancing or inhibiting resident's independence, mobility, and social interaction (Cater et al., 2021; Cooney, 2012; Johnson & Bibbo, 2014).

## 5.4  Resources for Theory Application

### 5.4.1  Evidence-Based Design Meaningful Environments

The resources to assist in designing a dwelling where older adults have positive life experiences that are full and rich and meaningful are ever-increasing and widely available.

As we examine the resources, it is essential to note that not all organizations will be able to fully adopt new buildings or all elements of the small house model of care. However, the links provided in Fig. 1 list many resources that provide information for designers, staff, residents, and their families to use in planning the design, operating plan, and education that will yield the positive elements of at-homeness.

By no means have we reached the pinnacle of success in design. Green House®/small house dwellings resulted from thinking that was once labeled risky, unable to be licensed, only applicable to high-functioning individuals, and more. The Hogeweyk Dementia Village in the Netherlands is a more recent example of a new concept and design underway. Risk-taking and bravery combined with willing funders and creative thinking have benefited older adults. Areas that remain under-researched or visibly absent include incorporating art, music, and complementary and alternative therapies, especially aromatherapy, nooks or rooms for sacred spaces, fitness spaces, proper transportation systems to enable community engagement, places and opportunities for meaningful work, and more. Architects, designers, planners, and organizational leaders need to mobilize caring intention and reach beyond the traditional to intentionally test new ideas.

### 5.4.2　Resources for Enabling At-Homeness During Transition

Evidence-based relocation guidelines have been published to guide best practices before, during, and immediately after relocation to residential LTC (Hertz et al., 2016). Qualitative data from persons with high levels of *at-homeness* before and after transition provide insight into the importance of identifying "what matters" and building an intentional, caring, transition plan (Molony et al., 2011; Johnson & Bibbo, 2014; Sullivan & Williams, 2017).

Balancing physical and physiological safety while not trampling dignity, emotional, social, or psychological safety requires skillful consideration and planning related to risk. The Rothschild Foundation has provided tools for risk mitigation and planning that recognize that risk is part of being human (Behrens et al., 2018). At the same time, physical and cognitive vulnerability may warrant more attentive strategies to maximize freedom while striving for holistic safety (Calkins et al., 2015). Guidelines for whole-person dementia care have also been published (Fazio et al., 2018; Wolverson & Clarke, 2016).

## 6　Theory in Action

*At-homeness* is not provided by a fancy hotel, high-amenity cruise ship, or a stage set of domesticity. There is a risk of creating superficial simulation homes if the voices (including verbal and nonverbal communication) of those who actually dwell in the long-term environment are not truly heeded.

If the purpose of the small house and other new models of care is to create a place that creates a sense of *at-homeness*, then one might measure the implementation's success by asking individuals for their input and thoughts at regular intervals. During the design phase, it is imperative to include future residents in discussions and meetings not just once or twice but as members of the planning team who regularly attend and contribute to the discussions. Including them as participants in planned mock-ups, materials and furnishing selection, landscaping, and other aspects of the project is a productive way to incorporate their voices and, in doing so, to demonstrate their empowerment in the new lifestyle they will be experiencing. In addition, regular post-occupancy interviews with residents, staff, and families are a strong indicator of how close designers have come to meeting their objectives.

In a longitudinal mixed method study that followed a group of nursing home dwellers moving from a traditional model to a small house model nursing home, all 16 residents demonstrated an increase in at-homeness after the move. Qualitative findings revealed that at-homeness was supported by enhanced freedom, privacy, friendship, and increased opportunity for self-care (Molony et al., 2011). The second author has provided consultation, training, and project leadership for numerous small house nursing home dwellings as they transitioned from planning to post-occupancy. The following statements are from field notes and interviews conducted with residents who transitioned to these sites (Rabig, 2003–2020). They illustrate components of *at-homeness* as defined by a range of residents.

> My, it's good to be home again after all of these years. *88-year-old woman with advanced cognitive impairment immediately after moving into a Green House*

> Yes, I can tell you what I like. I like cuddling with my husband when he comes to visit, walking out of the front door without asking for permission, having a chance to really get to know the people around our family table, and speaking up at listening sessions. I couldn't do any of those things before at the other place. Here, I don't need my depression pills. I'm happy. Life is good. *89-year-old woman, four months after transition to a small house*

> She's my best friend. We spend our time together. It's wonderful. I lived in the same hall as her back there, and I never met her. We could have been best friends long ago. *84-year-old small house resident, three months post-transition, describing her housemate*

> I never had choices, and now I choose everything. It's not perfect, but I feel relaxed like I used to feel at home. *79-year-old male six-month resident of a small house*

> I helped to give the tours around here. When outsiders are thinking about coming to live in our house, I show them around. I tell what it's like to live here. It's my job, and I feel useful again. *65-year-old female resident with multiple sclerosis who uses a wheelchair*

> So, this is a small house, and we call the old place the big house. The best part here is that I have privacy, and I have a say in my schedule. *86-year-old male resident of a small house*

# 7  Future Research and Policy Implications

## 7.1  Hypothesis Testing

More longitudinal studies are needed to evaluate the role of caring environments *on at-homeness* and thriving. In addition, Green House® and small house model environments require further studies that incorporate measures of satisfaction, quality of life, and well-being and standards of intervention fidelity that assure that the built environment is not the sole component of attempts at deinstitutionalization. Evaluation of model outcomes is complicated by varying degrees of implementation that are inconsistent with design (Zimmerman et al., 2016; Bowers et al., 2016).

The use of the caring plan template provided here has not been empirically tested. This would provide critical data for theory analysis. A key component of theory evaluation is outcome measurement. Quantitative measures should include multidimensional indicators of thriving, measures of at-homeness such as the Experience of Home Scale (Molony et al., 2007), and quality-of-life measures that include questions not only about satisfaction but also about the importance of various aspects of life, such as those provided by the Ferrans and Powers Quality of Life Index (Ferrans & Powers, 1985). A homelike atmosphere is conducive to better outcomes for persons with dementia, but self-report and observational measures of well-being and *at-homeness* need further development and validation in this population (Chaudhury et al., 2018).

When a tipping point of at-homeness is achieved, the person in the situation uses the word "love" to describe the experience (Molony et al., 2011). *At-homeness* is also indicated by the desire to return to the place or experience. At-homeness is communicated using atmospheric words such as warmth, peace, or harmony, and may be described as an ineffable whole (Hammer, 1999). Qualitative and mixed methods are therefore needed to fully capture these outcomes.

The goal of the theory is not intended to create a "home" or to replace or recreate a place-based experience created over a lifetime of dwelling. In some ways, the theory is simple to operationalize by keeping the construct of *"experiences of home"* at the forefront of every design, service, caregiving action, and interaction. Each leader, carer, and service provider must reflect on experiences of *at-homeness* and ask themselves, "When we strive to help others feel at home, how do we do this? How do we know and honor what really matters to that unique person? How do we convey that the other person is respected, heard, and valued? How do we provide comfort, hospitality, shared experiences, and sought-for privacy?" Leaders must ask these questions first, with residents in mind, and then with staff in mind, as the recipients of caring.

The theory is also complex because it necessitates identifying "what matters" on an ongoing, dynamic basis and requires recognition that while empowerment, refuge, and meaningful relationship are universally valued, they are experienced or threatened in unique and very personal ways. There is no static algorithm or protocol to produce *at-homeness*. Caring environments require the authentic selves of carers to fulfill the enduring intention to authentically know and be with those cared for and act on the illuminated meaning of *what matters* to enable experiences of at-homeness.

It is important to note that caring actions are rarely limited to a single domain or construct. For example, providing opportunities to share stories about a cherished possession may enhance the relationship with the possession, the relationship with the loved others who may be characters in the story of how the possession was first encountered or used, the relationship with the carers or listeners to the story, empowerment by acknowledging possession and ownership, and self-reconciliation as the object reinforces one's sense of personal narrative.

## 7.2 Overcoming Barriers

Long-term care staff need education, support, positive validation, and reinforcement to implement the caring plan. E. Rogers and Shoemaker (1971), considered the father of Innovation Theory, identified five participant categories in adopting change: the innovators, early adopters, early majority, late majority, and laggards. He defined innovators are the first 2.5% of participants adopting a change. Unfortunately, there were 15,600 nursing homes in the USA in 2015 (Harris et al.,

2019), and fewer than 250 nursing homes have adopted the deinstitutionalized model of care, which represents a slow pace of adoption. This is likely attributable to the various barriers to the implementation that discourage organizations from adopting the model of care.

Most organizations have experienced change. Typically, these are adaptive changes narrowly focused on a single characteristic or element of the organization, such as introducing new technology, equipment, or a revised system. Usually small and of limited scope, they achieve their purpose despite the implementation methods utilized. However, the deinstitutionalization of a nursing home is a broad and far-reaching transformational change that requires a radical departure from the status quo for each stakeholder. Collective beliefs, ethics, values, assumptions, and working methods shift dramatically. Adoption is complex, costly, and time intense. It requires specialized financial, architectural, clinical, and change management support. The challenges include financing capital costs, land availability, transitional human resource requirements, and regulatory concerns. There is an absence of detailed information regarding implementation and few available change agents who have deep knowledge of the complete process.

Actions which might enhance adoption could include changes in Medicaid capital reimbursement policy. Miller et al. (2014) studied the effect of Medicaid capital reimbursement policy on culture change and found that higher reimbursement rates and pay for performance incentives were associated with more private rooms and small households (two artifacts of culture change). This begins to build the case for revised reimbursement and increased use of pay for performance programs.

Another helpful strategy would be the creation of in-depth materials on the details of the implementation of the model of care and the training of implementation support consultants who demonstrate proficiency in operationalizing the model of care and all its elements, perhaps by specialty examination.

Finally, a revision of the regulations, including creating a new category of nursing home with accompanying architectural guidelines and operating requirements and specifically trained surveyors who lead a new survey approach that includes collaborative evaluation by all stakeholders, could provide a fresh motivation for facilities to embrace the change. Case studies, individual testimony, and longitudinal qualitative research about the lived experience of moving into one of these innovative environments will inspire others to adopt these new models.

# 8 Conclusion

This chapter envisions a future of LTC characterized by meaningful living in meaningful environments. Applying the Theory of Caring to enable *at-homeness* requires caring buildings that enlarge situational possibilities and support functional competence, caring plans that prioritize what truly matters to the individual, and caring actions to bring those plans to fruition. Being with adults inhabiting LTC dwellings, knowing what matters, and maintaining belief in their wholeness and potential for

| Resources for Designing Environments that Enable At-Homeness | | |
| --- | --- | --- |
| **Item** | **Description** | **Location** |
| A repository for evidence-based design planning, designing, and constructing health care and residential health care. | FGI *Guidelines* document how to consolidate minimum program space requirements perform risk assessment, infection prevention, architectural detail, surface, and built-in furnishing requirements. | The Facility Guidelines Institute's (FGI) *https://fgiguidelines.org/guidelines/purchase-the-guidelines/read-only-copy/* |
| Evidence-based design implementation tools | Houses research papers, checklists, planning tools, third-party assessments, workshops, research, collaboration opportunities, interactive design diagrams, Functional program process guides, houses. | The Center for Health Design *https://www.healthdesign.org* |
| Conceptual models showing the relationship between environmental variables and outcomes relating to seven topics | 1. Healthcare-Associated Infections 2. Medical errors 3. Patient Falls 4. Patient Satisfaction 5. Patient Waiting 6. Staff Efficiency 7. Staff Satisfaction | Center for Health Design Knowledge Depository Search  *https://www.healthdesign.org/knowledge-repository-0/knowledge-repository-resources* |
| Incorporating technology that enables and supports at-homeness | Current research and partnering opportunities in various areas. Mission: creatively translate technologies into practical solutions that improve people's health and enable them to "do things" throughout their lifespan. | MIT AgeLab *https://agelab.mit.edu/* |
| | Technology selection tools for shared care planning & coordination, social connectedness and engagement tools, safety technology, functional assessment, and activity monitoring, medication management | Leading Age (CAST) Center for Aging Services Technology https://leadingage.org/center-aging-services-technologies |
| AGNES (Age Gain Now Empathy System) | A high-tech suit that enables the wearer to experience many inherent changes in the aging process. Enables designers, architects, builders, and providers to engage in the caring, empathetic processes that may inspire new possibilities. | MIT Age Lab https://agelab.mit.edu/methods/agnes-age-gain-now-empathy-system |

**Fig. 2** Resources for designing environments that enable at-homeness

growth will illuminate situational possibilities for *at-homeness* and promote thriving (Fig. 2). Calling to mind Taniguchi's philosophy, there is a strong moral imperative to create a new and richer interdisciplinary collaboration that values and listens deeply to each of the stakeholders, not about planning a building or executing a project but examining what kind of tea they want to make for the people who live in the houses (Yoshio Taniguchi, n.d.).

# References

Alexander, C. (1996). *The origins of pattern theory, the future of the theory, and the generation of a living world,* Keynote speech to the 1996 OOPSLA convention https://www.patternlanguage.com/archive/ieee.html

Alexander, C., Ishikawa, S., Silverstein, M., Jacobson, M., Fiksdahl-King, I., & Shlomo, A. (1977). *A pattern language: Towns, buildings, construction.* Oxford University Press.

American Geriatrics Society (AGS) Expert Panel on Person-Centered Care. (2016). Person-centered care: A definition and essential elements. *Journal of the American Geriatrics Society, 64*(1), 15–18. https://doi-org.libraryproxy.quinnipiac.edu/10.1111/jgs.13866

Baldurrson, S. (2002). *The nature of at-homeness.* Phenomenology Online A Resource for Phenomenological Inquiry. https://www.phenomenologyonline.com/sources/textorium/

Benner, P., & Wrubel, J. (1989). *The primacy of caring: Stress and coping in health and illness.* Addison-Wesley Publishing.

Behrens, L., Van Haitsma, K., Brush, J., Boltz, M., Volpe, D., & Kolanowski, A. M. (2018) Negotiating Risky Preferences in Nursing Homes: A Case Study of the Rothschild Person-Centered Care Planning Approach. *Journal of Gerontological Nursing, 44*(8):11–17. https://doi.org/10.3928/00989134-20171206-02. Epub 2018 Jan 23. PMID: 29355878.

Bollnow, O. (1961). Lived-space. *Philosophy Today, 5,* 31–39.

Bowers, B., Nolet, K., Jacobson, N., & THRIVE Research Collaborative. (2016). Sustaining culture change: Experiences in the green house model. *Health Services Research, 51*(Suppl 1), 398–417. https://doi-org.libraryproxy.quinnipiac.edu/10.1111/1475-6773.12428

Calkins, M., Schoeneman, K., Brush, J., & Mayer, R. (2015). *A process for care planning for resident choice.* Rothschild Foundation.

Carboni, J. T. (1990). Homelessness among the institutionalized elderly. *Journal of Gerontological Nursing, 16*(7), 32–37. https://doi.org/10.3928/0098-9134-19900701-08

Cater, D., Tunalilar, O., White, D. L., Hasworth, S., & Winfree, J. (2021). "Home is home": Exploring the meaning of home across long-term care settings. *Journal of Aging and Environment,* 1–18. https://doi.org/10.1080/26892618.2021.1932012

Chaudhury, H., Cooke, H. A., Cowie, H., & Razaghi, L. (2018). The influence of the physical environment on residents with dementia in long-term care settings: A review of the empirical literature. *The Gerontologist, 58*(5), e325–e337. https://doi.org/10.1093/geront/gnw259

Cooney, A. (2012). 'Finding home': A grounded theory on how older people 'find home' in long-term care settings. *International Journal of Older People Nursing, 7*(3), 188–199. https://doi.org/10.1111/j.1748-3743.2011.00278.x

Cottam, H., & Leadbeater, C. (2004). *RED paper 01: Health: Co-creating services.* Design Council.

Coulter, A. (2002). Involving patients: Representation or representativeness? *Health Expectations: An International Journal of Public Participation in Health Care and Health Policy, 5*(1), 1–1.

Cutchin, M. P. (2012). The complex process of becoming at-home in assisted living. In G. D. Rowles & M. Bernard (Eds.), *Environmental gerontology: Making meaningful places in old age* (pp. 105–122). Springer.

Fazio, S., Pace, D., Flinner, J., & Kallmyer, B. (2018). The fundamentals of person-Centered Care for Individuals with dementia. *The Gerontologist, 58*(Suppl 1), S10–S19. https://doi-org.libraryproxy.quinnipiac.edu/10.1093/geront/gnx122

Ferrans, C. E., & Powers, M. J. (1985). Quality of life index: Development and psychometric properties. *ANS. Advances in Nursing Science, 8*(1), 15–24. https://doi.org/10.1097/00012272-198510000-00005

Gawande, A. (2014). *Being mortal: Medicine and what matters in the end.* Metropolitan Books/Henry Holt and Company.

Goffman, E. (1990). *Asylums: Essays on the social situation of mental patients and other inmates.* Doubleday.

Haight, B. K., Barba, B. E., Tesh, A. S., & Courts, N. F. (2002). Thriving: A life span theory. *Journal of Gerontological Nursing, 28*(3), 14–22. https://doi.org/10.3928/0098-9134-20020301-05

Hammer, R. M. (1999). The lived experience of being at home. A phenomenological investigation. *Journal of Gerontological Nursing, 25*(11), 10–18. https://doi.org/10.3928/0098-9134-19991101-07

Harris-Kojetin, L., Sengupta, M., Lendon, J. P., Rome, V., Valverde, R., & Caffrey, C. (2019). Long-term care providers and services users in the United States, 2015–2016. National Center for Health Statistics. *Vital Health Statistics, 3*(43), p. 6.

Hertz, J. E., Koren, M. E., Rossetti, J., & Tibbits, K. (2016). Management of relocation in cognitively intact older adults. *Journal of Gerontological Nursing, 42*(11), 14–23. https://doi.org/10.3928/00989134-20160901-05

Johnson, R. A., & Bibbo, J. (2014). Relocation decisions and constructing the meaning of home: A phenomenological study of the transition into a nursing home. *Journal of Aging Studies, 30*, 56–63. https://S0890-4065(14)00027-9.

Kane, R. A., Lum, T. Y., Cutler, L. J., Degenholtz, H. B., & Yu, T. C. (2007). Resident outcomes in small-house nursing homes: A longitudinal evaluation of the initial green house program. *Journal of the American Geriatrics Society, 55*(6), 832–839. https://JGS1169.

Kolanowski, A., Zhu, S., Van Haitsma, K., Resnick, B., Boltz, M., Galik, E., Behrens, L., Eshraghi, K., & Ellis, J. (2021). 12-month trajectory and predictors of affect balance in nursing home residents living with dementia. *Aging & Mental Health*, 1–7. Advance online publication. https://doi-org.libraryproxy.quinnipiac.edu/10.1080/13607863.2021.1947964

Lewin, K. (1951). *Field theory in social science: Selected theoretical papers* (D. Cartwright, Ed.). Harpers.

Lieberman, M. A., Prock, V. N., & Tobin, S. S. (1968). Psychological effects of institutionalization. *Journal of Gerontology, 23*(3), 343–353. https://doi.org/10.1093/geronj/23.3.343

Lum, T. Y., Kane, R. A., Cutler, L. J., & Yu, T. C. (2008). Effects of green house nursing homes on residents' families. *Health Care Financing Review, 30*(2), 35–51. https://hcfr-30-02-035.

Merleau-Ponty, M. (1962). *The phenomenology of perception*. Routledge/Kegan-Paul.

Miller, S. C., Miller, E. A., Jung, H. Y., Sterns, S., Clark, M., & Mor, V. (2010). Nursing home organizational change: The "culture change" movement as viewed by long-term care specialists. *Medical Care Research & Review, 67*(S4), 65S–81S. https://doi-org.libraryproxy.quinnipiac.edu/10.1177/1077558710366862

Miller, S. C., Cohen, N., Lima, J. C., & Mor, V. (2014). Medicaid capital reimbursement policy and environmental artifacts of nursing home culture change. *Gerontologist, 54*(Suppl 1), S76–S86. https://doi.org/10.1093/geront/gnt141. PMID: 24443609; PMCID: PMC3894793.

Miller, S. C., Mor, V., & Burgess, J. F., Jr. (2016). Studying nursing home innovation: The green house model of nursing home care. *Health Services Research, 51*(Suppl 1), 335–343. https://doi-org.libraryproxy.quinnipiac.edu/10.1111/1475-6773.12437

Molony, S. L. (2010). The meaning of home: A qualitative meta-synthesis. *Research in Gerontological Nursing, 3*(4), 291–307. https://doi.org/10.3928/19404921-20100302-02

Molony, S. L., McDonald, D. D., & Palmisano-Mills, C. (2007). Psychometric testing of an instrument to measure the experience of home. *Research in Nursing & Health, 30*(5), 518–530. https://doi.org/10.1002/nur.20210

Molony, S. L., Evans, L. K., Jeon, S., Rabig, J., & Straka, L. A. (2011). Trajectories of at-homeness and health in usual care and small house nursing homes. *The Gerontologist, 51*(4), 504–515. https://doi.org/10.1093/geront/gnr022

Norris, C. (1990). Stories of paradise: What is home when we have left it? Phenomenology + *Pedagogy, 8*(1990), 237–244. https://doi.org/10.29173/pandp15141.

Rabig, J., Thomas, W., Kane, R. A., Cutler, L. J., & McAlilly, S. (2006). Radical redesign of nursing homes: Applying the green house concept in tupelo, Mississippi. *The Gerontologist, 46*(4), 533–539. https://doi-org.libraryproxy.quinnipiac.edu/10.1093/geront/46.4.533.

Reinhard, S. & Hado, E. (2021, January 6). *LTSS choices: Small-house nursing homes*. AARP Public Policy Institute. https://doi.org/10.26419/ppi.00126.001

Rogers, E. M., & Shoemaker, F. F. (1971). *Communication of innovation*. The Free Press.

Rowles, G. D., & Bernard, M. (2012). The meaning and significance of place in old age. In G. D. Rowles & M. Bernard (Eds.), *Environmental gerontology: Making meaningful places in old age* (pp. 3–23). Springer Publishing Company.

Salingaros, N. (2000). The structure of pattern language. *Architectural Research Quarterly volume, 4*, 149–161. © Cambridge University Press. https://doi.org/10.1017/s1359135500002591

Seamon, D. (1979). *A geography of the lifeworld: Movement*. Rest & Encounter.

Sharkey, S. S., Hudak, S., Horn, S. D., James, B., & Howes, J. (2011). Frontline caregiver daily practices: A comparison study of traditional nursing homes and the green house project sites. *Journal of the American Geriatrics Society, 59*(1), 126–131. https://doi.org/10.1111/j.1532-5415.2010.03209.x

Sullivan, G. J., & Williams, C. (2017). Older adult transitions into long-term care: A meta-synthesis. *Journal of Gerontological Nursing, 43*(3), 41–49. https://doi-org.libraryproxy.quinnipiac.edu/10.3928/00989134-20161109-07

Swanson, K. M. (1991). Empirical development of a middle range theory of caring. *Nursing Research, 40*(3), 161–166.

Wolverson, E., & Clarke, C. (2016). *Positive psychology approaches to dementia*. Jessica Kingsley Publishers.

Yoshio Taniguchi Quotes. (n.d.). BrainyQuote.com. Retrieved February 28, 2022, from BrainyQuote.com Web site: https://www.brainyquote.com/quotes/yoshio_taniguchi_177780

Zimmerman, S., Shier, V., & Saliba, D. (2014). Transforming nursing home culture: Evidence for practice and policy. *The Gerontologist, 54*(Suppl 1), S1–S5. https://doi-org.libraryproxy.quinnipiac.edu/10.1093/geront/gnt161

Zimmerman, S., Bowers, B. J., Cohen, L. W., Grabowski, D. C., Horn, S. D., Kemper, P., & THRIVE Research Collaborative. (2016). New evidence on the green house model of nursing home care: Synthesis of findings and implications for policy, practice, and research. *Health Services Research, 51*(Suppl 1), 475–496. https://doi.org/10.1111/1475-6773.12430

Zimmerman, S., Dumond-Stryker, C., Tandan, M., Preisser, J. S., Wretman, C. J., Howell, A., & Ryan, S. (2021). Nontraditional small house nursing homes have fewer COVID-19 cases and deaths. *Journal of the American Medical Directors Association, 22*(3), 489–493. https://www.jamda.com/article/S1525-8610(21)00120-1

# The Evolution and Rise of Robotic Health Assistants: The New Human-Machine Frontier of Geriatric Home Care

Alex J. Bishop, Weihua Sheng, Barbara W. Carlson, and Nadia Firdausya Jones

## 1 Introduction

The home healthcare industry has been under growing pressure to develop innovative ways to effectively and efficiently meet the geriatric care needs of nearly two million homebound older adults, aged 65 and older (Kim & Jang, 2018). Approximately 50% of functionally disabled homebound older adults live alone in households with mostly outdated technologies, resulting in a lack of oversight to lower the risk of social isolation, loneliness, and depressive symptomology, no monitoring of daily activities of living (ADLs), and not limiting hazards contributing to unintentional injury, need for emergency treatment, or death (Ankunda et al., 2020; Ankunda et al., 2021). Consequently, many homebound older adults age in place with unmet care needs, which contribute to the revolving door of hospital or long-term care admissions and readmissions (DePalma et al., 2013). Despite high

A. J. Bishop (✉)
Human Development and Family Science Department, Oklahoma State University, Stillwater, OK, USA
e-mail: alex.bishop@okstate.edu

W. Sheng
School of Electrical and Computer Engineering, Oklahoma State University, Stillwater, OK, USA
e-mail: weihua.sheng@okstate.edu

B. W. Carlson
Fran and Earl Ziegler College of Nursing, University of Oklahoma Health Sciences Center, Oklahoma City, OK, USA
e-mail: Barbara-Carlson@ouhsc.edu

N. F. Jones
Oklahoma Department of Mental Health and Substance Abuse Services, Oklahoma City, OK, USA

© The Author(s), under exclusive license to Springer Nature Switzerland AG 2023
F. Ferdous, E. Roberts (eds.), *(Re)designing the Continuum of Care for Older Adults*, https://doi.org/10.1007/978-3-031-20970-3_6

97

rates of healthcare admission, homebound older adults tend to remain noncompliant with physician orders, often refusing to appropriately follow a treatment regimen requiring prescription medication adherence or self-care of chronic conditions upon being discharged to home and returning home (Musich et al., 2015). This demands a greater need to passively and actively monitor the health functioning of older homebound care recipients so that they maintain personal levels of autonomy, safety, and security necessary to remain living at home alone for as long as possible. Yet, identifying preexisting care needs among homebound older adults will require major changes in how home health practitioners work to gather, analyze, and communicate information in the delivery of direct geriatric care services.

## 1.1   Transforming the Home Care Environment

To combat the impact of COVID-19, the Centers for Medicare & Medicaid Services (CMS, 2020) launched the "hospital without walls" program. Also known as the *Acute Hospital at Home Program* (AHHP), this program allows hospitals greater flexibility in providing in-home care to older at-risk patients diagnosed with 60 different health conditions, who have typically required overnight hospitalization, intermediate rehabilitation, or longer-term intervention yet have been deemed as appropriate for in-home care with proper monitoring protocols (Pericas et al., 2020; Nundy & Patel, 2020). The aim of AHHP is to provide an alternative to conventional hospitalization and to reduce COVID-19-related exposure, infection, and mortality. Initial evidence suggests that adoption and implementation of AHHP are cost-effective, help increase hospital capacity during seasonal outbreaks of influenza, and help curb the risk of infection that might otherwise require some form of intensive care (Pericas et al., 2020). However, AHHP requires daily rounding by physicians and around-the-clock monitoring of health functioning by a team of trained home health practitioners. In these times of significant shortages in geriatricians, these requirements create additional burden to the home healthcare industry, which is already facing a critical shortage of geriatricians (85% shortfall, Health Resources and Services Administration, 2017).

Implementation of the AHHP has initiated a transition of care delivery within the home healthcare industry. This ongoing process closely resembles what Ingold (1993) conceptually coined nearly three decades ago as "taskscape" or transforming the lives of those who dwell in place. Ingold (1993) posited that taskscape would necessitate an array of socially collaborative human and nonhuman interactions to facilitate performance and monitoring of daily activities within the built environment. Pino et al. (2015) hinted that deployment of robotic technologies would be at the forefront of transforming the built living environments into in-home care spaces. Of central importance of this transformation is the goal to extend the time persons are able to age in place despite functional health impairment or physical disablement.

## 1.2  Technifying Later Life

While AHHP has contributed to a transformative shift in home healthcare, there has been an ongoing movement to further modernize the home healthcare industry or what has been referred to as the "technification of later life" (Peine, 2019; p.53). This concept refers to the use of existing and evolving digital care technologies, including telehealth, mobile digital health applications, and artificially intelligent smart devices, to create a more efficient exchange of care between the care provider and the care recipient and improve access to care services among care recipients residing in geographically remote or technologically deprived environments (Poli et al., 2021; see Table 1). Of particular relevance is the integration of technologies to suppress the so-called digital divide or nonuse of technology often due to poor design quality, lack of accessibility, or inadequate literacy surrounding proper device operation (Neves & Vetere, 2019).

Alternatively, Peine et al. (2015) posited that the use of digital devices to monitor and record health functioning, such as smartphone apps, pedometers, fitness and sleep trackers, and other wearables, has already become so pervasive across all age groups that continued technological advancements are likely to eventually change the way how future generations of older adults will seek, acquire, and use healthcare services. Some experts have noted a growing number of *technogeneraians* or older adults who creatively integrate and adapt new and old technologies to facilitate continued independent living within the private and familiar confines of home (Joyce & Loe, 2010; Neven, 2015). Yet, many smart tools and devices rely on design paternalism or the idea that technology should be designed as a solution for age-associated disablement rather than serve as innovative and comprehensive tool that allows older adults to maintain appropriate levels of autonomy and health necessary to meet everyday tasks of living (Peine et al., 2014).

## 1.3  Core Barriers of Technology Use in Geriatric Home Health

Although advancement of smart intelligent technologies represents a promising way to modernize geriatric home healthcare service delivery, the adoption of such technologies will require initial adjustments involving the way home healthcare workers socially interact with and relate to older care recipients, perform work duties, and address quality of care through on-the-job training and learning.

**Table 1** Evolving home healthcare smart technologies

| Technology | Function | Source |
|---|---|---|
| **Digital applications** | | |
| Fall detection system | Cloud-based system for detecting falls in real time | Toda, K., and Shinomiya, N. (2021). A cloud-based fall detection system for elderly care with passive RFID sensor tags. *2018 IEEE 7th Global Conference on Consumer Electronics (GCCE)*, 475–478. https://doi.org/10.1109/GCCE.2018.8574720 |
| Dietary composition perception system | Social robot that uses audition to understand semantic information and perceive dietary composition based on family member conversation | Su, Z., Li, Y., and G. Yang, Y. Li and G. Yang (2020). Dietary Composition Perception Algorithm Using Social Robot Audition for Mandarin Chinese, IEEE Access, 8, 8768–8782. https://doi.org/10.1109/ACCESS.2019.2963560 |
| **Smart device** | | |
| GoSafe 2 | Wearable pendant that includes advanced locating technologies, fall detection capabilities, and two-way voice communication | https://www.lifeline.philips.com/medical-alert-systems/gosafe-2.html |
| Pill dispenser | A medicine dispenser designed with alerting module using alarm and a camera unit; patients are able to take medicine without close professional supervision; prevents the problems of un-timing, overdosage, etc. | Evangeline, S. (2020). Preprogrammed Pill Dispenser for Elderly Care in COVID-19 Pandemic, *International Journal on Emerging Technologies 11(4)*, 464–468 |
| Home care system | Integrated artificial intelligence and IoT technology to collect real-time environmental parameters in home to optimize the living environment | Wang, L., Jia, L., Chu, F., and Li, M. (2021). Design of home care system for rural elderly based on artificial intelligence. Journal of Physics: Conference Series, 1757(1). https://doi.org/10.1088/1742-6596/1757/1/012057 |
| QMedic | Wearable device that works as a 24/7 medical alert for high-risk patients at home | https://www.qmedichealth.com/ |
| Smart walking assistant (SWA) | Fall and posture detection system to monitor fall risk within a stipulated period of time | Bhattacharjee, P., and Biswas, S. (2021). Smart walking assistant (SWA) for elderly care using an intelligent realtime hybrid model. *Evolving Systems*, 1–15. https://doi.org/10.1007/s12530-021-09382-5 |
| **Robotics** | | |

(continued)

**Table 1** (continued)

| Technology | Function | Source |
|---|---|---|
| Lio | A mobile personal robot with a multifunctional arm; able to communicate and support healthcare professionals in their daily tasks | https://www.fp-robotics.com/en/care-lio/ |
| BUDDY | Emotional companion robot connecting, protecting, and interacting older adults with family members | https://buddytherobot.com/en/buddy-the-emotional-robot/ |
| Care-O-Bot | Conversational humanoid robot for performing household tasks, such as cooking, delivering food, providing drinks, and dispensing medications | https://www.care-o-bot.de/en/care-o-bot-4.html |
| ElliQ | Personal assistant robot providing personalized suggestions for activity, online access, and communication with family and friends | https://www.intuitionrobotics.com/ |
| iPal | Humanoid robotic caregiver designed as a social companion, educator, and safety monitor | https://www.ipalrobot.com/ |
| Low-cost smart elderly care robot | Robot capable of simultaneous localization and mapping (SLAM), computer vision, and natural language conversation with easy-to-use interfaces for older users | Hing, S., and Hung, C. C. (2020), "Smart elderly care robot," 2020 IEEE 2nd International Workshop on System Biology and Biomedical Systems (SBBS), 1–4. https://doi.org/10.1109/SBBS50483.2020.9314943 |
| PARO | A socially assistive or therapeutic robot used in a manner similar to pet therapy, especially for older adults diagnosed with dementia | http://www.parorobots.com/ |
| **Telehealth** | | |

(continued)

**Table 1** (continued)

| Technology | Function | Source |
|---|---|---|
| Context-awareness for elderly care (CARE) | Telehealth sensor infrastructure to quantify behavior monitor daily well-being (e.g., activity, mood, social and nurse interactions) of older adults | Klakegg, S., Opoku Asare, K., van Berkel, N. et al. (2021). CARE: Context-awareness for elderly care. Health Technology, 11, 211–226. https://doi.org/10.1007/s12553-020-00512-8 |
| Clinical screening interview system | Social robot for conducting regular clinical geriatric telehealth screening, such as cognitive evaluation, falls' risk evaluation, and pain rating | Do, H. M., Sheng, W., Harrington, E. E., and Bishop, A. J. Bishop, Clinical screening interview using a social robot for geriatric care (2021). IEEE Transactions on Automation Science and Engineering, 18 (3)1229–1242. https://doi.org/10.1109/TASE.2020.2999203 |
| GiraffPlus | Telehealth robotic system to monitor daily activities and physiological parameters of older adults in the home using a network of sensors | Coradeschi S. et al. (2014) GiraffPlus: A system for monitoring activities and physiological parameters and promoting social interaction for elderly. In Z. Hippe Z., J. Kulikowski,T. Mroczek T., & J. Wtorek (Eds) *Human-Computer Systems Interaction: Backgrounds and Applications 3. Advances in Intelligent Systems and Computing, Vol 300.* Springer. https://doi.org/10.1007/978-3-319-08491-6_22 |
| Integrated smart system | Integrated IoT and mobile technologies for acoustic-based and accelerometer-based fall detection, real-time remote video monitoring on mobile devices, voice commands, and heart rate monitoring for geriatric care | Saraubon, K., Anurugsa, K. and Kongsakpaibul, A (2018). A smart system for elderly care using IoT and mobile technologies. 2018 2nd International Conference on Software and e-Business, 59–63. https://doi.org/10.1145/3301761.3301769 |
| IoT-based health monitoring system | Health monitoring system for continuous medical monitoring and assessment of older adults with disablement | Hosseinzadeh M, Koohpayehzadeh J, Ghafour MY, Ahmed AM, Asghari P, and Souri A et al. (2020) An elderly health monitoring system based on biological and behavioral indicators in internet of things. Journal of Ambient Intelligence and Humanized Computing, 1–11. https://doi.org/10.1007/s12652-020-02579-7 |
| Medication reminder system | Integrated companion robot with the cloud to create medication reminders and check medication adherence | Su, Z. Liang, F., Do, H. M., Bishop, A., Carlson, B., and Sheng, W. (2021). Conversation-based medication management system for older adults using a companion robot and cloud, *IEEE Robotics and Automation Letters*, 6, 2, 2698–2705. https://doi.org/10.1109/LRA.2021.3061996 |

(continued)

**Table 1** (continued)

| Technology | Function | Source |
|---|---|---|
| Robot-integrated smart home | Smart home for telehealth, including activity recognition, human localization and tracking, and fall detection | Do, H. M., Pham, M., Sheng, W., Yang, D., and Liu, M., RiSH: A robot-integrated smart home for elderly care, Robotic and Autonomous Systems, 101, 74–92 https://doi.org/10.1016/j.robot.2017.12.008 |
| VOLI | Personalized and context-aware voice-based digital telehealth assistant to improve the quality of care to older adults | http://voli.ucsd.edu/ |

### 1.3.1　Privacy

Privacy represents a prevalent barrier of technological integration within the home health industry. Although a high proportion of homebound older adults generally accept in-home monitoring as unobtrusive and are willing to have health data and information shared with a trusted physician and immediate family caregivers, most remained concerned with the privacy and security of personal information that may be placed or mutually shared on a technological device (Boise et al., 2013). Of particular worry is the potential for unauthorized access by a third party who might hack into and misuse personal health information (Elueze & Quan-Haase, 2018; Harrington et al., 2021). This often presents a conundrum pertaining to the enforcement of privacy and security standards under the Health Insurance Portability and Accountability Act (HIPPA), which legally requires healthcare providers to meaningfully regulate and limit communication and accessibility to patient health records, data, and communication of other healthcare information (Wang & Huang, 2013; Freundlich et al., 2017). Therefore, protecting patient privacy while implementing innovative digital and smart health technologies to benefit patient care represents a core challenge and barrier for the technification of home healthcare service delivery.

### 1.3.2　Human-Machine Interface Design

A second key barrier to adoption of technological advancement in home healthcare involves the design of the human-machine interface (HMI). Usability of design of technological tools is vital for timely delivery of home health services to geriatric patients. Usability of medical-based technologies is associated with patient protection and safety (Carayon & Hoonakker, 2019). In some cases, flaws in the usability of design can contribute to undue stress, anxiety, and frustration among healthcare workers engaged in the timely gathering and interpretation of patient health data, ultimately compromising the quality of patient care (Carayon & Hoonakker, 2019; Gardner et al., 2019). HMI designs that allow home health practitioners to rapidly learn and monitor geriatric patient symptomology, acquire and retain basic clinical skills, and reduce rate of human error in patient care delivery are advantageous.

Meanwhile, HMI designs for patients must remain sensitive to normative age-associated functional limitations, including sensory, cognitive, and motor ability limitations, which can impact detection and diagnosis. Johnson and Finn (2017) advocated for universal design interfaces that can be used interchangeably by young and old alike. They suggested several changes for advancing ease of use in HMI designs, including maximizing legibility of essential text; using consistent graphical language and numerical data; using click, tap, or swipe targets to help minimize the use of a keyboard; maximizing audio quality of the device with adjustable sound controls; and providing simple video demonstration of interactive elements.

### 1.3.3 Workforce Training and Education

A third barrier surrounding the technification of home healthcare delivery involves workforce training and education. According to the US Bureau of Labor Statistics (2021), home health occupations, including nurse practitioners, home health personal care aides and certified nursing assistants, and healthcare case managers represent some of the fastest-growing employment opportunities in the United States. In fact, it is projected that the direct care workforce will add nearly one million home care jobs, more than any other occupation in the country (PHI, 2020). Over half of all home health workers are women and persons of color who possess a high school education or less, with one-quarter who are immigrants (PHI, 2020). Unfortunately, health employees are typically paid lower wages, receive limited on-the-job training, report disproportionately higher rates of on-the-job injuries, and experience high employment turnover (McCaughey et al., 2013; Stone et al., 2013; Walton & Rogers, 2017). This has contributed to a crisis-level shortage of workers, particularly those seeking healthcare jobs that offer higher wages, a stable work schedule, less taxing work duties, and training and advancement opportunities, needed to meet the care needs of homebound older adults (Scales, 2021). Consequently, it is time to retool the home health workforce by leveraging new technical training and work opportunities to attract and develop the next-generation home health worker.

## 1.4 Evolution of Socially Assistive Robots in Geriatric Care

Recent circumstances surrounding the COVID-19 pandemic made clear that direct care supports cannot be substituted with remote technologies, such as telehealth, alone (Gajarawala & Pelkowski, 2021; Scales, 2021). Despite considerable risk of virus exposure during the height of the pandemic, home health workers continued to visit and provide essential "direct patient" care to vulnerable homebound patients. Many of these homebound patients are socially isolated, and the direct patient care may be the primary means to provide social contact and to detect problems early. Such experiences have revealed that smart technological tools and devices that incorporate sensing, computation, and communication, along with a broad spectrum of technological interventions, are needed to maximize personal safety in the delivery and reception of home healthcare services.

Multitasking socially assistive robots (SARs) evolved in the late 1990s as artificially intelligent smart devices designed to provide autonomous or semiautonomous assistance using both passive and active capabilities to assist with remote medical triage, direct patient care, and basic social companionship (Van Aerschot & Parviainen, 2020; Engelberger, 1997). SARs also have the capability to audio and video record health-related behaviors using advanced sensor technologies and then automatically code and process recorded observations into data for purposes of advancing personalized advice or producing automated actions and reactions (Liu et al., 2016). SARs provide greater comprehensive monitoring and can free home health workers of time needed to address more complex aspects of their work, which contributes to more effective delivery of care, greater worker resilience, and increased satisfaction for both care provider and homebound care recipient (Christoforou et al., 2020; Johnson et al., 2014; Kachouie et al., 2014). Below is a brief description of notable advancements in the evolution of SAR applications.

One of the earliest robotic healthcare applications involved the Nursebot Project. This was a collaborative project between the University of Pittsburgh and Carnegie Mellon University (Montemerlo et al., 2003) and focused on the use of a SAR as a platform for medication and appointment reminding, telepresence via video connection to healthcare providers, surveillance alert of emergencies, mobile manipulation matching robot intelligence with human sensation and intellect, and social interaction for older home care patients.

Meanwhile, Johnson et al. (2007) created the Robot/CAMR suite featuring a conventional force-reflecting joystick, a modified therapy joystick, and a steering wheel platform with embedded software to assess stroke rehabilitation among homebound patients. Similar SAR testing across various laboratories has reported modest reductions in the severity of stroke-associated impairments (Volpe et al., 2002).

Rehabilitative health benefits of SARs, particularly robotic pets, have also been examined with older adults in long-term care situations who are at risk for social isolation and loneliness. One of the more well-known SAR pets is PARO (Wada & Shibata, 2007), a therapeutic robot designed as a baby harp seal to elicit calming emotional responses among older adults and their caregivers. The PARO SAR application includes five types of sensors, (1) tactile, (2) light, (3) audio, (4) temperature, and (5) posture, which are used to perceive the environment for interpersonal interaction. The PARO is able to detect light from dark, being touched or stroked, and being lifted and held. Furthermore, it has the ability to detect sound in the form of voices and words, including its name, greetings, and praise. PARO pets have been tested in a variety of clinical care settings with encouraging findings pertaining to diminished feelings of agitation and anxiety, reductions in physiological markers of stress, and improvements in overall mood states among healthy and dementia care recipients, as well as their direct caregivers (Aminuddin et al., 2016; Kang et al., 2020; Yu et al., 2015). Similarly, SAR pets have been reported to alleviate feelings of loneliness among community-dwelling older adults. For instance, Banks et al. (2008) tested a robotic dog as part of animal-assisted therapy for loneliness. When compared with interventions using actual living dogs, each group was found to have statistically significant and comparable outcomes relative to reductions in reported loneliness. Meanwhile, Hudson et al. (2020) reported that SAR pets facilitate improved communication by fostering social connections among community-dwelling older adults who are homebound and live alone.

Usefulness of telepresence SARs has also been explored by many researchers. For instance, a tele-operated SAR named Giraff (Liu et al., 2016) enables older adults to make video calls to their caregivers, who can then remotely control the robot from a distance to inspect the older adult's living situation or environment from a distance. Recent advances in smart intelligent design application led to the development of the GiraffPlus robot (Coradeschi et al., 2014).

Unlike its predecessor, the GiraffPlus is able to more actively move about the living environment to track human movement and location in the home and collect and monitor physiological parameters (e.g., body temperature, blood pressure, blood glucose). The GiraffPlus also gives caregivers greater flexibility to provide continuous and intervening patient care through alert detection capabilities that automate virtual patient consultations and visits in the event of a health episode or medical emergency. Furthermore, reported evidence has indicated that the telepresence design of the Giraff robotic system helps promote greater social interaction between care providers and geriatric care recipients (Coradeschi et al., 2014).

Recently, there has been increased empirical testing of humanoid robotics designed to provide companionship and care to older adults (Andtfolk et al., 2020). For instance, the humanoid Ludwig robot (Rudzicz et al., 2017) can interact with dementia patients by asking them questions, considering their answers, and reporting back to caregivers on their condition. However, this robot is mainly targeted for use with dementia patients residing in long-term care facilities.

## 2 Research Objectives

Robotic technologies remain far from revolutionizing current home healthcare practices. This can be attributed to two major barriers: (1) existing SAR systems lack sufficient intelligence to replace and fulfill many of the physical and emotional work-related duties performed by human home health staff, especially those requiring a combination of health monitoring, in-person observation, and direct human intervention, and (2) current SAR systems are not yet properly designed or suited for long-term human-machine partnerships, therefore reducing patient and healthcare provider's willingness to accept and adopt them. Human-friendly and user-tailored interfaces should be designed by considering the needs and concerns of both the care recipient and their respective caregivers. Although most persons perceive the use of social robots to be more beneficial than personal privacy concerns (Lutz & Tamó-Larrieux, 2020), the incorporation and integration privacy, human-machine interface design, and human-machine learning have remained major obstacles in establishing a more prominent human-machine partnership in home health industry (Lin et al., 2014; Van Wynsberghe, 2015; Villaronga et al., 2018). Yet, few research efforts have addressed such barriers from the perspectives of clinical nurse practitioners, case managers, or outreach coordinators vital to the home health industry. Therefore, our aim was to explore and better understand the technology use and work-related needs of home health professionals to formulate a strategy for addressing core barriers to human-machine integration.

# 3  Methods

We conducted three separate 60-min focus group sessions in Oklahoma with stakeholders representing three different workforce areas within home healthcare: (1) clinical registered nurse case managers (e.g., medically trained formal caregivers), (2) social service caseworkers (e.g., trained social worker and aging service providers), and (3) rural community outreach coordinators (e.g., community volunteers, spousal caregivers). We purposefully identified and invited ten representatives from each group to participate. Participants across all groups were currently involved with providing care services to homebound older adults with expertise ranging from less than 1 year to over 20 years of professional service. With the exception of one participant who had completed some college, all participants had earned a baccalaureate degree. None of the participants had prior experience operating a socially assistive robot. Stakeholder participants were identified through the Oklahoma State University Center for Family Resilience, the Fran and Earl Ziegler College of Nursing within the University of Oklahoma Health Science Center, aging service network contacts (e.g., Oklahoma Aging Services Division, Area Agencies on Aging, and senior nutrition projects), and the Oklahoma State University Family and Consumer Science Cooperative Extension network.

Focus group participants were first asked to spend a few minutes reviewing a photo of the primary design features of a stationary robotic health assistant (RoHA), the Elder Life Smart Assistant (ELSA), being developed and tested within our lab (see Fig. 1). We then asked focus group participants to review a conceptual model of the robotic health assistant home healthcare system (see Fig. 2). We then engaged focus group participants in a deliberative brainstorming session. Focus group questions were designed to elicit insights into how stakeholders define their work duties, address the types of assistance and data one may need to effectively complete on-the-job tasks, and determine how their work might be done with and without robotic technology in the home (Table 2).

Focus group sessions were moderated by a lead investigator who also took notes of the key discussion points. To diminish prospect of analysis bias, undergraduate and graduate research assistants with no preexisting knowledge or expertise in the

**Fig. 1** Primary design features of the ELSA robot prototype

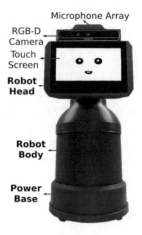

Microphone Array
RGB-D Camera
Touch Screen
**Robot Head**
**Robot Body**
**Power Base**

**Fig. 2** Home-based robot health assistant concept

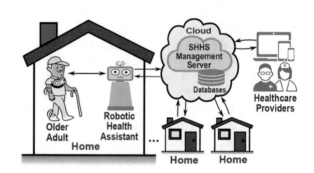

Older Adult
Robotic Health Assistant
**Home**
Cloud
SHHS Management Server
Databases
Healthcare Providers
... Home  Home

field of gerontechnology or familiarity with the current investigation voluntarily served as scribes. The scribes wrote detailed notes about primary focus group discussion comments, topics, and points. All scribed notes were transcribed verbatim, and the two scribes met to reach consensus with the notes from the lead investigator. An inductive approach was used to code the data (i.e., codes were data-driven rather than reflective of preexisting codes; Braun & Clarke, 2006). We implemented Lincoln and Guba's (1985) recommended criteria for establishing trustworthiness in conducting a qualitatively derived thematic comparison and consensus of scribed and transcribed data. These criteria included (1) credibility (e.g., first author coded and analyzed transcribed notes and shared findings with other co-authors who compared findings to the originally scribed notes), (2) transferability (e.g., a detailed synopsis of the focus groups including descriptions of participants and their occupational roles was summarized), (3) dependability (i.e., the authors double-checked and compared their work, including revisiting scribed notes and coding in developing the comparative themes), and (4) confirmability (i.e., the authors met several times for discussion and interpretation of unclear data pieces in finalizing the themes and categories).

**Table 2** Summary of focus group themes

| Theme | Nurse case managers | Social service case workers | Rural outreach providers |
|---|---|---|---|
| Vital functions | Collection of key vital signs, blood glucose, pacemaker activations, weight | Triage conditions indicative of risk to older adult's physical or mental health | Medication-dispensing, vital sign screening, and connection to health resources |
| Mental health | Provisions of companionship to manage feelings of loneliness | Serve as a companion for mental health prevention and intervention to manage risks such as loneliness, anxiety, or agitation | Screen for agitation, anxiety, and depression, and validating and reporting of emotional status |
| Privacy | Need strict limitation on when, what, and where to record daily routines and health data in private residence | Maintain privacy and identity of vulnerable, at-risk and highly targeted older adults | Create secure firewall to reduce invasion of personal privacy and intrusive access to physical and mental health data |
| Monitoring | Keep watch over what the older care recipient is doing in the home environment: mobility, hydration, eating, and medication adherence | Tracking daily routines in home such as medication use, mood, eating and sleeping patterns, and falls risk hazards in the home | Track and monitor food preparation and handling, water intake, and medication adherence within the home environment |
| Telehealth accessibility | Improved access and notification for emergency assistance | Telehealth access to a mental health counselor for counseling, coaching, or one-to-one therapy sessions | Expand connection with specialist(s) in nearby or larger towns for better health consultation and delivery of resources |
| Communication | Direct reporting and consultation of change in prescribed medication listings from care recipient's doctor and ease accessing record of recent medical appointments | Emergency alert option designed for better communication, reporting, and consultation between case manager and care recipient | Two-way communication between caregiver and care recipient including news, education, and translation of healthcare policies and regulations |

# 4 Results

## 4.1 Focus Group Results

Six themes were identified across the three focus group sessions: vital functions, mental health, privacy, monitoring, telehealth accessibility, and communication.

### 4.1.1 Theme 1: Vital Functions

Under the theme "vital functions," several clinical nurse case managers similarly stated that they preferred that the RoHA assist with the "collection and determination of patient vital signs." Others maintained that the RoHA also have the capacity to conduct weight and blood glucose screenings and pacemaker activations. Rural outreach providers maintained similar perspectives yet noted additional needs for the RoHA to help dispense medicine and provide ease of connection to health resources for educating patients about normative vitals. As one outreach provider noted, "Medication adherence involving easy-to-follow instructions, a reminder, or dispensing of pills would help reduce critical medication errors among our older clients living in rural medically underserved communities." Meanwhile, social case workers expressed a greater desire for the RoHa to assist with medical triage for determination of patient physical and mental health risks. One social case worker admitted that a RoHa that could assist in "detecting depressive symptoms or mood disturbances among clients that live alone" would be helpful.

### 4.1.2 Theme 2: Mental Health

The theme "mental health" spanned all three focus groups. The most notable was a desire for the RoHA to provide some type of provision or interventions of companionship. One social service caseworker commented that a RoHA could potentially offer a tool "to help identify and combat feelings of social isolation and loneliness that many clients express during routine visits." Rural outreach providers also noted the value of the RoHa providing diagnostic screening of emotional conditions pertaining to agitation, anxiety, and depression as a way to "further validate and confirm current emotional status of homebound older adults who may otherwise benefit from some type of social intervention, activity, or engagement."

### 4.1.3 Theme 3: Privacy

"Privacy" emerged as a third theme of interest across all three focus groups. As one clinical nurse participant noted, "Of particular concern is the assurance that the SAR would be limited relative to when, what, or where it may record information within the older homebound patient's home or private residence." This sentiment was echoed by one of the social case workers who also suggested: "The RoHA must be particularly sensitive to maintaining the privacy and identity of highly vulnerable or at-risk older adults, particularly those who may represent an active abuse case or others who may have issues with hoarding." Rural outreach providers further noted a desire for the RoHA to have a secure firewall to reduce unwanted intrusion and invasion of personal information and privacy due to hacking.

### 4.1.4 Theme 4: Monitoring

Each focus group seemed to maintain agreement relative to the "monitoring capabilities" of the RoHA. Across focus groups, there was a clear indication that the RoHA would be most helpful in keeping watch over older homebound care recipients via the tracking of activities of daily living within the home environment. Most notable, was an interest in having the RoHA monitor nutritional health behaviors (e.g., hydration, food handling), track medication adherence, and provide surveillance of mobility and movement within the home. As one social caseworker suggested, "We could use a robot to ensure that our clients drink enough water during the day, eat regularly, and take the right medications at the right time so they don't put themselves at greater risk of injury or harm inside their home."

### 4.1.5 Theme 5: Telehealth Accessibility

"Improved access to telehealth resources" was a fifth theme demonstrated across all three focus groups. Several nurse case managers suggested that the RoHA "provide telepresence assistance during emergency health situations." Meanwhile, case managers viewed the RoHA as a promising technological tool for connecting homebound older adults to a mental health counselor. As one case manager stated, "The robot could improve better initiation or facilitation individual or group telehealth therapy sessions." Finally, rural outreach coordinators recommended that the RoHA have the capability to teleconnect geographically remote older homebound adults to medical specialists located in nearby or larger communities that typically have more expansive medical and mental health services. As one coordinator acknowledged, "Several of our older homebound adults live in counties where there are no medical specialties, and therefore they drive miles away from home."

### 4.1.6 Theme 6: Communication

"Communication" represented a final theme that transcended across all three focus groups. Of particular interest was the ability of the RoHA to maintain care plan transparency relative to providing direct and two-way communication of key patient health data. One nurse case manager mentioned a desire for the RoHA to assist with "communicating any update or change in the daily medication listings of older care patients." Among case managers, there was a desire for the RoHA to provide improved communication of emergency or crisis situations in which the case manager or other care team members could then immediately contact and communicate the older homebound care recipient. Finally, rural outreach coordinators suggested that the RoHA provide increased information and data concerning changes in state and national healthcare policies and regulations. As one outreach coordinated admitted, "Policies like Medicare or HIPPA tend to impart two-way communication and decision-making between the care provider and care recipient, but our knowledge of policy changes or new information is not always the best or up to date."

## 5 Discussion

Focus group results in this study confirmed literature support of three notable underlying barriers, privacy protection, human-machine interface design, and learning, which create challenges for immediate integration of advanced robotic technology within geriatric home healthcare. The results further indicated agreement across various home health professionals concerning the utility of a Robotic Health Assistant (RoHA) for homebound older adults. In particular, it appears that a RoHA would serve a purposeful function if able to enhance monitoring, intervening, and healthcare literacy capabilities. Based on input collected across focus group sessions, we created a concept model of human-machine design for a home health RoHA (see Fig. 3).

### 5.1 Privacy Concerns

Relative to the engineering, design, and application of a RoHA tailored for geriatric care, three core challenges persist. The most pressing concern among home health professional appears to be privacy protection. Issues of privacy have been a longstanding problem with no easy solution in the engineering of geriatric healthcare robots. Testing and deployment of healthcare robots involve prevailing legal implications that warrant sensitivity to HIPPA regulations in order to minimize environmental intrusion of patient privacy and maximize introduction of artificially intelligent robots to compensate workforce shortages and sustain quality of care (Simshaw et al., 2016). Of particular interest has been how to best design a robot to passively and actively monitor human health while capturing and extracting sounds, images, and other environmental anomalies without disrupting behavioral autonomy necessary for intervention, prevention, and treatment adherence (Demiris et al., 2009; Berridge, 2017). Privacy of the individual in conjunction with the use of robotics represents trade-off with costs and benefits. It is common for most older adults to possess a degree of naiveté in the operation of artificially intelligent smart technologies and to experience technical uncertainties that put their personal identity and security at risk. Caine and et al. (2012) reported that older adults engage in more privacy-enhancing behaviors when interacting with robotic devices supported with a camera function for monitoring. Filtering the detection and limiting the release of videos or images that might unknowingly expose unwarranted health vulnerabilities, daily behavioral routines, and living conditions inside the private confines of one's living environment are vital steps toward protecting and preserving the privacy of older adults (Butler et al., 2015; Fernandes et al., 2016).

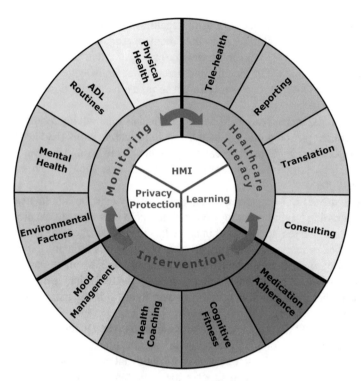

**Fig. 3**  Conceptual model for robot health assistant (RoHA) design

## 5.2  Intervening Robotic Care Benefits

Focus group results also provided key insights regarding the intervening roles of robots could in geriatric home healthcare delivery. Robotic pets, such as PARO, were previously detailed relative to intervening effects that help to manage and off-set age-associated cognitive impairment and negative changes in mood, particularly among dementia patients residing in nursing homes. However, one domain of shared interest acknowledged across the three focus groups concerned desire to improve medication management and adherence of homebound older adults. Most older adults are relatively open-minded about robotic-based assistive devices to help manage and take medication. In fact, Prakash et al. (2013) reported that older adults actually prefer a robot over a human to provide reminders of when to take medication; yet human assistance is still desired when it comes to deciding what appropriate medications should be administered or taken and verifying that medication has been ingested. Further evidence has also been reported that robotic health assistants significantly improve medication adherence among homebound older adults and increase patient safety through reduced dispensing and medication error (Rodriguez-Gonzalez et al., 2018). Medication-dispensing robotic prototypes within the marketplace, such as Pillo, offer a new technological tool for the future of personalized home care. Pillo has a number of positive features, including (1) facial recognition capabilities to identify multiple household members for accurately tracking and dispensing medication; (2) built-in reminders of when, what, and how medications should be taken; and (3) artificially intelligent-based knowledge regarding when a homebound patient may mistakenly forget to take a particular dose of medication (Tao et al., 2016).

Other robots, such as Autom™, were designed as mini talking robots to manage and direct care planning through health coaching interventions (Kidd & Breazeal, 2008). Autom™ engages users by encouraging healthy living and motivating dietary (e.g., tracking caloric intake) and exercise (e.g., demonstration) behaviors (Kidd & Breazeal, 2008).

Pillo and Autom™ are just two examples of many existing robotic health assistants undergoing lab-based testing and awaiting home deployment, where they will serve various intervening roles within home healthcare management and delivery of services. One primary goal of many of these robots is to shift a portion of the care burden away from home healthcare professionals and to place basic self-care responsibilities onto homebound patient, whereby the individual learns how to better manage their own health in order to remain living at home more independently (Dahl & Boulos, 2013).

Zheng et al. (2020) proposed a dialog system to collect medication information from patients, which obtains the necessary medication information in multiple rounds of conversation. However, it takes a significant amount of time to complete one medicine recording, and it ignores the important function of reminding the older adult to take medicine. Florence (https://florence.chat) is a text-based chatbot providing medication reminder and health-tracking functions. However, it does not offer audio input and cannot support natural language conversation. Only users can create reminders while caregivers cannot. Tiwari et al. [2011] developed a robotic medication assistant for the elderly. This robot ran a medication reminder application while the older adults took their medications. The interaction was followed by a questionnaire and structured interview to elicit their opinions and feedback.

## 5.3  Telehealth Communication

Communication was a final notable discovery from the focus groups. In particular, there was an expressed interest among focus group participants in enhancing how patient and healthcare information is learned and learning how to effectively engage in reporting, translation, and consultation using a telehealth presence. Human-machine learning is a collaborative effort facilitated by user-friendly interface designs that promote ease of use and motivate the initiation of positive human-to-machine and machine-to-human interactions (Neves & Vetere, 2019). Yet, there remains a knowledge gap among most professional care providers and care service managers regarding how to properly use care robots, as well as what types of information to seek regarding robotic functionality in the reporting, translation, and consultation of health data (Neves & Vetere, 2019). Formal care providers often have less experience and more negative attitudes and concerns about robots than do older adults for whom care is being provided (Turja et al., 2020; Johansson-Pajala et al., 2020). Many of these concerns stem from regular engagement within a non-technical work environment, low adoption and integration of technology within work-related tasks, ethical considerations surrounding user privacy, and cost-effectiveness and time efficiency (Dahl & Boulos, 2013). Closing the existing knowledge gap of robotic health assistants among future home health workers will most likely require basic training in what is referred to as *robot etiquette* or socially acceptable nonverbal and noncontact activation and human-guided navigation of service-based robots for the purpose of continued improved human-machine learning, translation, and prediction of human health (Qian et al., 2010).

## 5.4   Limitations

We must acknowledge some of the limitations in conducting this focus group research. First, we did not recruit or seek out a representative group of older home health patients or their respective family caregivers. Therefore, caution is advised in generalizing the results beyond geriatric home healthcare providers. Second, we conveniently and purposefully identified and recruited focus group participants. This may have contributed to selection bias, resulting in focus group participants who are more representative and invested in the administration and management of home healthcare programming. Third, frontline or essential home health employees who are not nursing and social service case workers, such as personal care aides and certified nursing assistants, were not represented in this focus group. Therefore, focus group results cannot be generalized to these types of home health employees.

# 6   Conclusions

## 6.1   Future Directions of Robotics in Geriatric Home Healthcare

Propelled in large part by the COVID-19 pandemic, a new human-machine frontier in geriatric care has evolved. Smart artificially intelligent technologies were brought front and center and called into action during the height of the COVID-19 outbreak. Telehealth tools, devices, and applications played a major role in helping geriatric health workers, and patients alike limit physical contact through proper social distancing and reduced COVID-19 transmission. Such applications typically relied on creative use and innovation involving one or a combination of three primary modalities: (1) synchronous (e.g., audio-video interaction via smartphone, tablet, or computer), (2) asynchronous (e.g., messaging, data, and images collected in real time and interpreted later), and (3) remote patient monitoring (e.g., direct transmission of clinical measurements and assessments from a distance) (Centers for Disease Control and Prevention, 2020). Although many healthcare providers found telehealth to be a suitable option for maintaining continuity of care with geriatric patients, most older adults remained underprepared and unready to use telemedicine. In addition to their inexperience with technology platforms, the complexity (multistep, multibutton, or even competing sounds and actions) of even the most "basic" self-assessment devices makes the collection of most vital measures (vital signs and body weight) difficult, particularly in clients who have significant hearing loss, poor communication skills, or dementia (Doraiswamy et al., 2021; Tan et al., 2020; Lam et al., 2020). Thus, telehealth technologies appeared to be widely used across geriatric care sectors, including home healthcare, but many older adults were unable to connect or even fully adhere to medical treatment interventions or guidelines.

Amid the COVID-19 surge, the Centers for Medicare and Medicaid Services (CMMS, 2020) introduced a comprehensive measure to increase the capacity of the American healthcare system to provide care to patients outside of a traditional hospital setting by placing such care back into the home. This effort, introduced on November 25, 2020, was designated as the Hospital Without Walls Program (HWWP) and granted hospitals greater flexibility in providing acute hospital care services within the homes of patients. This program was clearly differentiated from traditional home health services, which provides more skill-based nursing services. By comparison, the HWWP is for patients who require acute inpatient admission to a hospital and require at least daily rounding by a physician and a medical team responsible for continuous monitoring of care needs.

While current research and development are mainly focused on a single or a small number of robots for geriatric care, deployment of a large number of home healthcare robots is anticipated and will create many potential applications in the human-machine frontier and require research and refinement to interface designs, ethics of privacy, and solutions for implementation within varied home contexts. One practical scenario is to begin deploying healthcare robots into community-based household dwellings, such as senior retirement living communities, senior cohousing neighborhoods, or assisted living communities, so that each singular home or apartment dwelling has one robot, and together these devices are connected to form a robotic network capable of supporting a continuum of care necessary for humans to age independently and safely in place. We propose that the ongoing evolution and progression of robotic health assistants in the geriatric home health industry will present three future challenges in human-machine frontier: (1) how to use robots to improve social connectedness among communities of homebound geriatric care recipients, as well as their respective care providers, (2) how to facilitate inter-robot learning while providing care workers appropriate on-the-job training and advanced technology-based workforce skills, and (3) how to ethically protect individual users and ensure community-level privacy of monitored health information.

**Acknowledgments** This material is based upon the work supported in part by the National Science Foundation, FW-HTF-P, Robotic Health Assistants: A New Human-Machine Partnership in Home Health Care, under grant award #1928711.

# References

Ankunda, C. K., Husain, M., Bollens-Lund, E., Leff, B., Ritchie, C. S., Liu, S. H., & Ornstein, K. A. (2021). The dynamics of being homebound over time: A prospective study of Medicare beneficiaries, 2012–2018. *Journal of the American Geriatrics Society, 69*(6), 1609–1616. https://doi.org/10.1111/jgs.17086

Ankunda, C. K., Levine, D. A., Langa, K. M., Ornstein, K. A., & Kelley, A. S. (2020). Caregiving, recovery, and death after incident ADL/IADL disability among older adults in the United States. *Journal of Applied Geronotology, 39*(4), 393–397. https://doi.org/10.1177/0733464819826842

Aminuddin, R., Sharkey, A., & Levita, L. (2016). Interaction with the PARO robot may reduce psychophysiological stress responses. In *2016 11th ACM/IEEE International Conference on Human-Robot Interaction (HRI), 2016* (pp. 593–594). https://doi.org/10.1109/HRI.2016.7451872.

Andtfolk, M., Nyholm, L., Eide, H., & Fagerström, L. (2020). Humanoid robots in the care of older persons: A scoping review. *Assistive Technology.* https://doi.org/10.1080/1040043 5.2021.1880493

Ankuda, C. K., Freedman, V. A., Convinsky, K. E., & Kelley, A. S. (2020). Population-based screening for functional disability in older adults. *Innovation in Aging, 5*(1), 1–9. https://doi.org/10.1093/geroni/igaa065

Banks, M. R., Willoughby, L. M., & Banks, W. A. (2008). Animal-assisted therapy and loneliness in nursing homes: Use of robotic versus living dogs. *Journal of the American Medical Directors Association, 9*(3), 173–177.

Berridge, C. (2017). Active subjects of passive monitoring: Responses to a passive monitoring system in low-income independent living. *Ageing Society, 37*(3), 537–560. https://doi.org/10.1017/S0144686X15001269

Boise, L., Wild, K., Mattek, N., Ruhl, M., Dodge, H. H., & Kaye, J. (2013). Willingness of older adults to share data and privacy concerns after exposure to unobtrusive in-home monitoring. *Geron, 11*(3), 428–435. https://doi.org/10.4017/gt.2013.11.3.001.00

Braun, V., & Clarke, V. (2006). Unsing thematic analysis in psychology. Qualitative Research in Psychology, 3 (2), 77–101.

Butler, D. J., Huang, J., Roesner, F., & Cakmak, M. (2015). *The privacy-utility tradeoff for remotely controlled robots.* HRI 2015. https://doi.org/10.1145/2696454.2696484.

Caine, K., Šabanović, S., & Carter, M. (2012). The effect of monitoring by cameras and robots on the privacy enhancing behaviors of older adults. In *HRI '12: Proceedings of the seventh annual ACM/IEEE International Conference on Human-Robot Interaction* (pp. 343–350). https://doi.org/10.1145/2157689.2157807.

Carayon, P., & Hooakker, P. (2019). Human factors and usability for health information technology: Old and new challenges. *Yearbook of Medical Informatics, 28*(1), 71–77. https://doi.org/10.1055/s-0039-1677907

Centers for Disease Control and Prevention. (2020). *Using telehealth to expand access to essential health services during the COVID-19 Pandemic.* https://www.cdc.gov/coronavirus/2019-ncov/hdp/telehealth.html

Centers for Medicare & Medicaid Services. (2020). *Additional background: Sweeping regulatory changes to help U.S. Healthcare System address COVID-19 Patient Surge.* https://www.cms.gov/newsroom/fact-sheets/additional-backgroundsweeping-regulatorychanges-help-us-healthcare-system-address-covid-19-patient

Christoforou, E. G., Abgousti, S., Ramdani, N., Novales, C., & Panayides, A. S. (2020). The upcoming role for nursing and assistive robotics: Opportunities and challenges ahead. *Frontiers in Digital Health, 2*, Article 585656. https://doi.org/10.3389/fdgh.2020.585656

Coradeschi, S., Cesta, A., Cortellessa, G., Coraci, L., Galindo, C., Gonzalez, J., et al. (2014). GiraffPlus: A system for monitoring activities and physiological parameters and promoting social interaction for elderly. In Z. S. Hippe et al. (Eds.), *Human-computer systems interaction: Backgrounds and applications 3, Advances in intelligent systems and computing* (pp. 261–271). Springer.

Dahl, T. S., & Boulos, M. N. K. (2013). Robots in health and social care. A complementary technology to home care and telehealthcare? *Robotics, 3*(1), 1–21. https://doi.org/10.3390/robotics3010001

Demiris, G., Oliver, D. P., Giger, J., Skubic, M., & Rantz, M. (2009). *Technology and Health Care, 17*, 41–48. https://doi.org/10.3233/THC-2009-0530

DePalma, G., Xu, H., Covinsky, K. E., Craig, B. A., Stallard, E., Thomas, J., & Sands, L. (2013). Hospital readmission among older adults who return home with unmet need for ADL disability. *Gerontologist, 53*(3), 454–461. https://doi.org/10.1093/geront/gns103

Doraiswamy, S., Jithesh, A., Mamtani, R., Abraham, A., & Cheema, S. (2021). Telehealth use in geriatrics care during the COVID-19 Pandemic – A scoping review and evidence synthesis. *International Journal of Environmental Research and Public Health, 18*, 1755. https://doi.org/10.3390/ijerph18041755

Elueze, I., & Quan-Haase, A. (2018). Privacy attitudes and concerns in the digital lives of older adults: Westin's privacy attitude typology revisited. *American Behavioral Scientist, 62*(10), 1372–1391. https://doi.org/10.1177/0000276421878026

Engelberger, J. (1997). A gauntlet thrown down for elder care. *Industrial Robot, 24*(3), 202–206.

Fernandes, F. E., Yang, G., Do, H. M., & Sheng, W. (2016). Detection of privacy-sensitive situations for social robots in smart homes. *2016 IEEE International Conference on Automation Science and Engineering*, 727–732. https://doi.org/10.1109/COASE.2016.7743474

Freundlich, R. E., Freundlich, K. L., & Drolet, B. C. (2017). Pagers, smartphones, and HIPPA: Finding the best solution for electronic communication of protected health information. *Journal of Medical Systems, 43*(9). https://doi.org/10.1007/s10916-0170870-9

Gardner, R. L., Cooper, E., Haskell, J., Harris, D. A., Poplau, S., Kroth, P. J., et al. (2019). Physician stress and burnout: The impact of health information technology. *Journal of Informatics in Healthcare and Biomedicine, 26*(2), 106–114. https://doi.org/10.1093/jamia/ocy145

Gajarawala, S. N., & Pelkowski, J. N. (2021). Telehealth benefits and barriers. Journal for Nurse Practitioners, 17, 218-221. https://doi.org/10.1016/j.nurpra.2020.09.013.

Harrington, E. E., Bishop, A. J., Do, H., & Sheng, W. (2021). Perceptions of socially assistive robots: A pilot study exploring older adults' concerns. *Current Psychology.* https://doi.org/10.1007/s12144-021-01627-5

Health Resources and Services Administration (2017). National and regional projections of supply and demand for geriatricians: 2013-2025. https://bhw.hrsa.gov/sites/default/files/bureau-health-workforce/data-research/geriatricsreport-51817.pdf

Hudson, J., Ungar, R., Albright, L., Tkatch, R., Schaeffer, J., & Wicker, E. R. (2020). Robotic pet use among community-dwelling older adults. *The Journals of Gerontology. Series B: Psychological sciences and Social Sciences, 75*(9), 2018–2028.

Ingold, T. (1993). The temoproality of the landscape. World Archaeology. (Vol. 25) Conceptions of Time Ancient Society, 152–174.

Johansson-Pajala, R. M., Thommes, K., Hoppe, J. A., Tuisku, O., Hennala, L., Pekkarnen, S., et al. (2020). Care robot orientation: What, who and how? Potential users perceptions. *International Journal of Social Robotics, 12*, 1103–1117. https://doi.org/10.1007/s12369020-00619-y

Johnson, D. O., Cuijpers, R. H., Juola, J. F., Torta, E., Simonov, M., Frisiello, A., et al. (2014). Socially assistive robots: A comprehensive approach to extending independent living. *International Journal of Social Robotics, 6*, 195–211. https://doi.org/10.1007/s12369-0130217-8

Johnson, M., Feng, X., Johnson, L. M., & Winters, J. (2007). Potential of a suite of robot/computer-assisted motivating systems for personalized, home-based, stroke rehabilitation. *Journal of Neuroengineering and Rehabilitation, 4*, 6. https://doi.org/10.1186/17430003-4-6

Junior, F. E., Yang, G., Do, H. M., & Sheng, W. (2016). Detection of privacy-sensitive situations for social robots in smart homes. In *2016 IEEE International Conference on Automation Science and Engineering (CASE)* (pp. 727–732). https://doi.org/10.1109/COASE.2016.7743474.

Kachouie, R., Sedighadeli, S., Khosla, R., & Chur, M. T. (2014). Socially assistive robots in elderly care: A mixed-method systematic literature review. *International Journal of Human-Computer Interaction, 30*(5), 369–393. https://doi.org/10.1080/10447318.2013.873278

Kidd, C. D., & Breazeal, C. (2008). Robots at home: Understanding long-term human-robot interaction. In *Proceedings of the IEEE/RSJ International Conference on Intelligent Robots and Systems (IROS'08), Nice, France, 22–26* (pp. 3230–3235).

Liu, L., Stroulia, E., Nikolaidis, I., Miguel-Cruz, A., & Rios-Rincon, A. (2016). Smart homes and home health monitoring technologies for older adults: A systematic review. *International Journal of Medical Informatics, 91*, 44–59. https://doi.org/10.1016/j.ijmedinf.2016.04.007

Lutz, C., & Tamó-Larrieux, A. (2020). The robot privacy paradox: Understanding how privacy concerns shape intentions to use social robots. *Human-Machine Communication, 1*. https://doi.org/10.30658/hmc.1.6

Rodriguez-Gonzalez, C. G., Herranz-Alonso, A., Escudero-Vilaplana, V., Ais-Larisgoitia, M., et al. (2018). Robotic dispensing improves patient safety, inventory management, and staff satisfaction in an outpatient hospital pharmacy. *Journal of Evaluation in Clinical Practice, 25*(1), 28–35. https://doi.org/10.1111/jep.13014

Johnson, J., & Finn, K. (2017). *Designing user interfaces for an aging population: Towards universal design.* Morgan Kaufmann.

Joyce, K., & Loe, M. (2010). A sociological approach to ageing, technology, and health. *Sociology of Health & Illness, 32*(2), 171–180.

Kang, H. S., Makimoto, K., Konno, R., & Koh, I. S. (2020). Review of outcome measures in PARO robot intervention studies for dementia care. *Geriatric Nursing, 41*(3), 207–214. https://doi.org/10.1015/j-gerinurse.2019.09.03

Kim, C. O., & Jang, S. N. (2018). Home-based primary care for homebound older adults: Literature review. *Annals of Geriatric Medicine and Research, 22*(2), 62–72. https://doi.org/10.4235/agmr.2018.22.2.62

Lam, K., Lu, A. D., Shi, Y., & Covinsky, K. E. (2020). Assessing telemedicine unreadiness among older adults in the United States during the COVID-19 pandemic. *Journal of the American Medical Association, 180*(10), 1389–1390. https://doi.org/10.1001/jamainternmed.2020.2671

Lin, P., Abney, K., & Bekey, G. A. (2014). *Robot ethics: The ethical and social implications of robotics.* MIT Press.

Lincoln, Y. S., & Guba, E. G. (1985). Naturalistic inquiry. Newbury Park, CA: Sage Publications.

McCaughey, D., McGhan, G., Kim, J., Brannon, D., Leroy, H., & Jablonski, R. (2013). Workforce implications of injury among home health workers: Evidence from the national home health aid survey. *The Gerontologist, 52*(4), 493–505. https://doi.org/10.1093/geront/gnr133

Montemerlo, M., Roy, N., & Thrun, S. (2003). Perspectives on standardization in mobile robot programming: The Carnegie Mellon navigation (CARMEN) toolkit. *Proceedings 2003 IEEE/RSJ International Conference on Intelligent Robots and Systems (Cat. No 03CH37453), 2436–2441, vol 3.* https://doi.org/10.1109/IROS.203.1249235

Musich, S., Wang, S. S., Hawkins, K., & Yeh, C. S. (2015). Homebound older adults: Prevalence, characteristics, health care utilization, and quality-of-care. *Geriatric Nursing, 36*(6), 445–450. https://doi.org/10.1016/j.gerinurse.2015.06.013

Neven, L. (2015). By any means? Questioning the link between gerontechnological innovation and older people's wish to live at home. *Technological Forecasting and Social Change, 93*, 32–43.

Neves, B. B., & Vetere, F. (2019). Ageing and emerging digital technologies. In B. B. Neves & F. Vetere (Eds.), *Ageing and digital technology: Designing and evaluation emerging technologies for older adults* (pp. 1–14). Springer.

Nundy, S., & Patel, K. K. (2020). Hospital-at-home to support COVID-19 surge-Time to bring down the walls? *JAMA Health Forum, 1* (5): e200504. http://doi.org/10.10001/jamahealthforum.2020.0504.

Peine, A., Rollwagen, I., & Neven, L. (2014). The rise of the "innosumer" – Rethinking older technology users. *Technological Forecasting and Social Change, 82,* 199–214.

Peine, A., Faulkner, A., Jaeger, B., & Moors, E. (2015). Science, technology and the 'grand challenge' of ageing-Understanding the socio-material constitution of later life. *Technological Forecasting & Social Change, 93,* 1–15. http://doi.org/10.1016/j.techfore.2014.11.010

Peine, A. (2019). Technology and ageing – Theoretical propositions from science and technology studies (STS). In B. B. Neves & F. Vetere (Eds.), *Ageing and digital technology: Designing and evaluation emerging technologies for older adults* (pp. 51–64). Springer.

Pericas, J. M., Cucchiari, D., Torrallanrdona-Murphy, O., Calva, J., Serralabos, J., Alves, E. et al. (2020). Hospital at home for management of COVID-19: Preliminary experience of 63 patients. *Infection, 49* (2), 327–332. http://doi.org/10.1007/s15010-020-01527-z

PHI. (2020, September). *Workforce center data.* https://phinational.org/policyresearch/workforce-data-center/

Pino, M., Boulay, M., Jouen, F., & Rigaud, A. S. (2015). "Are we ready for robots that care for us?" Attitudes and opinions of older adults towards socially assistive robots. *Frontiers in Aging Neuroscience, 7,* Article 141. https://doi.org/10.3389/fnagi.2015.00141

Poli, A., Kostakis, I., & Barbabella, F. (2021). Receiving care through digital health technologies: Drivers and implications of old-age digital health exclusion. In K. Walsh, T. Scharf, S. Van Regenmortel, & A. Wanka (Eds.), *Social exclusion in later life. International perspectives on aging, vol 28.* Springer. https://doi.org/10.1007/978-3-030-51406-8_13

Prakash, A., Beer, J. M., Deyle, T., Smarr, C. A., Chen, T. L., Mitzner, T. L., Kemp, C. C., & Rogers, W. A. (2013). Older adults medication management in the home: How can robots help? *Proc ACM SIGCHI, 2013,* 283–290. https://doi.org/10.1109/HRI.2013.6483600

Rudzicz, F., Raimondo, S., & Pou-Prom, C. (2017). Ludwig: A conversational robot for people with Alzheimer's. *Alzheimer's and Dementia, 13*(7), 167. https://doi.org/10.1016/j.jalz.2017.06.2611

Qian, K., Ma, X., Dai, X., & Fang, F. (2010). Robot etiquette: Socially acceptable navigation of service robots with human motion pattern learning and prediction. *Journal of Bionic Engineering, 7,* 150–160.

Scales, K. (2021). It is time to resolve the direct care workforce crisis in long-term care. *The Gerontologist, 61*(4), 487–504. https://doi.org/10.1093/geront/gnaa1116

Simshaw, R., Terry, N., Hauser, K., & Cummings, M. L. (2016). Regulating healthcare robots: Maximizing opportunities while minimizing risks. *Richmond Journal of Law & Technology, 22*(2), 1–38. http://scholarship.richmond.edu/jolt/vol22/iss2/1

Stone, R., Sutton, J. P., Bryant, N., Adams, A., & Squillace, M. (2013). The home health workforce: A distinction between worker categories. *Home Health Service Quarterly, 32*(4), 218–233. https://doi.org/10.1080/016211424.2013.851049

Tan, L. F., Teng, V. H. W., Seetharaman, S. K., & Yip, A. W. (2020). Facilitating telehealth for older adults during the COVID-19 pandemic and beyond: Strategies from a Singapore geriatric center. *Geriatrics & Gerontology International, 20*(10), 993–995. https://doi.org/10.1111/ggi.14017

Tao, V., Moy, K., & Amifar, V. A. (2016). A little robot with big promise may be the future of personalized health care. *Technology Forum, 22*(9), 38.

Tiwari, P., Warren, J., & Day, K. (2011). *Comprehensive support for self-management of medications by a networked robot for the elderly.* HiNZ Conference.

Turja, T., Van Aerschot, L., Särkikoski, T., & Oksansen, A. (2020). Finish healthcare professionals' attitudes towards robots: Reflections on a population sample. *Nursing Open, 5*(3), 300–309. https://doi.org/10.1002/nop2.138

United States Bureau of Labor Statistics. (2021). *Occupational outlook handbook, Home health and personal care aides.* https://www.bls.gov/ooh/fastest-growing.htm. Retrieved July, 21, 2021.

Van Aeershot, L., & Parvianinen, J. (2020). Robots responding to care needs? A multi-tasking care robot pursued for 25 years, available products offer simple entertainment and instrumental assistance. *Ethics and Information Technology, 22,* 247–256. https://doi.org/10.1007/s10676-020-09536-0

Van Wynsberghe, A. (2015). *Healthcare robots: Ethics, design, and implementation.* Routledge.

Villaronga, E. F., Tamo-Larrieux, A., & Lutz, C. (2018). Did I tell you my new therapist is a robot? Ethical, legal, and societal issues of healthcare and therapeutic robots. *SSRN Electronic Journal.* https://doi.org/10.2139/ssrn.3267832

Volpe, B. T., Ferraro, M., Krebs, H., & Hogan, N. (2002). Robotics in rehabilitation treatment of patients with stroke. *Current Atherosclerosis Reports, 4,* 270–276.

Wada, K., & Shibata, T. (2007). Living with seal robots – Its sociopsychological and physiological influences on the elderly at a care house. *IEE Transactions on Robotics, 23*(5), 972–980.

Walton, A. L., & Rogers, B. (2017). Workplace hazards faced by nursing assistants in the United States: A focused literature review. *International Journal of Environmental Research and Public Health, 14*(5), 544. https://doi.org/10.3390/ijerph14050544

Wang, C. J., & Huang, D. J. (2013). The HIPPA conundrum in the era of mobile health and communications. *Journal of the American Medical Association, 310*(11), 1121–1122.

Yu, R., Hui, E., Lee, J., Poon, D., Ng, A., et al. (2015). Use of a therapeutic socially assistive Pet Robot (PARO) in improving mood and stimulating social interaction and communication for people with dementia: Study protocol for a randomized controlled trial. *JMIR Research Protocols, 4*(2), e45. https://doi.org/10.2196/resprot.4189

Zheng, J., Finzel, R., Pakhomov, S., & Gini, M. (2020). Spoken dialogue for medication management. Studies in Computational Intelligence. In A. Shaban-Nejad & M. Michalowski (Eds.), *Precision health and medicine: A digital revolution in healthcare* (pp. 119–127). Springer-Verlag. https://doi.org/10.1007/978-3-030-24409-511

# Rehabilitation Clinics that Enhance Stroke Recovery: Rethinking the Same-for-All Design Approach

Maja Kevdzija

## 1 Introduction

The current COVID-19 global health crisis has put a spotlight on the design of healthcare environments. This provides an opportunity to rethink established design practices and develop new concepts for improving patient well-being and recovery. Because stroke is a significant concern for the future and the aging population, it is urgent to identify which physical aspects of the built environment might help support and improve their recovery process. This chapter explores rehabilitation clinics as these facilities are where a large part of inpatient recovery after a stroke takes place.

### 1.1 Aging and Stroke

Stroke is one of the leading causes of disability in the adult population and the third most common cause of disability-adjusted life years lost globally (Feigin et al., 2017). It is also primarily a condition characteristic for older age, more specifically for the population aged at least 65 years (Kim et al., 2020). In the following decades, it is expected that the aging population will outweigh the overall declining numbers in age-standardized incidence rates (Stevens et al., 2017). The projections predict that there will be around 12 million stroke deaths, 70 million stroke survivors, and more than 200 million disability-adjusted life years lost globally by 2030 (Feigin et al., 2014).

M. Kevdzija (✉)
Faculty of Architecture and Planning, Institute of Architecture and Design, TU Wien, Vienna, Austria
e-mail: maja.kevdzija@tuwien.ac.at

© The Author(s), under exclusive license to Springer Nature Switzerland AG 2023
F. Ferdous, E. Roberts (eds.), *(Re)designing the Continuum of Care for Older Adults*, https://doi.org/10.1007/978-3-031-20970-3_7

Aside from a large number of persons affected by stroke, this condition is also accompanied by the widest range of impairments (Adamson et al., 2004). Around a third of affected people experience moderate to severe impairments requiring special care (Lyden et al., 2014). Stroke survivors are a diverse group with various poststroke conditions such as hemiparesis (weakness in one side of the body) or hemiplegia (one-sided paralysis) (Langhorne et al., 2009); diverse cognitive impairments involving memory, orientation, language, and attention (Tatemichi et al., 1994); speech impairments (Flowers et al., 2016); vision impairments (Rowe et al., 2009); and others. Depending on the nature of the stroke, these impairments can range from severe to mild, and no two strokes are alike. The largely individual character of stroke makes structured care and the design of rehabilitation facilities challenging.

Older adults are at a higher risk of stroke and at the risk of limited functional recovery and the reduced ability to live independently after a stroke. Younger stroke survivors are more likely to recover, with this probability gradually declining until the age of 75 and steeply declining afterward (Knoflach et al., 2012; Kugler et al., 2003). One of the main reasons for poor outcomes could be the additional age-related impairments and comorbidities common in the advanced age (Ween et al., 1996). Consequently, older individuals frequently fail to regain independence and, in some cases, require long-term care due to the decreased likelihood of recovery. Because of this, rehabilitation after a stroke is crucial for the recovery of lost functions, improving independence in the activities of daily living and regaining independence for returning home.

Since stroke is a complex health condition, each person's recovery path is unique. The recovery process can also greatly vary among different countries, depending on the accessibility of healthcare, availability of resources, and disparities in treatment systems (Norrving & Kissela, 2013). Although minor variations might be present, the overall features of the recovery process of stroke survivors in developed countries are comparable. On their path toward recovery, the majority of people that suffer a stroke go through several stages. The recovery usually starts in a hospital, where acute care is received. The recovery then continues through rehabilitation in different kinds of environments, depending on the country, healthcare system, and severity of the stroke, and ends by returning to their home (when rehabilitation took place in a healthcare facility) or, in some cases, being transferred to a long-term care facility. As one of the most important links in the stroke care chain, rehabilitation usually takes place in a hospital (stroke unit), a specialized rehabilitation clinic (inpatient or outpatient), or at home, with, in some cases, all of these environments being used for rehabilitation at different times as the recovery progresses.

This chapter will focus on rehabilitation clinics, large free-standing facilities with a complex program, and typical locations for stroke inpatient rehabilitation in many European countries (e.g., Austria, Belgium, Germany) and the United States.

## 1.2  Rehabilitation Clinics as Facilities

Rehabilitation clinics are buildings where stroke patients undergo rehabilitation as inpatients (and occasionally outpatients) after their hospital stay. The length of stay in these environments can vary from several weeks to several months, depending on the severity of the stroke and the health insurance coverage. During recovery, various poststroke symptoms are addressed by a multidisciplinary team that provides an organized care package (Clarke & Forster, 2015). Patients' rehabilitation is structured around the prescribed individual therapy plan and may include a variety of different forms of therapy, the most frequent of which are physiotherapy and occupational therapy (Hempler et al., 2018). Studies indicate that the majority of functional recovery after a stroke occurs within 3–6 months after the stroke onset (Branco et al., 2018; Lee et al., 2015). This is why an inpatient stay in a rehabilitation clinic, where the patient receives therapies from professionals from various disciplines multiple times per day for several weeks, is a setting where the patient can receive the highest intensity of therapies to regain lost functions in the months following a stroke.

The usual spatial organization of a rehabilitation clinic is divided into two main functions: patient wards (individual units where patients sleep and receive immediate care from nurses) and therapy areas (spaces where patients receive different kinds of therapy). These two functions can be completely separated (e.g., therapy rooms on the ground floor and patient wards on the upper floors) or mixed on the same floor. Most commonly, there are several patient wards on one floor of the clinic, each with a nurses' station. The number of patient rooms per ward can usually vary from 15 bedrooms to 30 bedrooms, depending on the organization of the clinic. Patients' rooms are mostly single occupancy or double occupancy bedrooms. Each of the therapies included in the program of a rehabilitation clinic usually requires a specific type of space ranging from a large sports hall to small office rooms, depending on the therapy type, necessary equipment, and the number of patients treated at the same time. Since rehabilitation clinics are places where patients stay for several weeks to several months, they are equipped with many other necessary facilities, such as a cafeteria, diagnostic facilities, medical and administrative staff offices, and patient communal spaces.

## 1.3  Stroke Patients' Experiences of Rehabilitation

While staying in rehabilitation clinics as inpatients, stroke patients' daily lives consist of scheduled meals and therapies and free time and family visits between and after daily therapies and during weekends. Even though patients have substantial time between and after therapies for their free time activities, they are often inactive and alone during their free time. Nothing has significantly changed since the first studies on the time use of stroke patients in various rehabilitation environments were conducted in the 1980s (Keith, 1980; Keith & Cowell, 1987). Stroke patients are consistently found inactive and alone during their free time between therapies during their rehabilitation stay (Anåker et al., 2018; Janssen et al., 2014a; Kārkliņa et al., 2021; Kevdzija & Marquardt, 2021b). This directly contradicts the recommendations for stroke care which suggest the avoidance of bed rest and increased activity (Billinger et al., 2014). Still, all the factors contributing to patients' low activity levels are not yet thoroughly investigated. General fatigue (Duncan et al., 2015; MacIntosh et al., 2017), various stroke-related motor and cognitive impairments (Van De Port et al., 2006), and exhaustion from therapies are the factors that certainly limit patients' mobility and activity. In addition, the inadequately designed built environment of rehabilitation facilities might be affecting patients' behavior and contributing to patients' low activity levels during rehabilitation.

In the interviews with healthcare professionals in stroke units, the physical environment was identified as a limiting factor to patients' exercises and daily activities (Nordin et al., 2021). In another study investigating the walking activity of stroke patients in rehabilitation, the authors identified the inadequate facility layout and lack of space as some of the reasons why individuals in inpatient stroke rehabilitation have limited capacity to increase their overall walking time (Mansfield et al., 2015). Some studies also indicate that common rooms' visibility, size, and location might influence patients' activity levels during free time (Anåker et al., 2017; Kevdzija & Marquardt, 2021b). The built environment of rehabilitation units is often reported as hindering (Anåker et al., 2017; Kevdzija & Marquardt, 2018) and not offering enough opportunities for activities and additional exercise (Eng et al., 2014). Furthermore, during rehabilitation, patients report feelings of loneliness (Anåker et al., 2019) and boredom (Cowdell & Garrett, 2003) and express wishes to pursue more recreational and social activities in their free time (Luker et al., 2015). Despite the relevance of the built environment being frequently emphasized, the relationship between stroke patients' activity and well-being and the built environment remains insufficiently explored.

## *1.4 Strategies for Increasing Patient Activity*

The low activity levels of stroke patients have been widely acknowledged as a challenge during rehabilitation. The significance of the environment in patients' activities is being investigated in the latest studies. There has been a growing interest in employing a concept of an enriched environment to increase patients' activity levels. In the context of rehabilitation, environmental enrichment implies the provision of an environment with different materials for exercising patients' cognitive capacities and motor skills, usually without altering the built environment. Several recent studies show mixed results on the efficiency of this intervention on patients' activity levels.

A pilot study in a mixed rehabilitation unit (Janssen et al., 2014b) tested the effect of the enriched environment (a common room with easy access to a computer with different kinds of content and games, a Wii console, reading material, various types of board games and recreational activities) on the activity levels of patients. Stroke patients exposed to the enriched environment were 1.2 times more active than the control group (Janssen et al., 2014b). In another study conducted in a stroke unit (Rosbergen et al., 2017), public areas were transformed into communal areas where participants had access to a variety of equipment to enhance activities away from the bedside. The equipment included iPads, books, puzzles, newspapers, games, music, and magazines available during and outside therapy hours. The patient group exposed to the enriched environment group spent a significantly higher proportion of their day engaged in any activity compared to the standard care patient group (Rosbergen et al., 2017). These pilot studies testing the influence on patients' activity levels were individual studies including a small number of participants ($n = 15$ and $n = 30$ in the experimental group, respectively), and they showed promising results. A recent larger cluster trial study ($n = 91$ in the experimental group) on the effect of environmental enrichment (communal area with interactive gaming, a computer with an Internet connection, reading material, jigsaw puzzles, board games, and a dining area for eating meals) identified a negligible effect on the activity levels of patients (Janssen et al., 2021). The important statement to highlight is the authors' conclusion that environmental enrichment might not be enough without altering the built environment, reorganizing the wards and therapy areas, and creating an activity-promoting culture in the rehabilitation facility (Janssen et al., 2021). Therefore, the importance of the built environment for stroke patients' activities in rehabilitation is being acknowledged even in the most recent studies, but not yet thoroughly investigated.

Since the influence of the built environment is still largely unexplored, the following empirical study aims to provide insights into the everyday lives of stroke patients during their inpatient stay in rehabilitation clinics and contribute to a better understanding of their spatial experiences.

## 2 How Stroke Patients Interact with the Built Environment: An Empirical Study

A research study was conducted in seven German stroke rehabilitation clinics to investigate how patients interacted with their built environment during their inpatient stay.

## 2.1 Research Methods, Settings, and Participants

The shadowing method (Mcdonald, 2005; Quinlan, 2008) was chosen to directly observe stroke patients during their daily life in rehabilitation clinics. The researcher was accommodated in each rehabilitation clinic (in the same building or one of the adjacent buildings in the rehabilitation complex) for 2 weeks and spent 1 whole day with a different patient. Throughout the day, patients were observed by the researcher in all public and semipublic areas of the clinics (corridors and common areas). Seventy patients were shadowed in total, each for 12 consecutive hours. The rehabilitation clinics were large multistory buildings, ranging from 188 to 250 beds.

The patients included in the research study had different mobility levels and used different mobility aids to move around due to various motor impairments after a stroke. They were all over the age of 60. Sixteen patients relied on the use of a wheelchair, 23 patients used a walker, and 31 patients could walk independently without using a mobility aid. Patient shadowing was done using the previously prepared floor plans and recording patients' paths, time logs of all activities, and notable encounters with the built environment, occasionally accompanied by sketches.

During the data collection, it was observed that using a mobility aid greatly affected how patients interacted with the built environment. The use of a particular mobility aid changed the way patients used the space, the dimensions they needed for being mobile, and the mobility issues they encountered. Consequently, patients were divided into three mobility level groups according to the used mobility aid in the data analysis phase. All the collected observational data were analyzed to explore the barriers and facilitators that patients encountered in the built environment of rehabilitation clinics. The explanation of each observed barrier is provided for clarity in the result presentation (Table 1). The following section summarizes the main findings of this multicenter shadowing study.

**Table 1** Explanation of the observed barriers in the built environment

| Barrier category | Explanation |
|---|---|
| Wayfinding | Difficulties with finding a way to the therapy, mistaking the corridor or the floor, asking other patients/or staff which way to go. This does not apply to patients visiting therapy for the first time or looking for the room number in the correct corridor |
| Dimensions | Not enough space to pass through a corridor, no room to park a wheelchair or a walker in the corridor |
| Distance | Stopping to rest on the way, asking a staff member or the researcher to push their wheelchair |
| Floor | Difficulties with controlling a wheelchair/walker on a floor slope, rolling a wheelchair backward on the carpet flooring/slope |
| Physical obstacles | Difficulties with overcoming various physical obstacles such as a heavy door, high door threshold, or equipment/furniture in the corridor |

**Table 2** Number of events when patients were observed to encounter a barrier

| Barrier category | Number of events per clinic | | | | | | | Total number of events | Prevalence |
|---|---|---|---|---|---|---|---|---|---|
| | A | B | C | D | E | F | G | | |
| Wayfinding | 7 | 2 | 7 | 6 | 3 | 6 | 11 | 42 | 40.8% |
| Dimensions | 1 | 0 | 0 | 5 | 9 | 2 | 1 | 18 | 17.5% |
| Distance | 1 | 0 | 0 | 0 | 4 | 1 | 12 | 18 | 17.5% |
| Floor | 4 | 0 | 0 | 3 | 2 | 0 | 4 | 13 | 12.6% |
| Physical obstacles | 2 | 0 | 0 | 3 | 3 | 0 | 4 | 12 | 11.6% |

## 2.2   Results

### 2.2.1   Barriers in the Built Environment

Out of 70 observed patients, 39 encountered at least one mobility barrier in the built environment during the observation day. A total of 103 events when a patient encountered a barrier in the built environment was observed in seven participating clinics (Table 2). The number of observed events varied in each clinic.

Wayfinding was the most common challenge that patients encountered in their daily life in rehabilitation. Since patients are encouraged to attend several therapies per day on their own, they need to find a way from their patient ward to the therapy rooms located in different parts of the building. Out of 42 observed events when the wayfinding issue occurred, the patient was going from their room to therapy or vice versa in 37 cases. In most cases, patients made a wrong turn in a corridor and used backtracking and asking for directions as the strategies to find the right way. Patients had difficulties finding their way on the paths that had multiple decision nodes and where they had to choose between going left or right, continuing straight, or changing a direction to left or right (Kevdzija, 2022). Most cases occurred in corridors that were very similar on both sides of the decision point, not only in floor plan dimensions but also in identity, color, and materials. The degree of corridor symmetry was likely a major factor in patients' decreased ability to find their way. Furthermore, in seven cases, a patient mistook the correct floor when exiting the elevator. These clinics had a central core with elevators, and each floor had the same spatial configuration. As a result, when looking out from the elevator, each floor appeared identical, making it difficult for patients to find their way around. Encountering a wayfinding challenge increased patients' traveled distances by around 26% over what they would have covered if they had not gotten lost (Kevdzija, 2022).

Long distances between the two most important areas, patient wards and therapy rooms, were also challenging for stroke patients (18 events). Patients were more dependent on staff members to bring them to therapies over greater distances, and they also encountered more barriers in the built environment (Kevdzija & Marquardt, 2021a). This was especially the case for patients using a wheelchair. Staff members often brought these patients to therapy rooms since they were located far away from their wards. This likely contributed to patients' feelings of loss of control and denied them the opportunity to exercise independent mobility. The average distance traveled by patients when they were independent and did not encounter barriers in the built environment was about 60 m, compared to 110 m when they required assistance from staff or encountered a mobility barrier (Kevdzija & Marquardt, 2021a). Daily distances that patients covered in rehabilitation clinics ranged from 912.4 m to 2107.9 m, depending on the rehabilitation clinic (Kevdzija & Marquardt, 2021a). As a result, distances between spaces had a major impact on the built environment experience for patients of all mobility abilities. When the distances were longer, there was a greater chance that patients would encounter a barrier and/or seek help from medical staff.

Another observed barrier for stroke patients in the built environment was the width of corridors (18 events). Corridors leading to therapy rooms were particularly challenging since numerous patients attended therapies at the same times of the day. The corridor width problems were observed in areas with increased patient traffic. This was most common in clinics where the patient wards were vertically separated from the therapy area or where the therapy rooms were all in the same section of the building, far away from the patient wards. An unexpected observation was that all the corridors in the clinics were dimensioned adequately according to the German DIN 18040-1 standard (DIN 18040-1, 2010), with enough space for two people in a wheelchair to pass each other (1.8 m). What was not accounted for was the way the dimensions of the corridors changed with their actual daily use and the amount of patient traffic that specific corridors would be receiving. For example, a main corridor in the therapy area would have additional waiting chairs, with patients keeping their walkers in front of them and patients in wheelchairs waiting for therapy (see Fig. 1). These factors, along with the usual number of about 200 patients using this corridor at similar times of day, notably shrink the corridor width. This causes considerable problems for patients who cannot reach their therapy on time and have limited space to maneuver their wheelchairs and walkers. Another example is the lack of space in front of elevators in clinics with a vertical separation between patient wards and therapy rooms and only one vertical core. Since patients need to use this vertical core when going to therapies at similar times of the day, this creates significant patient traffic. Because many patients require a wheelchair or a walker to get around, they take up more room when waiting in front of the elevators. This

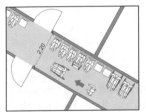 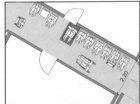 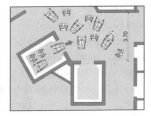

**Fig. 1** Observed issues with corridor widths and spaced in front of elevators (2021). (Diagram by the author)

creates a constant issue where patients cannot enter or exit the elevators due to insufficient space (see Fig. 1).

Floor surfaces, specifically carpet flooring and sloped floors, were another barrier identified in the built environment. All of the observed issues with floor surfaces (13 events) were encountered by patients using a wheelchair. Carpet flooring used in some clinics in the wards or common areas created friction between the wheelchair wheels and the floor surface. This was a challenge for wheelchair users suffering from hemiplegia or hemiparesis. The patients adopted one of two techniques to get around the issue: driving the wheelchair backward or making a detour to avoid the area with carpet flooring. A similar strategy of going backward was used when the patients encountered a corridor that was on a slope. These slopes were usually the result of the clinic's growth over time, where different sections were subsequently connected, resulting in the sloping connecting corridors. Another strategy that patients used to overcome this barrier was asking staff members to push their wheelchairs.

Physical obstacles in corridors were identified as another barrier for stroke patients in the built environment (12 events). It was also observed that the categories of physical obstacles and dimension issues were often intertwined. Physical items added to corridors might limit the width of the corridors, causing dimension issues. At the same time, corridors with dimensions that were not planned for the addition of particular items (such as waiting chairs) might cause these objects to be physical obstacles for patients. As a result, these two categories might occasionally act as a mobility barrier simultaneously, but only in the case of various temporary or permanent items in the corridors. These items in the corridors were most commonly the unused medical equipment, patient beds, and furniture (waiting chairs or a seating area). The observed individuals had insufficient control of their mobility aids and hit them in the corridors with their wheelchair or walker. Aside from items in the corridors, patients encountered other physical obstacles when traveling the clinics' corridors, specifically heavy nonautomatic doors. These doors were especially challenging for wheelchair and walker users.

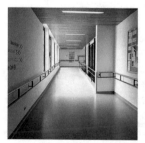 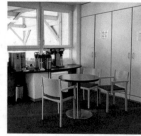 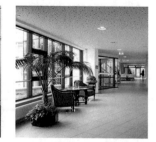

**Fig. 2** Observed activity and mobility facilitators: wall handrails, informal seating area with a beverage station in the corridor, rest stop on the way to therapy (2017). (Photos by the author)

## 2.2.2 Facilitators in the Built Environment

Several specific spatial elements were identified as the facilitators to the mobility of patients (Fig. 2). Patients, particularly those in wheelchairs, were observed utilizing the handrails on the walls to pull themselves along corridors where there were too many people. It was difficult for them to operate the wheelchairs due to insufficient space. The same was the case in corridors that were on a slope. The presence of automated doors was also a significant help for patients, particularly those who used a walker or a wheelchair. The availability of rest stops (i.e., small seating areas in the corridors) enabled patients to stop and rest on their way to and back from therapies. During patient shadowing in this research study, patients were often observed visiting places with a directed view of nature. Another frequently visited type of space was the corridor widenings where a seating area was located, sometimes together with a beverage station (i.e., coffee machine, kettle, and tea selection). They provided a more informal socializing space than standard common rooms, making them more approachable. These examples illustrate that even minor changes to the physical environment may positively impact patients' mobility and activity. Most of them are small-scale interventions that might enhance patients' quality of life in rehabilitation clinics.

Few activity facilitators were found when examined on a larger scale of the patient wards and the entire clinic. Patients were generally very inactive and spent 50% of their free time in their rooms (Kevdzija & Marquardt, 2021b), which is consistent with all previous studies on the time use of stroke patients during rehabilitation. The most often visited locations were corridors, with activities including socialization, exercise, enjoying the view, sitting alone, and many others (Kevdzija & Marquardt, 2021b). As previously mentioned, seating areas in the corridor widenings and a beverage station were attractive for patients and commonly visited. Another commonly visited space was the common room on the ward, when it existed. Some of the participating clinics lacked a common room or seating space on the wards. More mobile patients would leave the wards in those clinics to visit common spaces in other clinic areas, while the less mobile patients would stay in their rooms.

**Table 3** Comparison of numbers of encountered barriers for each mobility level ($n = 70$)

| Barrier category | Mobility level[a] | | | |
| | Wheelchair versus walker | Walker versus walking | Wheelchair versus walking | Significance[b] |
|---|---|---|---|---|
| Wayfinding | $p = 0.918$ | $p = 0.926$ | $p = 0.841$ | $p = 0.980$ |
| Dimensions | $p = 0.046$ | $p = 0.184$ | $p = 0.001$ | $p = 0.002$ |
| Distance | $p = 0.039$ | $p = 0.097$ | $p < 0.001$ | $p = 0.001$ |
| Floor | $p = 0.001$ | $p = 1.000$ | $p < 0.001$ | $p < 0.001$ |
| Physical obstacles | $p = 0.948$ | $p = 0.101$ | $p = 0.173$ | $p = 0.237$ |

[a]Mann-Whitney U test, comparison between two mobility level groups at a time
[b]Kruskal-Wallis Test, comparison between all three mobility level groups

### 2.2.3   Differences Between Patients with Different Mobility Levels

Patients who used wheelchairs were the most dependent on the built environment of rehabilitation clinics and most vulnerable to barriers. Five categories of barriers were previously discussed, and some differences were identified among patients using (or not) a different mobility aid (Table 3). These differences were the most significant in the categories of dimensions (corridor width), distance, and floor (covering, slopes) between patients using a wheelchair and the other two patient groups (using a walker and independently walking). This stark difference between patients using a wheelchair and other patients is most likely due to their health condition. Stroke patients utilizing a wheel chair are usually at the start of their rehabilitation and significantly impaired, especially in motor functions. Some of them are still getting used to driving a wheelchair and developing strategies to use them with one-sided muscle weakness or paralysis.

All observed groups of patients encountered issues related to wayfinding and physical obstacles, both common problems in healthcare facilities. Even patients who could walk independently and who were at the end of their rehabilitation still encountered an equal number of wayfinding issues as the other two patient groups. As a result, regardless of the patients' mobility level, solutions to wayfinding challenges and physical obstacles in rehabilitation clinics should be developed.

# 3   Discussion

This chapter provided an overview of the challenges in designing rehabilitation environments for stroke by looking at recent literature and presenting the results of an empirical research study. These key findings emerge from the conducted research study and the recent literature: (1) built environment is unsupportive to patients' activity and mobility; (2) wards within rehabilitation clinics are mostly designed in the same way, disregarding the patients' very different spatial needs in different rehabilitation stages; (3) the many physical barriers in the built environment limit patients' possibilities to be independent and to prepare for going back home adequately; and (4) primarily functional designs of these facilities do not provide enough motivating and inviting spaces for socializing or spending time alone outside of patient rooms. The empirical study's results were consistent with all previous studies on the time use of stroke patients (Anåker et al., 2018; Bernhardt et al., 2004; De Wit et al., 2005; Janssen et al., 2014a), finding them very inactive in their free time during rehabilitation. At the same time, the main results show the built environment of rehabilitation as hindering and promoting inactivity, similar to the research studies conducted in smaller settings of stroke units (Anåker et al., 2019; Nordin et al., 2021).

## 3.1   Physical Aspects of the Built Environment

The conducted research study offers insight into how stroke patients interact with the built environment during rehabilitation and the barriers and facilitators they encounter in this environment by observing each patient's activities over a whole day. The built environment of rehabilitation clinics was found to hinder the mobility of stroke patients significantly. Certain factors such as the unused medical equipment in the corridors, chair use in the therapy areas, distances between spaces, or heavy patient traffic should be better anticipated during the planning process. The important point to emphasize as one of the primary outcomes of this investigation is that while separating barriers makes it simpler to analyze specific elements of the built environment, many physical features of the built environment are interconnected and can impact each other and the patient's experience of the built environment. Therefore, the design of the rehabilitation environments is a challenge that requires careful coordination of various aspects to avoid creating a hindering environment for patients undergoing recovery.

Physical barriers are generally regarded as negative features of the built environment. However, they do not necessarily create limiting environments. Experiencing barriers and knowing how to overcome them may also be a practical rehabilitation approach. Hence, design elements that are barriers for some patients might be mobility facilitators for others. After rehabilitation, patients return home and resume regular life, where they will almost certainly encounter a variety of barriers in both their indoor (Marcheschi et al., 2017) and outdoor environments (Robinson et al., 2013). Certain physical obstacles can be used as exercise aids to help patients transition from life in a rehabilitation clinic to life at home by challenging them during recovery. They might also encourage patients to be active and exercise mobility outside of treatment sessions. As a result, physical barriers are not necessarily negative aspects of the built environment if they are intentionally designed for training and exercise rather than being the product of inadequate planning and construction.

Patients who rely on staff members to get around the clinic and patients with very limited mobility abilities cannot overcome barriers in the built environment without danger and risk of injury. If the environments are created for significantly impaired patients at the beginning of rehabilitation, fairly mobile individuals may not find enough opportunities to be more active and exercise their mobility. Patients in advanced rehabilitation phases and those ready to return home could potentially train their mobility by overcoming various types of barriers in a controlled manner. These barriers must be intentionally designed for patients' mobility training, and existing physical obstacles in the built environment should not be considered appropriate for mobility training. At the same time, patients using a wheelchair who are still getting used to their impairments and exercising to reach independence already face many challenges in their recovery, even without the barriers in the built environment. This highlights the very different needs of patients who are in different rehabilitation phases and use various mobility aids. Therefore, the "same-for-all" design approach does not create equal opportunities for stroke patients' independence, exercise, and activity in rehabilitation. Patients in different stages of rehabilitation face diverse challenges and are likely to benefit from tailored environments planned to support their rehabilitation goals much more than from the "same-for-all design."

Another critical aspect to consider is the common rooms' design and allocation inside and outside the wards for different ward types. Some wards did not have any designated common spaces in the clinics participating in the empirical study, which likely did not promote patients' activity. In this study, corridors emerged as important informal spaces in rehabilitation clinics. Similar to studies in other healthcare contexts (Colley et al., 2018; González-Martínez et al., 2016), corridors were spaces where many activities other than circulation occurred. In this study, the particularly interesting spaces were seating areas in the wider parts of corridors combined with a beverage station. They were one of the most commonly visited spaces during observations. Corridors have a great potential to be designed as attractive spaces for patients since they are less formal than classic common rooms and immediately available as the patient steps out of their room. The patient can easily see what is happening and decide whether they will join the activities. Further investigation of communal spaces as mobility facilitators is necessary to encourage and support patients' activities.

## 3.2 A New Perspective to Rehabilitation Clinic Design

If rehabilitation clinics are viewed as patients' temporary homes during recovery, they must accommodate the treatment procedures that are taking place and the patients' daily activities. In contrast, the study results and the recent literature show that existing design strategies for rehabilitation clinics do not meet the needs of patients and do not fully contribute to their recovery.

Stroke survivors with the most severe poststroke impairments can progress through various stages of rehabilitation, depending on their recovery potential. Their recovery path would start in a hospital bed (sometimes even needing mechanical ventilation) and, ideally, progress to walking without mobility aid devices. The recovery stages taking place in rehabilitation clinics also differ in terms of rehabilitation goals, such as stabilization, mobilization, and activation, achieving independence in the activities of daily living (ADLs) and improving everyday life and work skills (Fig. 3). Patients in rehabilitation have varying levels of dependence on mobility aids and nursing staff. Some might require a wheelchair to move around, while others can walk and perform the majority of their ADLs unassisted. As their needs are changing during the rehabilitation process, the built environment should also have the ability to adapt and accommodate these changes to offer the best possible environment for the patients' well-being and recovery. The design goals of these environments could also differ to support each rehabilitation goal/recovery stage (Fig. 3), resulting in a tailored design approach.

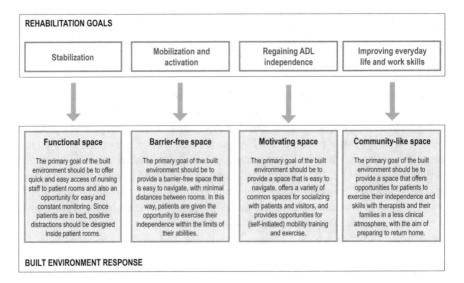

**Fig. 3** Proposed built environment responses to rehabilitation goals (2021). (Diagram by the author)

A simple design exercise was undertaken by the author on a typical patient ward to demonstrate the possible accommodation of these different rehabilitation goals. This exercise was carried out after the study results were obtained, and it is based on these results and the observations of daily life in the clinics made throughout the 3.5 months of data collecting. The intention was to attempt to provide diverse environments with minimal alterations to a typical rehabilitation ward structure. These ideas and concepts could be further explored and translated to various ward configurations. For the clarity of presentation, a similar ward configuration is used for all environments. Three of the rehabilitation goals were explored in this ward design exercise. The first goal of stabilization was omitted since this phase usually takes place in a hospital and outside of rehabilitation clinics.

Some differences in considerations regarding wayfinding, dimensions (corridor width), and distances are presented (Fig. 4). The ward for mobilization and activation is a ward with fewer beds, wider corridors to allow for enough space for patients in a wheelchair, and a clear central area with a nurses' station. Recessed storage areas are planned in the ward's corridor for storing unused wheelchairs and other necessary equipment such as transfer lifts. Since these patients have very limited mobility, a dining room is placed on the ward to encourage them to leave their rooms. This dining room is directly in front of the nurses' station for easy monitoring. Another vital element to plan for is the distance to therapy rooms. Since these patients have limited mobility, therapy areas should be located close to their wards, ideally in a radius of 50–60 m. In this way, patients are given an opportunity to exercise their independence. The next ward type is slightly larger and has similar central zone principles with nurses' station, wider corridor, and less recessed

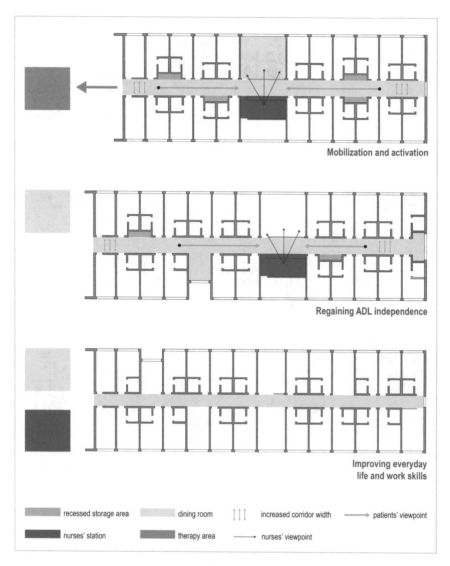

**Fig. 4** Schematic floor plans of wards for patients in different rehabilitation stages wayfinding, dimensions, and distances (2021). (Diagram by the author)

storage areas. What is different is that there is no dining room on the ward. These patients are already much more mobile and should be encouraged to have meals in the main cafeteria. The third ward type is very different. It is organized on a principle of a shared apartment with single bedrooms and several common rooms and with the nurses' station outside of the ward for increased independence and a non-clinical atmosphere. These patients would also have meals in the main cafeteria.

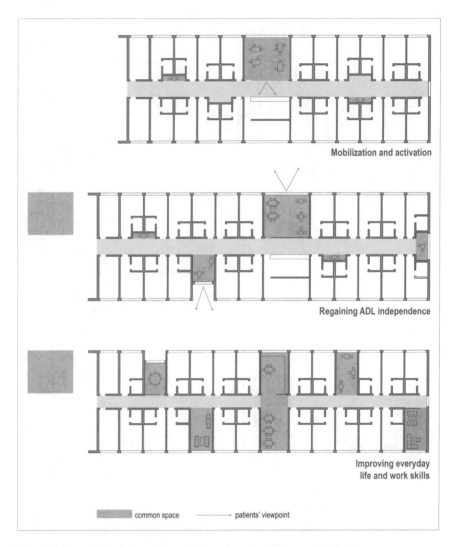

**Fig. 5** Schematic floor plans of wards for patients in different rehabilitation stages: common spaces (2021). (Diagram by the author)

Another essential element identified in the empirical study was the common rooms/spaces, often nonexistent on the wards. An attempt was made to create a concept for common spaces for each of these ward environments (Fig. 5). In the first ward type, the main common room is in the center of the ward, and it doubles as a dining room. The aim is to provide an opportunity for patients to get familiar with each other from mealtimes and be more comfortable leaving their rooms for socializing in their free time. Some recessed wall areas can also be used as small common spaces if not used to store the equipment. The second ward type has a wider variety of common spaces, both as rooms and open seating areas in the corridor. Other kinds of common areas with different activities outside of the wards should be easily reachable for these patients, where they could meet patients from other wards and exercise to improve everyday life and work skills. Views could be provided from some of these common spaces toward therapy areas. According to the medical staff, seeing other people exercising and progressing might motivate stroke patients in this stage. The last ward type is created with a communal kitchen in the center equipped with facilities necessary for patients to practice their daily activities with the therapists or their families. This kind of shared space is intended to replace the clinical atmosphere of the ward with a more homelike environment.

Many more aspects should be considered when designing environments tailored for patients in particular rehabilitation stages, such as sizes of the spaces, window heights, furniture type, activities that can be performed in a specific space or a room, etc. The presented examples illustrate that even a classic ward design could provide different environments and atmospheres with minimal changes. The reconfiguration of rooms to fit the needs of different patients could also be one of the strategies for designing common spaces in the clinics. This could provide a flexible and supportive environment for patients in different stages of recovery. The division into rehabilitation goals could also be looked at differently: the wards could be designed for rehabilitation of particular functional deficits, such as a ward for lower extremities (gait, balance, stairs), a ward for the upper extremities (fine motor skills, use of tools, ADL skills), a ward for swallowing and speech impairments, etc. This kind of organization would be a radical departure from the usual ways rehabilitation clinics are designed but might greatly benefit patients' recovery process. The described ideas and concepts need to be further explored for their applicability in practice. Thus, there is still much room for improvement in rehabilitation clinics' design strategies.

## 3.3   Limitations

This research study has several limitations that need to be mentioned. The sample size was limited to 70 patients due to the time-consuming nature of the shadowing method. Because stroke is predominantly a condition occurring in older adults and because the participants were recruited from available patients during the 2 weeks of field study in each clinic, the sample was also limited in age representation. Furthermore, the research study was conducted in Germany. The discussed characteristics of stroke care and the built environment might not be completely comparable to the context of the United States.

Finally, the illustrated ward examples are not presented as perfect solutions. Instead, they are used for starting a conversation about the possibility of designing specifically tailored environments for different rehabilitation goals rather than creating the same-for-all wards. The presented examples are limited to only looking at the patient wards and not considering the accommodation of the new developments, such as telerehabilitation, enriched environment, the use of robotics in rehabilitation, and the influence of the COVID-19 pandemic. All these aspects will have implications for the future design of the built environment of rehabilitation clinics and need to be further examined. At the same time, this new way of looking at the ward design for rehabilitation clinics asks for the reorganization of care and potentially higher initial investments. Nevertheless, these illustrated examples can facilitate a discussion about how to depart from the "same-for-all" design and start developing new design concepts for better rehabilitation environments.

# 4 Conclusion

Rehabilitation clinics need to be seen as important environments where patients stay for an extended period and exercise to become more independent and return home. Their built environment can greatly impact patients' recovery and should aid rehabilitation rather than hinder it. Therefore, the design of rehabilitation clinics should provide an environment that enriches the daily life of patients and offers them opportunities for exercising independence and for various activities, with the company or alone. The lack of independent activity resulting from inadequately designed environments can considerably limit the recovery of patients, potentially creating the added costs of healthcare, increased burden on the caregivers, and the need for additional long-term care after rehabilitation. Hence, future designs should start departing from the purely functional "same-for-all" approaches and developing new concepts for rehabilitation clinics that support and enhance stroke patients' recovery.

**Acknowledgments** This work was supported by the Sächsische Aufbaubank and the European Social Fund (Grant Number 100235479) and the Graduate Academy at the Technische Universität Dresden (Completion Grant Number 0051155915).

# References

Adamson, J., Beswick, A., & Ebrahim, S. (2004). Is stroke the most common cause of disability? *Journal of Stroke and Cerebrovascular Diseases, 13*(4), 171–177. https://doi.org/10.1016/j.jstrokecerebrovasdis.2004.06.003

Anåker, A., von Koch, L., Heylighen, A., & Elf, M. (2019). "It's Lonely": Patients' Experiences of the Physical Environment at a Newly Built Stroke Unit. *Health Environments Research and Design Journal, 12*(3), 141–152. https://doi.org/10.1177/1937586718806696

Anåker, A., Von Koch, L., Sjöstrand, C., Bernhardt, J., & Elf, M. (2017). A comparative study of patients' activities and interactions in a stroke unit before and after reconstruction – The significance of the built environment. *PLoS One, 12*(7), 1–12. https://doi.org/10.1371/journal.pone.0177477

Anåker, A., Von Koch, L., Sjöstrand, C., Heylighen, A., & Elf, M. (2018). The physical environment and patients' activities and care. A comparative case study at three newly built stroke units. *Journal of Advanced Nursing*, 1–33. https://doi.org/10.1111/jan.13690

Bernhardt, J., Dewey, H., Thrift, A., & Donnan, G. (2004). Inactive and alone: Physical activity within the first 14 days of acute stroke unit care. *Stroke, 35*(4), 1005–1009. https://doi.org/10.1161/01.STR.0000120727.40792.40

Billinger, S. A., Arena, R., Bernhardt, J., Eng, J. J., Franklin, B. A., Johnson, C. M., Mackay-Lyons, M., Macko, R. F., Mead, G. E., Roth, E. J., Shaughnessy, M., & Tang, A. (2014). Physical activity and exercise recommendations for stroke survivors: A statement for healthcare professionals from the American Heart Association/American Stroke Association. *Stroke, 45*(8), 2532–2553. https://doi.org/10.1161/STR.0000000000000022

Branco, J. P., Oliveira, S., Sargento-Freitas, J., Laíns, J., & Pinheiro, J. (2018). Assessing functional recovery in the first 6 months after acute ischaemic stroke: A prospective, observational study. *European Journal of Physical and Rehabilitation Medicine.* https://doi.org/10.23736/S1973-9087.18.05161-4

Clarke, D. J., & Forster, A. (2015). Improving post-stroke recovery: The role of the multidisciplinary health care team. *Journal of Multidisciplinary Healthcare, 8*, 433–442. https://doi.org/10.2147/JMDH.S68764

Colley, J., Zeeman, H., & Kendall, E. (2018). "Everything happens in the hallways": Exploring user activity in the corridors at two rehabilitation units. *Health Environments Research and Design Journal, 11*(2), 163–176. https://doi.org/10.1177/1937586717733149

Cowdell, F., & Garrett, D. (2003). Recreation in stroke – Rehabilitation part two: Exploring patients' views. *International Journal of Therapy and Rehabilitation, 10*(10).

DIN 18040-1:2010-10, Construction of accessible buildings – Design principles – Part 1: Publicly accessible buildings.

De Wit, L., Putman, K., Dejaeger, E., Baert, I., Berman, P., Bogaerts, K., Brinkmann, N., Connell, L., Feys, H., Jenni, W., Kaske, C., Lesaffre, E., Leys, M., Lincoln, N., Louckx, F., Schuback, B., Schupp, W., Smith, B., & De Weerdt, W. (2005). Use of time by stroke patients: A comparison of four European rehabilitation centers. *Stroke, 36*(9), 1977–1983. https://doi.org/10.1161/01.STR.0000177871.59003.e3

Duncan, F., Lewis, S. J., Greig, C. A., Dennis, M. S., Sharpe, M., MacLullich, A. M. J., & Mead, G. E. (2015). Exploratory longitudinal cohort study of associations of fatigue after stroke. *Stroke, 46*(4), 1052–1058. https://doi.org/10.1161/STROKEAHA.114.008079

Eng, X. W., Brauer, S. G., Kuys, S. S., Lord, M., & Hayward, K. S. (2014). Factors affecting the ability of the stroke survivor to drive their own recovery outside of therapy during inpatient stroke rehabilitation. *Stroke Research and Treatment, 2014.* https://doi.org/10.1155/2014/626538

Feigin, V. L., Forouzanfar, M. H., Krishnamurthi, R., Mensah, G. A., Connor, M., Bennett, D. A., Moran, A. E., Sacco, R. L., Anderson, L., Truelsen, T., O'Donnell, M., Venketasubramanian, N., Barker-Collo, S., Lawes, C. M. M., Wang, W., Shinohara, Y., Witt, E., Ezzati, M., & Naghavi, M. (2014). Global and regional burden of stroke during 1990–2010: Findings from the Global Burden of Disease Study 2010. *The Lancet, 383*(9913), 245–255. https://doi.org/10.1016/S0140-6736(13)61953-4

Feigin, V. L., Norrving, B., & Mensah, G. A. (2017). Global burden of stroke. *Circulation Research, 120*(3), 439–448. https://doi.org/10.1161/CIRCRESAHA.116.308413

Flowers, H. L., Skoretz, S. A., Silver, F. L., Rochon, E., Fang, J., Flamand-Roze, C., & Martino, R. (2016). Poststroke aphasia frequency, recovery, and outcomes: A systematic review and meta-analysis. *Archives of Physical Medicine and Rehabilitation, 97*(12), 2188–2201.e8. https://doi.org/10.1016/j.apmr.2016.03.006

González-Martínez, E., Bangerter, A., Lê Van, K., & Navarro, C. (2016). Hospital staff corridor conversations: Work in passing. *Journal of Advanced Nursing, 72*(3), 521–532. https://doi.org/10.1111/jan.12842

Hempler, I., Woitha, K., Thielhorn, U., & Farin, E. (2018). Post-stroke care after medical rehabilitation in Germany: A systematic literature review of the current provision of stroke patients. *BMC Health Services Research, 18*(1), 1–9. https://doi.org/10.1186/s12913-018-3235-2

Janssen, H., Ada, L., Bernhardt, J., McElduff, P., Pollack, M., Nilsson, M., & Spratt, N. (2014a). Physical, cognitive and social activity levels of stroke patients undergoing rehabilitation within a mixed rehabilitation unit. *Clinical Rehabilitation, 28*(1), 91–101. https://doi. org/10.1177/0269215512466252

Janssen, H., Ada, L., Bernhardt, J., McElduff, P., Pollack, M., Nilsson, M., & Spratt, N. J. (2014b). An enriched environment increases activity in stroke patients undergoing rehabilitation in a mixed rehabilitation unit: A pilot non-randomized controlled trial. *Disability and Rehabilitation, 36*(3), 255–262. https://doi.org/10.3109/09638288.2013.788218

Janssen, H., Ada, L., Middleton, S., Pollack, M., Nilsson, M., Churilov, L., Blennerhassett, J., Faux, S., & New, P. (2021). Altering the rehabilitation environment to improve stroke survivor activity. *A Phase II Trial, 0*(0), 1–9. https://doi.org/10.1177/17474930211006999

Kārkliņa, A., Chen, E., Bērziņa, G., & Stibrant Sunnerhagen, K. (2021). Patients' physical activity in stroke units in Latvia and Sweden. *Brain and Behavior, 11*(5), 1–8. https://doi.org/10.1002/brb3.2110

Keith, R. A. (1980). Activity patterns of a stroke rehabilitation unit. Social Science & Medicine. *Medical Psychology & Medical Sociology, 14A*(6), 575–580. http://www.pubmedcentral.nih. gov/articlerender.fcgi?artid=3760181&tool=pmcentrez&rendertype=abstract

Keith, R. A., & Cowell, K. S. (1987). Time use of stroke patients in three rehabilitation hospitals. *Social Science & Medicine, 24(ENGLAND PT-Journal Article LG-English DC-19870626)*, 529–533.

Kevdzija, M., & Marquardt, G. (2018). Physical barriers to mobility of stroke patients in rehabilitation clinics. *Breaking Down Barriers*, 147–157. https://doi.org/10.1007/978-3-319-75028-6_13

Kevdzija, M., & Marquardt, G. (2021a). Impact of distance on stroke inpatients' mobility in rehabilitation clinics : A shadowing study. *Building Research & Information, 0*(0), 1–15. https://doi.org/10.1080/09613218.2021.2001302

Kevdzija, M., & Marquardt, G. (2021b). Topics in Stroke Rehabilitation Stroke patients' non-scheduled activity during inpatient rehabilitation and its relationship with the architectural layout : A multicenter shadowing study. *Topics in Stroke Rehabilitation, 00*(00), 1–7. https://doi. org/10.1080/10749357.2020.1871281

Kevdzija, M. (2022). "Everything looks the same": wayfinding behaviour and experiences of stroke inpatients in rehabilitation clinics. *International Journal of Qualitative Studies on Health and Well-being 17*(1) 2087273 https://doi.org/10.1080/17482631.2022.2087273

Kim, J., Thayabaranathan, T., Donnan, G. A., Howard, G., Howard, V. J., Rothwell, P. M., Feigin, V., Norrving, B., Owolabi, M., Pandian, J., Liu, L., Cadilhac, D. A., & Thrift, A. G. (2020). Global stroke statistics 2019. *International Journal of Stroke, 15*(8), 819–838. https://doi. org/10.1177/1747493020909545

Knoflach, M., Matosevic, B., Rücker, M., Furtner, M., Mair, A., Wille, G., Zangerle, A., Werner, P., Ferrari, J., Schmidauer, C., Seyfang, L., Kiechl, S., & Willeit, J. (2012). Functional recovery after ischemic stroke – A matter of age: Data from the Austrian Stroke Unit Registry. *Neurology*. https://doi.org/10.1212/WNL.0b013e31824367ab

Kugler, C., Altenhöner, T., Lochner, P., & Ferbert, A. (2003). Does age influence early recovery from ischemic stroke? A study from the Hessian Stroke Data Bank. *Journal of Neurology, 250*(6), 676–681. https://doi.org/10.1007/s00415-003-1054-8

Langhorne, P., Coupar, F., & Pollock, A. (2009). Motor recovery after stroke: A systematic review. *The Lancet Neurology, 8*, 741–754. https://doi.org/10.1016/S1474-4422(09)70150-4

Lee, K. B., Lim, S. H., Kim, K. H., Kim, K. J., Kim, Y. R., Chang, W. N., Yeom, J. W., Kim, Y. D., & Hwang, B. Y. (2015). Six-month functional recovery of stroke patients: A multi-time-point study. *International Journal of Rehabilitation Research, 38*(2), 173–180. https://doi. org/10.1097/MRR.0000000000000108

Luker, J., Lynch, E., Bernhardsson, S., Bennett, L., & Bernhardt, J. (2015). Stroke Survivors' Experiences of Physical Rehabilitation: A Systematic Review of Qualitative Studies. *Archives of Physical Medicine and Rehabilitation, 96*(9), 1698–1708e10. https://doi.org/10.1016/j. apmr.2015.03.017

Lyden, P., Amir, K., & Tidus, I. (2014). Cerebrovascular diseases in geriatrics. In A. K. Nair & M. N. Sabbagh (Eds.), *Geriatric neurology* (pp. 302–312). Wiley Blackwell. https://doi.org/10.1002/9781118730676.ch11

MacIntosh, B. J., Edwards, J. D., Kang, M., Cogo-Moreira, H., Chen, J. L., Mochizuki, G., Herrmann, N., & Swardfager, W. (2017). Post-stroke fatigue and depressive symptoms are differentially related to mobility and cognitive performance. *Frontiers in Aging Neuroscience, 9*(OCT), 1–7. https://doi.org/10.3389/fnagi.2017.00343

Mansfield, A., Wong, J. S., Bryce, J., Brunton, K., Inness, E. L., Knorr, S., Jones, S., Taati, B., & McIlroy, W. E. (2015). Use of accelerometer-based feedback of walking activity for appraising progress with walking-related goals in inpatient stroke rehabilitation: A randomized controlled trial. *Neurorehabilitation and Neural Repair, 29*(9), 847–857. https://doi.org/10.1177/1545968314567968

Marcheschi, E., Von Koch, L., Pessah-Rasmussen, H., & Elf, M. (2017). *Home setting after stroke, facilitators and barriers: A systematic literature review* (pp. 1–9). Health & Social Care in the Community. https://doi.org/10.1111/hsc.12518

Mcdonald, S. (2005). Studying actions in context: A qualitative shadowing method for organizational research. *Qualitative Research, 5*(4), 455–473.

Nordin, S., Swall, A., Anåker, A., Von Koch, L., Elf, M., Nordin, S., Swall, A., Anåker, A., Von Koch, L., Elf, M., Nordin, S., Swall, A., & Anåker, A. (2021). Does the physical environment matter ? – A qualitative study of healthcare professionals' experiences of newly built stroke units professionals' experiences of newly built stroke units. *International Journal of Qualitative Studies on Health and Well-Being, 16*(1). https://doi.org/10.1080/17482631.2021.1917880

Norrving, B., & Kissela, B. (2013). The global burden of stroke and need for a continuum of care. *Neurology, 80*(3 SUPPL.2), 5–12. https://doi.org/10.1212/wnl.0b013e3182762397

Quinlan, E. (2008). Conspicuous invisibility: Shadowing as a data collection strategy. *Qualitative Inquiry, 14*(8), 1480–1499. https://doi.org/10.1177/1077800408318318

Robinson, C. A., Noritake Matsuda, P., Ciol, M. A., Shumway-Cook, A., Matsuda, P. N., Ciol, M. A., Shumway-Cook, A., Noritake Matsuda, P., Ciol, M. A., & Shumway-Cook, A. (2013). Participation in community walking following stroke: The influence of self-perceived environmental barriers. *Physical Therapy, 93*(5), 620–627. https://doi.org/10.2522/ptj.20110217

Rosbergen, I. C., Grimley, R. S., Hayward, K. S., Walker, K. C., Rowley, D., Campbell, A. M., McGufficke, S., Robertson, S. T., Trinder, J., Janssen, H., & Brauer, S. G. (2017). Embedding an enriched environment in an acute stroke unit increases activity in people with stroke: A controlled before–after pilot study. *Clinical Rehabilitation, 31*(11), 1516–1528. https://doi.org/10.1177/0269215517705181

Rowe, F., Brand, D., Jackson, C. A., Price, A., Walker, L., Harrison, S., Eccleston, C., Scott, C., Akerman, N., Dodridge, C., Howard, C., Shipman, T., Sperring, U., Macdiarmid, S., & Freeman, C. (2009). Visual impairment following stroke: Do stroke patients require vision assessment? *Age and Ageing, 38*(2), 188–193. https://doi.org/10.1093/ageing/afn230

Stevens, E., Emmett, E., Wang, Y., McKevitt, C., & Wolfe, C. (2017). The burden of stroke in Europe: The challenge for policy makers. In *The Burden of Stroke in Europe: The challenge for policy makers*. Stroke Alliance for Europe.

Tatemichi, T. K., Desmond, D. W., Stern, Y., Paik, M., Sano, M., & Bagiella, E. (1994). Cognitive impairment after stroke: Frequency, patterns, and relationship to functional abilities. *Journal of Neurology, Neurosurgery & Psychiatry, 57*(2), 202–207.

Van De Port, I. G. L., Kwakkel, G., Schepers, V. P. M., & Lindeman, E. (2006). Predicting mobility outcome one year after stroke: A prospective cohort study. *Journal of Rehabilitation Medicine, 38*(4), 218–223. https://doi.org/10.1080/16501970600582930

Ween, J. E., Alexander, M. P., D'Esposito, M., & Roberts, M. (1996). Factors predictive of stroke outcome in a rehabilitation setting. *Neurology, 47*(May 1994), 388–392. https://doi.org/10.1212/WNL.47.2.388

# Exploring the Role of the Built Environment in Person-Centered Care During Mealtimes in an Ethno-specific Long-Term Care Home

**Shreemouna Gurung and Habib Chaudhury**

## 1 Ethnic Minority Aging Population and Long-Term Care

According to the 2016 census in Canada, older immigrants consisted of 31% of the total older adult population aged 65 and over (Statistics Canada, 2019); among the total population in Canada, more than 22% represented visible minorities (Statistics Canada, 2017). Visible minorities are defined by the Employment Equity Act as "persons, other than Aboriginal peoples, who are non-Caucasian in race or non-white in colour" (Statistics Canada, 2020, para. 1). The change in Canada's immigration policy since the 1960s and the rapid globalization of international migration have led to increased foreign-born populations from Asia, Africa, and the Middle East, thereby making Canada a multicultural nation with diverse ethnocultural populations (Statistics Canada, 2018). Individuals whose culture, race, ethnicity, or religion differ from the Caucasian population are referred to as ethnocultural minorities, often also known as ethnic minority and ethnically diverse groups (Statistics Canada, 2018). In the province of British Columbia (BC), 20% of the population aged 65 and over are visible minorities; among this group, Chinese-Canadians were the most prevalent (9%) visible minority (Statistics Canada, 2016).

In the forthcoming years, the population of older immigrants and aging visible minorities is expected to grow. As a result, there is an increased recognition of the need to provide culturally responsive care and support services, such as long-term care (LTC) for ethnocultural minority older adults. The term *LTC* refers to wide-ranging services that include personal, social, and medical care for people with physical and/or cognitive disabilities for a short or long period of time (Barrass, 2012; Koehn et al., 2018; Mold et al., 2005). The provision of LTC services can occur in various settings (e.g., community centers, nursing homes, and institutional

S. Gurung (✉) · H. Chaudhury
Department of Gerontology, Simon Fraser University, Vancouver, BC, Canada
e-mail: Shreemouna_gurung@sfu.ca; chaudhury@sfu.ca

© The Author(s), under exclusive license to Springer Nature Switzerland AG 2023
F. Ferdous, E. Roberts (eds.), *(Re)designing the Continuum of Care for Older Adults*, https://doi.org/10.1007/978-3-031-20970-3_8

145

care homes) and is often catered to older adults who require care and assistance with activities of daily living (ADLs), such as eating, medication intake, bathing, and dressing (Banerjee, 2007; Brotman, 2002). In BC, the average age of older adults living in LTC is 84 years old, with 31% requiring full assistance with ADLs from care staff (Office of the Seniors Advocate, 2021).

Older adults in ethnically diverse communities have traditionally relied on family members and generally avoided relocation to care homes. However, the combination of labor demands (Wright & Mindel, 1993), ever-shifting cultural values (Chappell, 2003; Lee & Mjelde-Mossey, 2004), and lifestyle changes in general have deterred family members from undertaking the primary caregiver role (Barrass, 2012; Ujimoto, 1995). This has required more ethnic minority individuals and families to rely on LTC settings that are not always tailored to addressing their diverse and unique needs. Empirical literature on ethnically diverse older adults' needs in such care settings, however, has been limited in Canada. Lack of emphasis on ethno-specific care can be ascribed to wide-ranging factors, such as false notions about the care needs of ethnic groups (e.g., assumptions that ethnic older adults rely on family and, as a result, do not require LTC) (Barrass, 2012; Brotman, 2003). Other factors include challenges of conducting ethnicity-related research (e.g., utilization of appropriate methods to avoid homogenizing ethnic groups and their experiences) (Torres, 2015) and diverse cultural preferences on the care delivery to different ethnic minority population groups (Brotman, 2003).

The rapid growth of ethnic minority aging population in Canada with care needs warrants an examination of their experiences and challenges in LTC homes. Literature on ethnocultural minority older adults in broader terms has largely focused on social determinants of health, access to healthcare (Brotman, 2002), and the challenges experienced by family and informal caregivers (Barrass, 2012; Brotman, 2002; Deri, 2005). Additionally, the decision-making in aging in place in the community versus care homes (Kaida et al., 2009), implications of cultural values and norms on older immigrants' living arrangements, and adjustment to new care settings have been explored in various research studies (Barrass, 2012; Brotman, 2003). A particular area of interest is the quality of life (QoL) and models of care provided to ethnic minority older adults in LTC homes. Person-centered care (PCC) has been widely recognized to increase the QoL of older adults living in care homes (Li & Porock, 2014); this care approach is described in the following section.

## 1.1 Built Environment and Person-Centered Care During Mealtimes

Person-centered care is increasingly used as a guiding approach to enhance the delivery of health and social services globally. The philosophical underpinning of person-centeredness follows a holistic approach to care that integrates the diverse aspects of well-being by primarily placing people at the center (McCormack &

McCance, 2010; Santana et al., 2017). Person-centered model takes the perspectives of individuals into consideration while viewing them as equal partners in establishing and facilitating care that responds to their needs and preferences (Brownie & Nancarrow, 2013; Kitwood & Bredin, 1992; McCormack & McCance, 2006). This approach recognizes the unique values and beliefs of individuals, along with fostering care that promotes respect, dignity, and autonomy (Cingel et al., 2016; McCormack & McCance, 2006). PCC encompasses a healthful collaboration between individuals, their relatives, and care professionals to achieve the best care practices and outcomes (Kitwood & Bredin, 1992; McCormack & McCance, 2010).

As a fundamental concept that challenges the traditional biomedical framework, PCC models adopt a humanistic and holistic approach to provide more responsive quality of care for older adults (Kitwood & Bredin, 1992; Li & Porock, 2014). Some of the key components of PCC include promoting choice and independence, respecting the individual, understanding the importance of personhood, fostering interpersonal relationships, and delivering supportive organizational and physical settings (Kitwood & Bredin, 1992; McGilton et al., 2012). Responsive built environments of care settings have been shown to significantly impact the facilitation of PCC, particularly in supporting and enhancing positive experiences for the residents (e.g., increased autonomy and independence) and reducing adverse behaviors (e.g., social withdrawals and spatial disorientation) among older adults living in LTC homes (Chaudhury et al., 2018; Geboy, 2009; Hung & Chaudhury, 2011). The built environmental features of the dining room are commonly viewed as an important factor in contributing to the quality of the residents' mealtime experiences, which is shaped by their personal preferences, habits, and life history (Chaudhury et al., 2013; Geboy, 2009). In addition to the nutrient intake, mealtimes are often linked to social, cultural, and psychological aspects that can promote and meet the unique preferences and needs of older residents in care homes (Chaudhury et al., 2013). Hence, appropriate built environmental features of dining spaces are considered an integral component of implementing PCC approaches in care homes.

The existing empirical research on the role of the built environment for mealtimes suggests that dining features such as small, intimate, and homelike atmosphere created opportunities for increased social interactions, personalized care, and sense of belonging, which can lead to optimal mealtime experiences for both residents and staff in LTC settings (Chaudhury et al., 2013; Hung & Chaudhury, 2011; Van Hoof et al., 2010). Having appropriate lighting (e.g., minimum level of ambient light), contrasting color (e.g., for tabletops and dishware), sensory cues (e.g., smell of cooking and presence of signage), and accessibility (e.g., accessible pathways to and within dining spaces) lead to increased functional ability, orientation, and feelings of safety and security during mealtimes (Chaudhury et al., 2013; Nolan & Mathews, 2004; Passini et al., 2000). Further, minimizing institutional features using family-style foodservice, personal and homelike décor, and smaller and intimate dining rooms provided optimal sensory stimulation, familiarity, privacy, and higher level of social interactions, all of which enhanced quality of care and QoL of older residents in care homes (Chaudhury et al., 2013; Roberts, 2011).

## 2   Objectives

The increase in ethnically diverse older adult population in care homes, as well as the concerns with the quality of care practices, necessitates an in-depth examination of the role of the built environment on the provision of PCC for minority older adults in LTC settings. This chapter explores how the built environment influences mealtime care practices in an ethno-specific care home that promotes PCC. Using the integrative conceptual framework of person-environment (P-E) exchange by Chaudhury and Oswald (2019), the findings from this chapter are contextualized to understand the role of the built environment on the mealtime processes and outcomes for ethnically diverse residents.

## 3   Theoretical Context

The integrative conceptual framework of P-E exchange by Chaudhury and Oswald (2019) present an exhaustive and integrative conceptual understanding of P-E exchange occurring in the latter part of an individual's life by addressing two emerging issues. The first being the urgency to link current theoretical understanding founded on the wide-ranging idea of ecology of aging with a more explicit reporting on the role of the physical or built environment as a tangible and definite reality and the second being the need for concrete integration of the cognitive-affective-behavioral aspects to the conceptual understanding of P-E exchange process that indicate the primary reason for any interchange, such as independent functioning, social interaction, and mobility (Chaudhury & Oswald, 2019). By addressing the two aforementioned points, Chaudhury and Oswald's (2019) framework aims to incorporate discounted aspects of the physical environment (e.g., land use, neighborhood, interior design) and contextualize the theoretical understanding of P-E interchange process in daily living and lifestyle behaviors for improved applicability to empirical research.

The conceptual framework by Chaudhury and Oswald (2019) consists of three interconnected segments, referred to as (1) components of P-E interaction, (2) P-E processes, and (3) environment-related outcomes. The first segment, P-E interaction, characterizes four distinct components that interact with one another at a basic level; they are identified as *individual characteristics, social factors, physical/built environment*, and *technological systems*. In the context of mealtimes, these would include the residents' functional capacity (physical and cognitive), staff care and support interactions, characteristics of the built environment of the dining room, and any technological systems to support dining experience. The second segment, P-E process, points to the interaction between *agency* and *belonging*. In this framework, the specific dimensions of P-E interaction that transpire from the preceding segment are addressed to better comprehend agency-belonging (A-B) dynamics. Residents' *agency* during mealtimes can be manifested in their autonomy in independent or assisted dining, choice of food, seating option, etc., whereas their *belonging* in mealtimes can be represented by homelike and familiar dining space, familiar food, and meaningful social connections, among others. These dimensions of environmental exchange are rooted in the functions or goals of an interaction, such as pleasurable mealtime experience, mobility, independent functioning, and social interaction. The third segment, environment-related outcomes, is recognized with the extensive notions of *identity* and *autonomy* as interdependent binary outcomes, without neglecting other prospective outcomes such as well-being or social participation. This framework offers conceptualization and understanding of the P-E interaction, processes, and outcomes of ethnic minority older adults living in care homes. More specifically, the built environmental component in the framework has significant influence on the way broader P-E interactions transpire in a given care setting.

## 4    Ethnographic Observations

The findings presented in this chapter are based on non-participant ethnographic observations conducted in an ethno-specific care home in metro Vancouver, Canada. Ethnography in broader terms involves the use of in-depth observation of groups and individuals and encapsulates how social interactions are influenced by their cultural and historical contexts (Hammersley & Atkinson, 2007; Jones & Smith, 2017). This approach provides researchers with the perspectives of those under study when viewing social events and activities that are entrenched within a socially organized domain (Jones & Smith, 2017; Nixon & Odoyo, 2020). Since ethnography entails the process of engaging in the real-world context and comprehensive analysis, it allows researchers to explore and explain the complexities and shared cultural understandings of the social world, along with construing the meaning of the concerned phenomenon (Hammersley & Atkinson, 2007; Jones & Smith, 2017). Non-participant observation, in particular, offers researchers the opportunity to immerse in a culture and observe, learn, and interpret reality without actively interacting or participating in the study setting (Hammersley & Atkinson, 2007; Jones & Smith, 2017; Nixon & Odoyo, 2020).

Ethnographic observations provide an effective means to examine the care practices and experiences of those involved in LTC settings while accounting for structural and sociopolitical contexts that contribute to the production of inequalities (Baumbusch, 2011). LTC settings consist of residents and workers from diverse backgrounds; they also include collaborative dynamics among all involved parties, which are profoundly influenced by the interplay between individual, organizational, social, and physical contexts (Baumbusch, 2011). Ethnography enables the researcher to fully immerse in LTC cultures, policies, and procedures and engage with residents, family members, staff, and administrators in their everyday environments (Baumbusch, 2011; Hammersley & Atkinson, 2007; Jones & Smith, 2017). Through ethnography, the practical incongruency, interpersonal conflicts, and organizational issues that exist in LTC settings are brought to light and examined to improve the overall care practices (Baumbusch, 2011; Cudmore & Sondermeyer, 2007).

## 4.1 Setting and Sample

The selected ethno-specific LTC home is a nonprofit organization in Vancouver, specializing in delivering culturally oriented LTC services for Chinese older adults since the early 1980s. As an ethno-specific LTC home, this organization strives to provide the highest quality of individualized and professional care by fostering a homelike environment that promotes dignified and respectful care for older residents. This care home was selected as the observation site because it offers LTC services that not only cater to the needs of Chinese-Canadian older adults but also aims to deliver PCC. Almost all (99%) of the residents in the selected care home are ethnically Chinese, and just over half (50–60%) of the residents live with dementia. In total, the care home consists of 134 number of beds, housing 103 women and 30 men who range from 63 to 105 years in age. The professional healthcare team included ethnically Chinese registered nurses, licensed practical nurses, and registered care aides who worked closely with residents' physicians, occupational and physical therapists, and other healthcare providers. The executive director of the care home acted as a gatekeeper, informing the staff members about the study details and enabling the researcher to access the study site during mealtimes for ethnographic observations.

## 4.2 Data Collection and Analysis

Table 1 provides the observation schedule; approximately 9 h of ethnographic observations were conducted during lunch and dinner by the first author over the course of four visits in the month of October 2019. Observations during breakfast were omitted due to conflicts with accessing the LTC building at early hours. The approximate 9 h of observation captured variations in the type, frequency, and quality of interactions that occurred during mealtimes. Several aspects were observed and recorded by the researcher, beginning with the physical environmental features of the dining area, followed by observing the residents and staff members' behaviors and interactions and the events and activities that unfolded during mealtimes. The nuanced details, including the informal and impromptu engagements and activities, prevalence and length of events, as well as other relevant factors (e.g., nonverbal cues), were recorded to allow for a comprehensive observation of the social phenomenon of dining (Merriam, 1988). Following each mealtime observation,

**Table 1** Observation schedule

| Observation visits | 1 | 2 | 3 | 4 |
|---|---|---|---|---|
| Meal type | Lunch | Dinner | Lunch | Dinner |
| Time | 11:00 am–1:00 pm | 4:00–6:30 pm | 10:30 am–1:00 pm | 4:00–6:30 pm |
| Date | 10/18/2019 | 10/18/2019 | 10/19/2019 | 10/19/2019 |

additional contextual issues and reflections were recorded by the researcher to meaningfully capture the mealtime experiences of LTC residents.

Data collected from the ethnographic observations were analyzed using thematic analysis. According to Braun and Clarke (2008), thematic analysis enables the researcher to establish, analyze, and describe patterns within the data (p. 79). The process of thematic analysis as outlined by Braun and Clarke (2008) consists of familiarizing with the data, open coding, seeking patterns and themes, and reviewing and naming themes. For this study, field notes were recorded and reviewed by the first author, providing familiarity with the data. Using NVivo, a qualitative analysis software (Zamawe, 2015), field notes were open coded; subsequently, open codes were collated into categories to identify preliminary themes. The first draft of the potential themes was reviewed by the second author to validate and confirm the emerging findings. The themes were revised, defined, and named to accurately reflect the open codes and the overall data set.

# 5  Findings

The five emerging themes from the mealtime observations provide insight into how built environment of the dining room influences the mealtime experiences of residents and staff, key factors that play a role in shaping the experience of residents and staff during mealtimes, and how features of the mealtimes align with PCC practices. These five emerging themes are (1) space as the stage for mealtime, (2) mealtime routine as a primer for dining experience, (3) teamwork for institutional efficiency, (4) varied assistance, and (5) the lost meaning in interaction.

## 5.1  Space as the Stage for Mealtime

The dining space and its surrounding area in the observed ethno-specific care home were institutional in character – a large hall with multiple pillars, a television room, a kitchen, and two washrooms (see Fig. 1 for layout). Although the open plan of the space and the glass windows between the television and dining room supported the care staff in monitoring and supervising the residents, the large scale of the space created an unfamiliar and institutional setting for new residents or residents with cognitive disabilities. Devoid of any natural lighting, the dining space was illuminated by florescent light and, when combined with dull wall colors, created a somber atmosphere during mealtimes. The lack of cultural (e.g., color and symbols reflective of Chinese traditions) and homelike décor (e.g., personalized furniture, household objects, wall art) and the use of trays for food serving were unsupportive in creating a familiar environment and a sense of belonging for older residents. The wide hallways and ramps, along with the absence of stairs, doors, and uncarpeted floors, however, supported optimal mobility, particularly for residents who relied

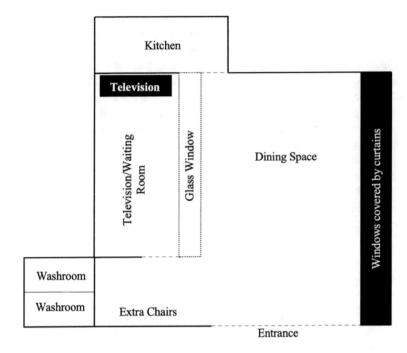

**Fig. 1** Layout of the dining space

heavily on assistive devices (e.g., canes, walkers, wheelchairs). The shape and the size of the table (e.g., round and accommodating height) enabled residents to safely navigate around the dining room and facilitated the use of wheelchairs and chair arms under the table. Other positive environmental features included placeholders in the dining tables with residents' name, photo, and dietary information which was described to help "staff members identify the meal choices and dietary restrictions while [also] helping residents identify their seating" (care staff).

Further, the adjacent television room functioned positively in providing an opportunity for residents to wait while maintaining visual contact with the dining room and other residents. The television room being separated, yet visually linked with the dining room, as well as the display of Chinese shows on the television facilitated a sense of belonging to the mealtime activity without being affected by the full spectrum of stimulation in the dining space itself. Several care aides and nurses traversed in and out of the television and dining room during the mealtime, contributing to an institutional social atmosphere. The physical attributes of the dining room, along with the presence of staff members, set the stage for mealtime routines and care practices.

## 5.2   Mealtime Routines as a Primer for Dining Experience

Mealtime routines at the observed ethno-specific care home can be categorized by the following three segments: pre-meal, during the meal, and post-meal. The pre-meal routines consisted of kitchen staff preparing meals based on the care home's designated menu, accounting for residents' nutrition and dietary restrictions. Kitchen staff worked together to set up the dining tables, while care aides prepared residents by rallying them into the television room and assisting with clothing protectors. The routines during the meal comprised of food servings (e.g., appetizers, entrees, and desserts) by kitchen staff and care aides assisting residents with food intake. The post-meal routines included nurses supervising residents with medication intake, care aides directing and assisting residents out of the dining space, and kitchen staff sanitizing and clearing the dining hall.

The meal options available for residents extended beyond the cultural food preference of Chinese older adults as one care staff praised, "the menu is so good, it's almost like a restaurant. It also has a lot of nutritious value for the residents…." The meal selections adhered to the residents' dietary needs and depended on the available menu options for the day. On Saturdays, for example, the lunch menu comprised of dried bean curd soup as appetizer; braised pork or steamed pork slices served with rice, congee (i.e., rice porridge), or bread as entrées; and fresh fruits as dessert. Alternative meal options were also available according to individual needs of the residents (e.g., vegetarian and liquid diet).

A notable mention related to the mealtime routine was the timing and number of sittings for lunch and dinner. Mealtimes included two back-to-back sittings due to the dining hall's lack of capacity to hold more than 76 residents at a time. Consequently, lunch time for the first sitting was scheduled at 11:20 a.m., followed by the second sitting at 12:25 p.m. Similarly, dinner for the first group was set at 4:30 p.m., and the second group at 5:30 p.m. This directly impacted the duration of mealtimes, which lasted between 45 and 60 min each for both first and second sittings. Staff members also followed a rigid schedule to prevent delays with meal servings. Another key feature of the mealtime routine was the seating arrangements for the residents, which was based on the level of care needs and interactions. Residents who were capable of functioning independently and with partial care needs were seated in or around the same tables, while residents with high level of care needs were seated together. Since the dining tables could only seat up to four people, the grouping of residents was sometimes challenging and did not provide flexibility in seating arrangements. Overall, these mealtime routines observed at the LTC home served as a primer for residents and staff members' dining experience.

## 5.3   Teamwork for Institutional Efficiency

The facilitation of mealtimes at the ethno-specific care home involved a dynamic collaboration among kitchen staff, care aides, and nurses as part of and guided by an institutional efficiency approach. The care home staff shared similar ethnic backgrounds and languages (e.g., Cantonese and Mandarin) as the residents. Kitchen staff members were distinguishable by their green apron and white hairnets and played an integral part in the process of dining set up and meal preparation, which included understanding the meal preferences and dietary constraints of the residents. In order to avoid mishaps with dietary restrictions, kitchen staff used trolley carts to organize meals according to the seating arrangements. During each sitting, only three kitchen staff worked together to distribute beverages, appetizers, entrées, and desserts to approximately 60 residents at once. Following the first sitting, kitchen staff worked quickly to sanitize and prepare the dining tables for the second sitting.

Both care aides and nurses played a significant role in assisting the residents, as well as facilitating the overall mealtime routines. A care staff stated, "nurses are present if care is required and if medicine needs to be allocated to residents before and after lunch." Residents who required a partial or high level of care were closely supervised by nurses and care aides, providing one-on-one care throughout the mealtime. Nurses also assisted beyond the meal and medication consumptions; for example, when a resident appeared to be in distress and refused to consume their meal even after efforts were made by several care aides, nurses acted as the last point of resort. Similar to kitchen staff, care aides and nurses were identifiable by their uniform (e.g., care aides with flower patterned scrubs and nurses with neutral-colored scrubs).

Although kitchen staff, care aides, and nurses were assigned with distinct roles and responsibilities during mealtimes, facilitating mealtimes appeared to be a team effort. For instance, care aides and nurses regularly assisted kitchen staff with preparing, sanitizing, and clearing dining tables. Thus, mealtime outcomes were not a product of separate functions, but rather resulted from collaborations between kitchen staff, care aides, and nurses.

## 5.4   Varied Assistance

Three levels of care interaction or assistance, in particular, were observed between the residents and staff, based on the residents' varied physical and/or cognitive functioning levels: residents without care needs, with partial care needs, and with high level of care needs. Residents without care needs functioned independently; for example, they did not require prompts, cues, or help from care staff to wait in the television room, wear a clothing protector, and transfer in and out of the dining hall. There was minimal contact between the staff members and residents without care needs as they appeared to be self-sufficient with regard to the mealtime routine and engagement. The mealtime support and assistance from care aides for residents with partial care needs varied from day to day and depended on factors, such as residents' mood and fatigue levels. A care staff during mealtime explained, "we encourage residents to be as independent as possible...whatever they can do, we allow them to do...sometimes the residents feed themselves until they are tired or not capable and then a staff will step in to help them with the rest of the meal." This seems to indicate that efforts were made by care staff to promote and foster independence and autonomy of residents during mealtimes. For residents with high level of care needs – often those with physical and/or cognitive disability – care aides and nurses provided one-on-one care (e.g., emotional, social, and physical support) for the entirety of their mealtimes. Despite the differing levels of care needs, residents were dispersed in both first and second sittings which contributed to the individual and group experiences during mealtimes.

## 5.5   The Lost Meaning in Interaction

The nature and level of social interactions that occurred among the residents and between residents and staff were influenced by the level of care needs. Residents with high level of care needs were seated individually and away from the group tables. For these residents, meal and medication consumptions took precedence over meaningful social interactions. On the contrary, residents without and with partial care needs were grouped and seated together, which created opportunities for social engagements. The provision of support by care aides also prompted casual conversations with some of the residents. However, conversations between the staff and residents seemed to be functionally oriented and predominantly about meal intake. The social interaction between most of the residents and staff members were, for the most part, limited as they were more focused on residents with partial or high care needs. In instances where residents' relatives were present during mealtimes, social interactions appeared to remain low as visiting family and friends often belonged to residents with partial or high care needs who exhibited responsive behaviors. The institutional or systemic need for efficiency and a biomedical orientation loomed large in the social atmosphere.

The institutional physical environment of the dining space, in conjunction with the rigid mealtime schedule, also added to the lack of social interaction between residents and staff. The limited capacity of the dining hall, resulting in two successive sittings, incited care staff to primarily focus on facilitating efficient mealtimes. This resulted in residents to experience mealtime as a routinized and mechanical process rather than a social experience including conversations and interactions. Further, the large institutional and impersonal dining room did not encourage residents to linger and have a social time and instead gave a "psychological push" to leave the space and seek out private spaces with reduced level of environmental stimulation.

# 6  Discussion and Conclusion

Mealtimes in care homes serve as an important context to reinforce person-centered practices where residents' autonomy, preferences, biography, and interpersonal relations between staff and residents are respected. In order for mealtimes to be person-centered, it is essential for the care environment to embrace person-centered vision, planning, and interactions. The care environment consists of social, organizational, and physical contextual factors that impact the overall mealtime experience of the residents. While staff training and organizational policies are vital, the role of the built environment in the implementation of good quality care and interaction need to be better recognized. The relationship between the resident and staff members, along with the resident's characteristics, are also fundamental in facilitating PCC during mealtimes. The findings from the observations direct our attention to how the built environmental features of the dining space, mealtime routines, collaboration among staff members, levels of care needs, and the lack of social interactions influence the mealtime experiences of ethno-specific LTC residents and staff members.

Using Chaudhury and Oswald's (2019) integrative conceptual framework of P-E exchange, the findings from the ethnographic observations can be extricated to understand the influence of the built environment on the mealtime experiences of Chinese-Canadian residents and care staff. The findings of the observation point to the dynamic and complex interaction between the individual characteristics, such as residents' level of care needs, sociocultural background, and Chinese-Canadian ethnicity, as well as the social factors and physical/built environment, which contribute to the process of care practices and outcomes during mealtimes. Despite shared languages and ethnicity among residents and staff members, along with the presence of family and relatives, social interactions during dining hours were limited as a result of socio-organizational factors, such as the prioritization of food and medication intake, inflexible mealtime routine and schedule, and the various levels of care needs. These socio-organizational factors and the overall mealtime experience are influenced by the built environment of the dining hall. The implications of the built environment are also reflected in the observed mealtime ambiance and routines. For example, the fluorescent lighting, dark curtains, absence of natural light, lack of cultural and homelike décor, and prearranged seating created an institutionalized atmosphere. Limited capacity to hold residents in the dining hall resulted in a rigid schedule for the first and second sittings, which further added to the institutional feel and generated challenges with mealtime routines and care practices.

The infinite possibility and variability of individual, social, and physical components indicate a multifaceted and complex interaction process that influences LTC residents' behavior and experience during mealtimes. This chapter primarily focuses on the built environment, finding that aspects of the dining space, such as lighting, layout, and size, are critical in optimizing residents' agency and belonging as outlined in Chaudhury and Oswald's (2019) framework. The high level of sensory stimulation observed from the group size of the residents, noise, and lighting may have necessitated residents with dementia and other cognitive disabilities to heavily depend on the care staff for functioning and mobility. Residents with dementia were also likely to be more distracted and anxious by the high level of environmental stimulation in the dining room, resulting in social withdrawals and social anxiety and impacting their ability to participate in meaningful interactions. The lack of freedom for residents to decide where to sit and when to eat, along with the P-E interaction, may have further minimized their agency. However, having the option to choose from a menu that aligns with the meal preference of Chinese residents may have provided them with a sense of agency, as well as belonging. The shared languages, ethnicity, and cultural values among residents and care staff may have increased residents' feeling of belonging during mealtimes. Despite these shared characteristics, the dominance of institutional practices and lack of meaningful social interaction between staff and residents persisted, reflecting traditional LTC philosophy, policies and practices, and the traditional institutional nature of the built environment of the dining room.

By using Chaudhury and Oswald's (2019) framework, the residents' agency and belonging dynamics are examined through disentangling the individual, social, and, more specifically, physical component of the P-E exchange. The integrative conceptual framework of P-E exchange further underlines the need to consider both the objective and the subjective perspective of P-E interaction to have a holistic understanding (Chaudhury & Oswald, 2019). Future studies should aim to capture the ethno-specific LTC residents' subjective perception of these components of P-E interaction. The application of Chaudhury and Oswald's (2019) framework also makes it explicit that shared individual characteristics between residents and staff alone are not sufficient and rather involves the dynamic and synergistic interactions among social, organizational, and physical environment to create a person-centered mealtime experience. Future research should collectively consider the individual, social, organizational, and built environment of an ethno-specific LTC home. Further, the benefits and challenges of implementing person-centered approach during mealtimes should be explored. For instance, the undifferentiated open dining space was unhelpful to provide levels of physical separation among residents with differing physical and/or cognitive capacities. A person-centered approach would be supported by partitions or screens to subdivide the large dining space to provide visual and auditory separation among the groups and reduce the unwarranted environmental stimulation.

Finally, this chapter points to the built features that are foundational in optimizing as well as creating positive and person-centered mealtime experiences for Chinese older residents. Different table sizes (i.e., tables for two, four, six, or even eight people), for example, could provide both functional efficiency from the staffs' perspective and more homelike and variable choices for the residents. Perspectives from residents and their relatives, along with care professionals, are essential in providing a comprehensive picture of how the LTC built environment influences the way PCC is practiced and fostered in contexts beyond mealtimes. There remains an opportunity to understand PCC from the lived experience of ethnically diverse older adults, family members, and care providers using qualitative inquiries (e.g., photovoice, semi-structured interviews, art-based methods), specifically exploring the role of the physical environment on residents' functioning and well-being. Participatory methods for design solutions, such as co-design with residents and staff, can be effective in identifying meaningful and effective interventions, ensuring buy-in from staff and administration. As the provision of PCC necessitates collaborative and healthful relations among all parties involved in the care process, capturing the experiences of families and staff becomes critical to understand and develop effective implementation of PCC for ethnically diverse older adults in LTC settings.

**Acknowledgments** A very special thanks to the residents and care staff at the observed ethno-specific LTC home for welcoming me to be part of their mealtime experience.

# References

Banerjee, A. (2007). *An overview of Ontario long-term care in Canada and selected provinces and territories.* Women and Health Care Reform https://www.researchgate.net/publication/284652528_Long-term_care_in_Canada_An_overview

Barrass, S. (2012). *An ecological model for culturally sensitive care for older immigrants: Best practices and lessons learned from ethno-specific long-term care.* [Unpublished Major Research Paper]. Ryerson University.

Baumbusch, J. L. (2011). Conducting critical ethnography in long-term residential care: Experiences of a novice researcher in the field. *Journal of Advanced Nursing, 67*(1), 184–192. https://doi.org/10.1111/j.1365-2648.2010.05413.x

Braun, V., & Clarke, V. (2008). Using thematic analysis in psychology. *Qualitative Research in Psychology, 3*(2), 77–101. https://doi.org/10.1191/1478088706qp063oa

Brotman, S. (2002). The primacy of family in elder care discourse: Home care services to older ethnic women in Canada. *Journal of Gerontological Social Work, 38*(3), 19–52. https://doi.org/10.1300/J083v38n03_03

Brotman, S. (2003). The limits of multiculturalism in elder care services. *Journal of Aging Studies, 17*(2), 209–229. https://doi.org/10.1016/S0890-4065(03)00003-3

Brownie, S., & Nancarrow, S. (2013). Effects of person-centred care on residents and staff in aged-cared facilities: A systematic review. *Clinical Interventions in Aging, 8,* 1–10. https://doi.org/10.2147/CIA.S38589

Chappell, N. L. (2003). Correcting cross-cultural stereotypes: Aging in Shanghai and Canada. *Journal of Cross-Cultural Gerontology, 18*(2), 127–147. https://doi.org/10.1023/a:1025156501588

Chaudhury, H., & Oswald, F. (2019). Advancing understanding of person-environment interaction in later life: One step further. *Journal of Aging Studies, 51,* 1–9. https://doi.org/10.1016/j.jaging.2019.100821

Chaudhury, H., Hung, L., & Badger, M. (2013). The role of physical environment in supporting person-centered dining in long-term care: A review of the literature. *American Journal of Alzheimer's Disease and Other Dementias, 28*(5), 491–500. https://doi.org/10.1177/1533317513488923

Chaudhury, H., Cooke, H., Cowie, H., & Razaghi, L. (2018). The influence of the physical environment on residents with dementia in long-term care settings: A review of the empirical literature. *The Gerontologist, 58*(5), e325–e337. https://doi.org/10.1093/geront/gnw259

Cingel, M. V. D., Brandsma, L., Dam, M. V., Dorst, M. V., Verkaart, C., & Velde, C. V. D. (2016). Concepts of person-centered care: A framework analysis of five studies in daily care practices. *International Practice Development Journal, 6*(1), 1–17. https://doi.org/10.19043/ipdj.62.006

Cudmore, H., & Sondermeyer, J. (2007). Through the looking glass: Being a critical ethnographic researcher in a familiar nursing context. *Nurse Researcher, 14*(3), 25–35. https://doi.org/10.7748/nr2007.04.14.3.25.c6030

Deri, C. (2005). Social networks and health service utilization. *Journal of Health Economics, 24*(6), 1076–1107. https://doi.org/10.1016/j.jhealeco.2005.03.008

Geboy, L. (2009). Linking person-centered care and the physical environment: 10 design principles for elder and dementia care staff. *Alzheimer's Care Today, 10*(4), 228–231. https://doi.org/10.1177/1533317513488923

Hammersley, M., & Atkinson, P. (2007). *Ethnography: Principles in practice* (3rd ed.). Routledge. Chapters 1 and 7.

Hung, L., & Chaudhury, H. (2011). Exploring personhood in dining experiences of residents with dementia in long-term care facilities. *Journal of Aging Studies, 25*(1), 1–12. https://doi.org/10.1016/j.jaging.2010.08.007

Jones, J., & Smith, J. (2017). Ethnography: Challenges and opportunities. *Evidence-Based Nursing, 20*(4), 98–100. https://doi.org/10.1136/eb-2017-102786

Kaida, L., Moyser, M., & Park, S. Y. (2009). Cultural preferences and economic constraints: The living arrangements of elderly Canadians. *Canadian Journal of Aging, 28*(4), 303–313. https://doi.org/10.1017/S0714980809990146

Kitwood, T., & Bredin, K. (1992). Towards a theory of dementia care: Personhood and well-being. *Ageing and Society, 12*(3), 269–287. https://doi.org/10.1017/S0144686X0000502X

Koehn, S., Baumbusch, J., Reid, R. C., & Li, N. (2018). It's like chicken talking to ducks' and other challenges to families of Chinese immigrant older adults in long-term residential care. *Journal of Family Nursing, 24*(2), 156–183. https://doi.org/10.1177/1074840718774068

Lee, M. Y., & Mjelde-Mossey, L. (2004). Cultural dissonance among generations: A solution-focused approach with east Asian elders and their families. *Journal of Marital and Family Therapy, 30*(4), 497–513. https://doi.org/10.1111/j.1752-0606.2004.tb01258.x

Li, J., & Porock, D. (2014). Resident outcomes of person-centered care in long-term care: A systematic review of interventional research. *International Journal of Nursing Studies, 51*(10), 1395–1415. https://doi.org/10.1016/j.ijnurstu.2014.04.003

McCormack, B., & McCance, T. V. (2006). Development of a framework for person-centred nursing. *Journal of Advanced Nursing, 56*(5), 472–479. https://doi.org/10.1111/j.1365-2648.2006.04042.x

McCormack, B. G., & McCance, T. (2010). *Person-centred nursing: Theory, models and methods.* Wiley.

McGilton, K., Heath, H., Charlene, H., Bostrom, A. M., Mueller, C., Boscart, V. M., Mackenzie-Green, B., Moghabghab, R., & Bowers, B. (2012). Moving the agenda forward: A person-centred framework in long-term care. *International Journal of Older People Nursing, 7*(4), 303–309. https://doi.org/10.1111/opn.12010

Merriam, S. B. (1988). *Case study research in education: A qualitative approach.* Jossey-Bass Publishers.

Mold, F., Fitzpatrick, J. M., & Roberts, J. D. (2005). Minority ethnic elders in care homes: A review of the literature. *Age and Ageing, 34*(2), 107–113. https://doi.org/10.1093/ageing/afi009

Nixon, A., & Odoyo, C. O. (2020). Ethnography, its strengths, weaknesses and its application in information technology and communication as a research design. *Computer Science and Information Technology, 8*(2), 50–56. https://doi.org/10.13189/csit.2020.080203

Nolan, B. A., & Mathews, R. M. (2004). Facilitating resident information seeking regarding meals in a special care unit: An environmental design intervention. *Journal of Gerontological Nursing, 30*(10), 12–56. https://doi.org/10.3928/0098-9134-20041001-07

Office of the Seniors Advocate. (2021). *2020–21 annual report of the Office of the Seniors Advocate.* https://www.seniorsadvocatebc.ca/app/uploads/sites/4/2021/08/Annual_Report_2020_21-FINAL.pdf

Passini, R., Pigot, H., Rainville, C., & Tétreault, M.-H. (2000). Wayfinding in a nursing home for advanced dementia of the Alzheimer's type. *Environment and Behavior, 32*(5), 684–710. https://doi.org/10.1177/00139160021972748

Roberts, E. (2011). Six for lunch: A dining option for residents with dementia in a special care unit. *Journal of Housing for the Elderly, 25*(4), 352–379. https://doi.org/10.1080/0276389 3.2011.621862

Santana, M. J., Manalili, K., Jolley, R. J., Zelinsky, S., Quan, H., & Lu, M. (2017). How to practice person-centered care: A conceptual framework. *Health Expectation, 21*(2), 429–440. https://doi.org/10.1111/hex.12640

Statistics Canada. (2016). *Visible minority (15), generation status (4), age groups (12) and sex (3) for the population in private households of Canada, Provinces, territories, census metropolitan areas and census agglomerations, 2016 census-25% sample data.* Statistics Canada catalogue no.98-400-X2016190. https://www12.statcan.gc.ca/census-recensement/2016/dp-pd/dt-td/Rp-eng.cfm?TABID=2&Lang=E&APATH=3&DETAIL=0&DIM=0&FL=A&FREE=0&GC=0&GID=1341679&GK=0&GRP=1&PID=110531&PRID=10&PTYPE=109445&S=0&SHOWA LL=0&SUB=0&Temporal=2017&THEME=120&VID=0&VNAMEE=&VNAMEF=&D1=0 &D2=0&D3=0&D4=0&D5=0&D6=0

Statistics Canada. (2017). *Immigration and ethnocultural diversity: Key results from the 2016 census.* https://www150.statcan.gc.ca/n1/daily-quotidien/171025/dq171025b-eng.htm?indi d=14428-3&indgeo=0

Statistics Canada. (2018). *Ethnic diversity and immigration.* https://www150.statcan.gc.ca/n1/pub/11-402-x/2011000/chap/imm/imm-eng.htm

Statistics Canada. (2019). *Results from the 2016 Census: Examining the effect of public pension benefits on the low income of senior immigrants.* https://www150.statcan.gc.ca/n1/pub/75-006-x/2019001/article/00017-eng.htm

Statistics Canada. (2020). *Visible minority of person.* https://www23.statcan.gc.ca/imdb/p3Var.pl?Function=DEC&Id=45152

Torres, S. (2015). Ethnicity, culture and migration. In J. Twigg & W. Martin (Eds.), *Handbook of cultural gerontology* (pp. 277–284). Routledge.

Ujimoto, K. V. (1995). Ethnic dimensions of aging in Canada. In R. Neugebauer-Visano (Ed.), *Aging and inequality: Cultural constructions of difference* (pp. 3–29). Canadian Scholars' Press.

van Hoof, J., Kort, H. S., van Waarde, H., & Blom, M. M. (2010). Environmental interventions and the design of homes for older adults with dementia: An overview. *American Journal of Alzheimer's Disease and Other Dementias, 25*(3), 202–232. https://doi.org/10.1177/1533317509358885

Wright, R., & Mindel, C. (1993). Economic, health, and service use policies: Implications for long-term care of ethnic elderly. In C. Barresi & D. Stull (Eds.), *Ethnic elderly in long-term care* (pp. 247–263). Springer.

Zamawe, F. (2015). The implication of using NVivo software in qualitative data analysis: Evidence-based reflections. *Malawi Medical Journal, 27*(1), 3. https://doi.org/10.4314/mmj.v27i1.4

# Part III
# Memory Care and End-of-Life Care

# Designing for Dementia: An Approach that Works for Everyone

Jeffrey Anderzhon

## 1 Introduction

It has long been understood in the design community that the built environment can have a profound effect on the occupants of that environment. As early as the first century B.C., Roman Vitruvius wrote that architecture should resolve three values: functionality (utilitas; it should be useful and function for the people using it), durability (firmitas; it should stand up robustly and remain in good condition), and beauty (venustas; it should delight people and raise their spirits) (Pollio, 1914). Two millennia after Vitruvius' tome was published, it can be argued that following these design principles provides environments that mitigate the effects of dementia within the built environment. But understanding how to translate both large and small details of design for dementia into a holistic and inclusive community can often be problematic.

The recent COVID-19 pandemic has provided an increased focus on senior congregate living facilities and how their design can alleviate the spread of any disease providing a healthier environment. It has also offered an opportunity to consider how senior living environments can serve as partners in the quality of senior care, particularly for those with dementia. There have been numerous articles and white papers produced examining how designers can be more conscious of the spread of disease within the confines of a congregate living facility. Many of these approaches easily cross over as effective elements in designs that contribute to a higher quality of life and greater independence for those with dementia. The design community has collected a broad knowledge base from which to draw when considering environments for those with dementia. The design principles from this base, while

J. Anderzhon (✉)
Crepidoma Consulting, LLC, West Des Moines, IA, USA
e-mail: jeffa@crepidoma.com

F. Ferdous, E. Roberts (eds.), *(Re)designing the Continuum of Care for Older Adults*, https://doi.org/10.1007/978-3-031-20970-3_9

derived for those with dementia, can also effectively contribute to environments for any elderly congregate living facility.

Whether a design is meant specifically for those with dementia or for the broader elderly resident population, in the end, that design is meant to not only create a home for the residents but also, through that design, create a community (Cohen & Weisman, 1991). In order to be successful, that community's design needs to contribute to the residents' senses of place, purpose, independence, safety, and choice. This contribution must be telegraphed intuitively through the included design elements individually and their collective familiarity to the residents. Having followed the principles of completed gerontological environmental research, there are a number or completed senior living designs that have adhered to the tenets of "making home" and "making community" that can be utilized as examples to follow by designers for both environments for dementia and other senior living congregate designs. This chapter does not necessarily review the specific completed research, but rather how elements of that research have been successfully incorporated into completed environments.

## 1.1   A Design Vocabulary for Those with Dementia

Following a lengthy period when designers were little interested and did not understand designs for long-term care that were aimed at creating "home" for residents, several environmental gerontologists, led by M. Powell Lawton, began exploring and researching how built environments affect human behavior and in particular the aging and those with dementia (Lawton, 1980). As the presentment and recognition of dementia increased, perhaps due to the extension of life expectancy, designers and providers realized that the segregation of this group of residents might serve to improve their care. Basically, the newly created "dementia units" simply became a wing of those facilities that was secured by means of locked entrance doors to the wing. Of course, this tended to exacerbate the agitation of the residents in these "units" as the environment was certainly not a replication of the home from which they came.

Sometime following the middle of the twentieth century, academic interest in the cause of elderly dementia, and specifically Alzheimer's disease, rose significantly. The causes of cognitive disorders became clearer along with the manifestation dementia took in individuals. This knowledge and the accompanying interest by care providers to improve built environments for these individuals led to a significant increase by environmental gerontologists to research efficacious environmental design responses to elder cognitive losses. Academicians and practitioners alike began publishing their groundbreaking work, both in research and in-place environmental modifications and design (Lawton, 1980; Calkins, 1988; Cohen & Weisman, 1991).

However, this early work tended to focus on specific manifestations and efficacies of dementia such as incontinence, unproductive wandering, agitation, and rummaging, and not on the total effects on an individual. These design efficacies, which are so well documented in the seminal work by Margaret Calkins and further amplified by Elizabeth Brawley through specific discussion of age- and dementia-related physical deterioration, were and remain quite useful for designers. They provide insight into the physical manifestations of aging as well as the cognitive manifestations of dementia and how those manifestations affect an individual's relationship to the built environment (Calkins, 1988; Brawley, 1997; Brawley, 2006).

Although this research tends to discuss the environment as a whole, many designers have unfortunately tended to utilize it simply as a menu from which selections could be made, and they have not necessarily considered them as a holistic design approach. Applied in this way, the efficacies could lead to stereotyping individuals with dementia and to not treating residents as individuals. In addition, the resultant environments become specifically tailored to a group of residents rather than one that can serve all elderly residents.

The environmental interventions suggested by this research included some very simple and commonsense approaches. These included the following, as well as others:

- Clear visual access to bathrooms that reinforces their location and use in order to avoid incontinence incidents.
- Display areas for resident memorabilia to identify individual bedroom occupancy and spark long-term memories.
- Minimization of "dead-end" corridors to eliminate a wandering resident's anxiety when they are faced with no choice to continue.
- Open serving kitchens that replicate residents' homes and provide the aroma of food being prepared and served.
- Use of visual design and artwork landmarks to provide orientation cues for residents.
- Allowing residents to bring their own furniture into their bedrooms to add familiarity to the space.

While these are just a few of the proactive design elements, they, as well as others, have in the years since their publication been utilized effectively throughout the senior living design world.

In subsequent years, many designers began to understand that everyone with dementia was indeed an individual, one with individual physical needs, individual cognitive losses, and individual personalities. Bolstered by Uriel Cohen and Gerald Weisman's research (Cohen & Weisman, 1991), designs of congregate living facilities and care programs began to take shape which were more "homelike" while maintaining specific elements of design that assisted the cognitively impaired and designed more to accommodate the culture and personal history of the individual residents. Designers began to understand the individual need for a sense of place, belonging, and community. It would take the design thrust of the small house design movement to bring to light a more holistic approach to built environments for those with dementia.

## 2 Translating Research into Reality

One of the first dedicated dementia environments that was constructed following this initial research was Woodside Place of Oakmont in Oakmont, Pennsylvania. First occupied in 1991, this assisted living environment is divided into 3 small households of 12 residents each along with a large central community area. Each household has two shared occupancy resident rooms and eight private rooms along with a household great room and serving kitchen. The central community area provides back-of-house functions and spaces for large group activities and other spaces for smaller and individual activities. Each household has a "front porch" and front door defined through architectural elements reflecting single-family design and that clearly announced the entry to a "home."

The design incorporates the ability to display resident memorabilia on plate rails within the resident room and portrait photos of the resident as room signage. Dutch doors to the resident rooms are utilized so residents can feel secure but also visually recognize activities that may be taking place outside their rooms. Within the corridors, tactile artwork is hung to orient residents as they traverse to their rooms as well as heighten their sense of touch.

The three households are laid out in a manner that creates two secured courtyards accessible by the residents in good weather. Within the central common spaces, there are areas designed where residents can participate in individual art activities or simply sit in front of the fireplace, read a book from the library, or visit with a family member. The operational model is tailored to the individual allowing choice of mealtimes, access to areas outside the household, and interaction of visiting family members anywhere in the environment.

Throughout the built environment of Woodside Place, the design intentionally calls upon residential architectural elements which are at an individual human scale. From the moment of entry, the occupant feels comfortable and intuitively understands a feeling of home. This senior environment is built upon the evolving research of the time and has added its own research to the collective knowledge base while providing dementia care that allows residents safety of place and supports efficacies for their memory losses. A community of residents is created at Woodside Place through the environmental design and the care program that interacts with that design (Anderzhon et al., 2007).

## 2.1 The Small House Concept

Although the small house design concept, such as Woodside Place, emanated from a variety of sources as a response to the traditional medical model of senior congregate care, it was broadly brought to designers' attention in the early part of the twenty-first century by Dr. Bill Thomas' Green House® movement. This approach provides a significant move forward to creating an environment that respects and embraces the typology of home and, in particular, the principles espoused by Christopher Alexander's "*A Pattern Language*" (Alexander et al., 1977). The Green House® concept clearly delineates public, public-private, and private domains within the residential environment and thus allows for a more intuitive sense of place by the residents. The small number of residents within the environment, along with consistent staffing and encouragement of family members to participate in the care program, also provides a sense of belonging and continuity for the residents.

The first Green Houses® constructed in Tupelo, Mississippi, were a successful move forward toward community for dementia care and away from the traditional, staff-oriented, medical model of care. The objective was to create an appropriate environment in which residents could be as independent as possible and staff could be empowered to provide superior care. Additionally, the small house design intent was to enable the care environment to be translated into any residential location and to be an essential part of the surrounding community (Robert Wood Johnson Foundation, 2007).

These small houses are limited to 10 residents and foster the "family" experience through both physical environmental design and care operations. The house layout allows each private room visual access to the center public-private portion of the house where activity gathering takes place. Additionally, the open kitchen promotes resident participation, either actively or vicariously, in meal preparation, allowing the aroma of that preparation to invigorate resident's appetites. The large single community dining table where residents and staff dine together promotes social interaction around mealtimes.

Design of the Green Houses® includes all the elements that previous research had indicated would be efficacious for individuals with dementia, allowing them more independence, choice in life's activities, and a resultant-reduced anxiety. As such, it could be argued that this original design was one that was the complete package for senior congregate living specifically for those with dementia. Bringing these elements into a single design that also integrates a coordinated care program which fully involves residents in the decision-making process is a major step toward forward-thinking dementia care. In a study completed in 2007 to determine the effects of this built environment on residents' outcome and quality of care (Kane et al., 2007), it was found that residents achieved a higher level of satisfaction with their environment and had better emotional well-being, a lower incidence of decline in activities of daily living, and improvement in meaningful activities and relationships.

These first Green Houses® are unfortunately built in an area significantly remote from the remainder of the life plan community campus. Community integration beyond their enclave of small houses is somewhat difficult, and, as a result, residents are still faced with some segregation from an embedded larger community sense of place (Anderzhon et al., 2007). However, the concept has become a benchmark for all senior living design that provides residents with an intuitively familiar environment, continuity of the lifestyle, enhanced choice, and increased independence.

There are obvious benefits to small house senior living environments beyond those that have to do with dementia. Empirical evidence during the COVID-19 pandemic showed that spread of the virus was less in small house settings largely due to the ability to segregate the small number of residents and fewer staff within the small house. Consistent staffing and the ability to quickly test residents and staff along with restrictive control of vendors and visitors diminish the spread of COVID-19 or any other disease. These benefits combined with sensible design utilizing efficacious elements for those with dementia point to the logical consideration of small house design for any senior living congregate facility. One must keep in mind, however, how a small house or group of small houses can become a viable community outside of the house in the broader community.

As originally conceived, the Green House® concept was meant to be adaptable in any neighborhood as, architecturally, it is simply a large house and thus can be placed on any single-family lot assuming local zoning regulations allow. With this design approach and a collaborating programmatic approach, connection to the larger community could be expedited and celebrated (Fig. 1).

The Green House® approach, while somewhat regulated by the Green House® organization, allows freedom of architectural design depending on location. But each building, regardless of location, incorporates the principles and elements that best serve those with dementia as previous research conclusions provided. These first Green Houses® were designed to be specifically for individuals with dementia. But the small house design concept, following the typology of home, has spread widely throughout senior living design to serve the elderly regardless of acuity levels.

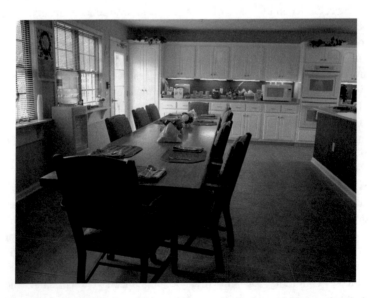

**Fig. 1** The large household dining table provides opportunity for social interaction during each meal. (Photo courtesy Jeffrey Anderzhon)

## 2.2   Adding to Community

Shortly after the Green Houses® in Mississippi opened, Park Homes, a life plan community in central Kansas, chose to replace their aging skilled nursing facility with the small house concept, but in a manner that would maintain the connection of the residents to the larger campus community. The campus in this small rural town sits amid a mid-century single-family housing development and is often the center of activity for community residents.

Understanding that while only a few residents are diagnosed with dementia, most of their resident population are of an age where their cognitive memory is at least partially diminished. The client's building program was to construct free-standing small houses that function well for their elderly population regardless of physical or mental acuity. It was also decided that when complete, the population would not be segregated according to memory loss but allow residents to maintain the social relationships they had established over the years within the community.

The design of the houses, along with the repurposing of the existing traditional nursing facility, provides both a sense of place for the residents and, through the built environment, a variety of opportunities for social interaction. It also creates a familiar setting for the residents by means of simple residential architecture surrounded by exterior spaces replicating those within the larger community.

The siting of the new houses around the repurposed skilled nursing building provides two distinct and secure courtyards or backyards to the houses. The smaller one is designed to be a "passive" courtyard with plantings that attract butterflies and small birds. Contemplative seating areas around the courtyard provide serendipitous social opportunities, and both sunny and shaded areas are included within the courtyard as a part of the houses' design. The larger courtyard serves as the "active" one with playground equipment for grandchildren and exercise stations for residents. These courtyards are fully secured allowing residents access without overt staff oversight (Fig. 2).

The small houses accommodate 12 residents, but the large private rooms are sized to allow two resident occupants when couples move in. Residents are strongly encouraged to bring their own familiar furnishings to their rooms. Extra storage space is accomplished by window seat benches in some rooms. Full bathrooms, including no-barrier showers and large vanities, are finished with ceramic tile, a finish with which most residents would be familiar. Visual access is provided to the bathrooms from most areas of the resident rooms. Electrical wiring in the rooms is done in a manner that allows easy change of overbed lights when the resident wants to rearrange their furniture.

The house design provides a layout that complies with a resident's home typology including a distinct front door that leads to the living room, or public-private space, complete with an iconic fireplace. Beyond this public-private space, there is an open plan serving kitchen, dining room, and family room that are fitted with a variety of natural and artificial lighting levels that allow staff to lower anxiety levels or assist in promoting resident circadian rhythms. The bedroom entry points are

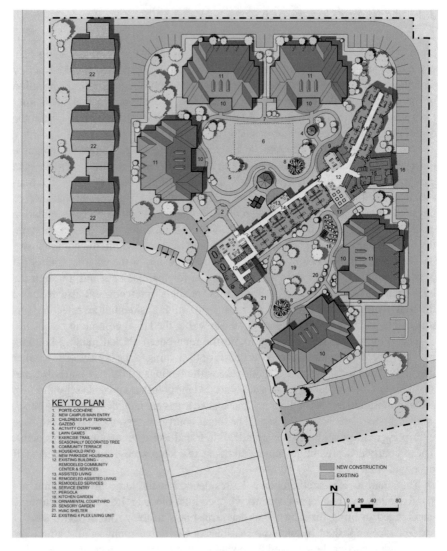

**Fig. 2** The siting of the Park Homes provides passive and active secured courtyards. (Image courtesy of Jeffrey Anderzhon)

clearly a part of the private space of the house with small transitional living or social spaces for each four-bedroom grouping. This transitional space introduces an additional layer of community for residents.

Residents can sit at the lower-level kitchen counter to assist staff in meal preparation or to simply observe the meals being prepared and enjoy the aromas of cooking that may serve to enhance their appetites. As meals are not served on a rigid schedule, this is where residents can take a late breakfast or a midday snack enjoying conversation with the staff or other residents.

In good weather, residents are free to leave the house to enjoy the outdoors. They can sit on the shaded patio or freely wander through the secured gardens. These have been specifically designed with surfaces and plantings that are appropriate for the level of cognition experienced by the resident. As a safety measure, staff has full and adequate visual access to these areas from most locations within the house and thus can provide covert oversight and rapid response, if necessary, of resident activities within the garden areas.

The built environment at Park Homes is completed with simple architectural design but in a manner familiar with that which the residents have known. The houses' layout complies with an intuitive residential one and staffing within the houses is consistent. The design includes elements that are efficacious for those with dementia as indicated in early research. The result is a modified institution more readily accepted not only by the residents and staff but also by the surrounding community (Anderzhon et al., 2012).

## 2.3   *Extending Community*

In 1692, Sir Christopher Wren, the well-known early British architect, completed the design for the Royal Hospital Chelsea on the banks of the Thames River in London, UK. This early senior living community was intended to be a retirement home for veteran non-officer pensioned soldiers who had no other living or care arrangement choice. For the following 300 years, the Royal Hospital struggled to provide care service for residents who, after living in the facility for many years, found their health deteriorating significantly. (Note: The terms "hospital" and "infirmary" as used in the United Kingdom do not always refer to acute care provided as it does in the United States and elsewhere but refer more to the resident living arrangement combined with some level of care.)

In 2009, the Royal Hospital completed the Margaret Thatcher Infirmary on the 67-acre in-town site adjacent to Wren's architecture. This building now houses residential care, nursing care, and dementia care residents. While these care levels are segregated within the building, there is little difference in design between each care level within the three-story-square donut-shaped structure.

Wren's original design of berths (small sleeping rooms) for the pensioners is rich with wood finishes and details, and each private berth includes a Dutch door enabling the pensioner to sit in his room and visually connect with activity occurring just outside the room. The design for the new infirmary replicates those attributes by extensive use of wood finishes. But more cleverly, the new design includes full doors with upper glass vision panels glazed with integral blinds controlled in a way that allows the resident to leave them open to view activity outside the room. Additionally, if the blinds are closed, staff can open them with a special key in order to briefly check on the resident without fully opening the door and disturbing them (Figs. 3 and 4).

**Fig. 3** Berths in Royal
Hospital Chelsea, designed
by Sir Christopher Wren in
1692. (Photo courtesy
Jeffrey Anderzhon)

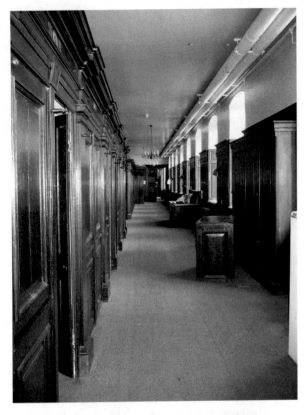

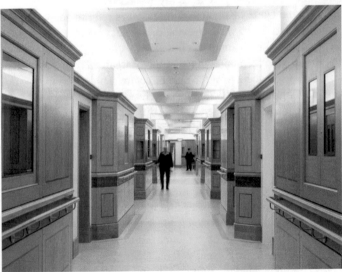

**Fig. 4** Replicated pensioner berths in Margaret Thatcher Infirmary. (Photo courtesy Jeffrey Anderzhon)

The care programs are divided into small houses that merge seamlessly with one another. Living and dining areas are conveniently located so residents have very little distance from their room to an activity or social area. The designers replicated the small gathering and seating areas from the main hospital in the infirmary but with a more contemporary feel. The dementia households have direct access to the center courtyard formed and secured by the building's shape. This also allows care staff to have continual visual access to this nicely landscaped exterior area from the centrally located social areas.

Each resident room is fitted with a "memory case" where residents generally display memorabilia from their time in the military service. This design touch replicates the Wren design of the resident berths where there was a small shelf at each berth for pensioner memorabilia. The original Wren hospital design has an oak-paneled covered colonnade with built-in benches facing the hospital parade ground where pensioners can sit and enjoy the view toward the Thames. As a clear reference to this design element, the infirmary has a wood paneled enclosed "colonnade," complete with built-in wood benches that allow residents to also sit and admire the views through large windows.

As most residents of the infirmary have spent several years on the Royal Hospital campus, the infirmary design required a continuation of the gained sense of place for both those with dementia and those who simply needed additional health care. This is accomplished by providing design elements with which residents are familiar but in updated, more contemporary ways. The pensioners are already accustomed to a level of socialization with each other which is well supported within the design layout of the building and building's exterior spaces. The dignity, independence, sense of place, and sense of community are clearly supported by the design.

In its exterior design as well as its interior layout and finishes, the Thatcher Infirmary completes the community of the Royal Hospital. It does so with respect to the Wren original but, more importantly, in a manner with which residents are familiar and comfortable regardless of their care level.

## 2.4 Replicating Community

Contemporaneously with the Green House® concept and the Park Homes design, The Village at Waveny Care Center in New Canaan, Connecticut, embarked on the construction of a new dementia care environment that includes assisted living residency and adult day care for those with dementia. These two programs are physically separated by a large "main street" space for activities, social events, and commercial replication of the New Canaan main street. The main street provides a meeting place for both programs and larger community events.

Understanding that the residents of the new environment would predominantly be from the New Canaan community in which they have resided most of their lives, the designers were tasked to provide a familiar environment. This was considered a way to ease resident move-in and orientation. Replicating the community's main street, complete with storefronts for a convenience store and ice cream parlor, would also provide residents opportunities for an outing away from their rooms and small house functions.

The new main street serves another purpose beyond simple familiarity: it has become a meeting place for residents and family members with spaces for both privacy of conversation and engagement with others. It is a popular location for birthday celebrations that involve the entire community, for concerts from local high school bands and choirs, and for simply taking a stroll from "home" to the garden at the end of the street. Simply put, the Waveny main street has become a broader center for community engagement allowing residents and day care clients a continuation of their community involvement.

Unlike other, subsequent design attempts at providing a "main street" experience for dementia residents, the Waveny design is neither contrived nor artificial. The design elements utilized are drawn directly from those present in New Canaan and with which the resident would be familiar. Their integration into the campus community becomes much easier and expedient. Their ability to understand the community and maneuver through it also becomes easier. Staff provides both active and passive activities on the main street that fully engage residents and day care clients and that promote independence and purpose and an enhanced sense of place and purpose.

The residential portion of the project is a two-story structure divided into two small houses on each floor of 13 residents each. Resident rooms are large, enabling residents to bring and arrange their own furniture to personalize their private space. Each small house has a living room and serving kitchen. Residents can choose to eat in their house or enjoy a meal in a larger restaurant-like dining room located just outside the small house.

Each resident room has ample built-in storage and display space for personalization as well as a full bathroom with barrier free access and easy visual access from the resident room. Within the small house, residents can easily access the many activities or social gatherings that take place in the common spaces. While the small house does not fully follow the tenets of household typology, each set of four resident rooms is accessed through a transitional space that residents can claim as their own, and not directly from a common corridor.

The Village at Waveny Care Center provides the New Canaan community with a dementia care environment that not only enhances the care for residents within a familiar environment but also adds a community gathering center for the entire town. It has easily become an integral part of the larger community and thus has extended the sense of community and belonging to residents.

## 2.5   Creating a New Community

In 2009, the not-for-profit Dutch senior living provider Vivium Hogewey had become dissatisfied with an older dementia environment they operated. They had extensive experience in dementia care for seniors and through that experience had amassed knowledge of better methods and better environments in which to provide dementia care. They thus began a journey to reinvent dementia care in the Netherlands and eventually created an approach that is now looked upon internationally and often studied as the benchmark for creation of dementia care program and environment that provides residents with familiarity of place, enhanced independence, and choice all within a complete community.

De Hogeweyk®, located in Weesp, Netherlands, is a result of Vivium's disruptive and forward-thinking desire to provide a deinstitutionalized setting for the care and housing of those with dementia. Simply put, De Hogeweyk® is built as a fully functioning community that meets the needs of the residents but is not segregated from the surrounding community.

Built with 23 small houses for residents, the community is inward looking without disassociating itself from its surroundings. The construction fills a site about a block square in a residential area and is two stories in height with the outside façade appearing to simply be a nice-looking residential block, not unlike any of its neighbors. The outer edges of the building reach the extent of the lot, and the façade design is varied in order to scale it to a residential level and to provide indication of differing uses beyond.

Within that façade, there is a vibrant and extensive use of courtyards, building layouts, main streets, and side alleys. Each of the households within the structure is a home for six residents and is entered off one of the interior streets, either at grade-level street or at the elevated level directly above the first. Households are self-contained complete with great room, kitchen, and private resident rooms. While the resident rooms do not have en-suite bathrooms, the arrangement of them is more like a small house with a shared bathroom off the corridor near all the bedrooms and becomes quite familiar to the residents' experience in their previous homes. Households have well-appointed private entry courtyards that are inviting and are often utilized by residents for their morning coffee.

The system of "streets" leads in a logical way to the main boulevard and then to a plaza around which is a small grocery, a restaurant with a bar and streetside dining, a post office, a theatre, and the main entrance for members of the surrounding community. The boulevard and plaza have resting benches, umbrella tables, information kiosks, water features, tricycles for anyone's use, and areas for concerts and art displays. Residents are completely free to navigate the small, complete village at their leisure (Fig. 5).

Staffing in the households is consistent, and, along with the residents, each household really becomes a family. Encouraged to assist in meal preparation, laundry, and other household chores, residents quickly are filled with a sense of purpose. The households are furnished and finished in traditional Dutch fashion with residents allowed to bring personal memorabilia and small furnishings into their rooms.

The inwardly focused design of De Hogeweyk® provides a sense of safety and security. The design also enhances the sense of belonging as the households are small, "family"-oriented, and closely adjacent to one another. This proximity encourages residents from adjacent households to socially congregate in the small entry courtyards for morning conversations.

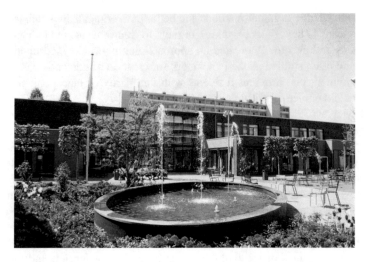

**Fig. 5** De Hogeweyk® interior streets lead to the plaza and offer many activities for the entire community. (Photo courtesy of Vivium Hogewey)

The belief that an individual's life does not occur solely within the confines of a home or a bedroom is the foundation of De Hogeweyk's® design. Understanding the principles of designing for those with dementia have, for the most part, been implemented within this environment. But to its credit, the design goes further. The project, simply put, created a full and vibrant community that allows residents a greater sense of independence without overt staff oversight. The design promotes social interaction among residents by providing that community with physical locations to socially interact in an unstructured manner, not unlike similar opportunities in the environments from which the residents came.

Vivium De Hogewey provided, within their building program, a design framework that by all standards has been accomplished:

- A favorable human-scaled and familiar physical surrounding where confusion and anxiety of place are minimized.
- Providing for life's pleasures and for a meaning and purpose of life.
- Experiencing a high quality of living and well-being.
- A favorable lifestyle, determined by the resident.
- An enjoyable and fulfilling place for caregivers and volunteers (Anderzhon et al., 2012; Godwin, 2015; Sodo & Winters, 2021).

## 3   Conclusion

As the twentieth century ended, senior living designers understood the built environment, as we had known it, was generally not providing the quality-of-care elders deserved, particularly for those with dementia. Part of that understanding was that most senior environments traumatized residents as they moved from a familiar home and community environment into an unfamiliar, regimented, and mostly homogenously designed congregate setting, one void of individuality and choice. It was also understood that most senior living environments were institutional in nature, were designed for staff efficiency rather than resident needs and comfort, and were unresponsive to specific needs of those with dementia, stereotyping the needs of the elderly. These underlying principles tended to lead to designs that ignored individuals' sense of purpose, sense of place, belonging, independence, dignity, and choice.

There is really no question that the understanding of dementia as well as the design of environments for dementia has significantly advanced over the past few decades. The knowledge base of how environments for those with dementia can affect residents has grown significantly, continues to increase, and is widely available to designers. Unfortunately, many designers are still focused on designing for a stereotype or with their own unsubstantiated perspective of how a building should function and look. Regardless of whether the design is for dementia or simply the elderly, ignoring the individuality of occupants is an unproductive and an antithetical approach to serving the occupants of the environment.

Current quality, sensible designs for dementia have also led the way in "crossover" senior living designs. Small houses have been shown to be operationally highly efficient with less staff turnover and a greater ease in maintaining full census. During the pandemic, small house residences have demonstrated less likelihood to spread virus to a wider audience and easier to isolate residents while even allowing a higher level of family visitations. They continue to demonstrate a higher level of resident wellness and physical and emotional well-being.

The fundamentals promulgated through research have, over time, been shown to assist in the independence of not only those with dementia but also any elderly individual in a congregate setting. Utilizing those principles, combined with the design typology of home, also allows providers the versatility of moving quickly from nonspecific dementia care to a household specifically for dementia without major financial outlay.

Providing design that is familiar to residents translates into faster orientation and an easing of trauma associated with moving into a new environment. Allowing residents to bring their own furnishings into that environment goes another step further in this process of orientation and independence. Utilizing visual cues and furnishings and finishes that enhance residents' visual and tactile senses promotes and stimulates individual intellectual well-being. Resident innate spatial layout familiarity of "home" is promoted with logical and familiar building layout.

It is neither difficult nor technically challenging for designers to apply the well-researched principles to new elderly design projects. The result, regardless of the level of care intended, will be more of a home for the residents and an extension of the community from which they have come. It is a design approach that works for everyone.

# References

Alexander, C., Ishikawa, S., & Silverstein, M. (1977). *A pattern language: Towns, buildings, construction*. Oxford University Press.

Anderzhon, J., Fraley, I., & Green, M. (Eds.). (2007). *Design for aging post-occupancy evaluations*. Wiley.

Anderzhon, J., Hughes, D., Judd, S., Kiyota, E., & Wijnties, M. (2012). *Design for aging international case studies of building and program*. Wiley.

Brawley, E. (1997). *Designing for alzheimer's disease*. Wiley.

Brawley, E. (2006). *Design innovations for aging and alzheimer's; creating caring communities*. Wiley.

Calkins, M. (1988). *Design for dementia, planning environments for the elderly and the confused*. National Health Publishing.

Cohen, U., & Weisman, G. (1991). *Holding on to home, designing environments for people with dementia*. The Johns Hopkins University Press.

Godwin, B. (2015). Hogewey: A "home from home" in the Netherlands. *The Journal of Dementia Care, 23*(3) https://www.researchgate.net/publication/283228026_Hogewey_A_'home_from_home'_in_the_Netherlands

Kane, R., Lum, T., Cutler, L., Degenholtz, H., & Yu, T. (2007). Resident outcomes in small-house nursing homes: A longitudinal evaluation of the initial green house program. *Journal of the American Geriatric Society, 55*(6), 832.

Lawton, M. (1980). *Environment and aging*. Wadsworth, Inc.

Pollio, V. (1914). *The ten books of architecture*. Harvard University Press.

Robert Wood Johnson Foundation. (2007). *Green houses provide a small group setting alternative to nursing homes – And a positive effect on residents' quality of life*. https://www.rwjf.org/en/library/research/2007/01/-green-houses%2D%2Dprovide-a-small-group-setting-alternative-to-nurs.html

Sodo, J. & Winters, M. (2021). *Missing Main Street: Reconnecting Older Adults with Dementia to the Fabric of Authentic Living*. https://www.perkinseastman.com/white-papers/missing-main-street-reconnecting-older-adults-with-dementia-to-the-fabric-of-authenticliving/

# Communication and Environmental Positioning in Dementia Care Units: Dialogues Through Space and Place

Kate de Medeiros

## 1 Introduction

Changes in communication with advancing dementia can cause unique challenges to the experience of home and place for people living in long-term care (LTC) settings. Communication includes more than just language and is affected by how one is positioned within the social and living spaces of a given environment. This chapter is guided by a social constructionist perspective and considers how position and place are socially constructed, negotiated, and performed by LTC dementia residents and care staff through various types of verbal and nonverbal positioning. Positioning theory addresses how identities and roles are enacted through language, often in conversations (Harre & van Langenhove, 1999; Sabat et al., 2011). Environmental positioning describes how identities and roles can be jointly constructed through dialogue and in relation to space and place (de Medeiros et al., 2013; de Medeiros & Sabat, 2016). Environmental positioning may be influenced by the rules that govern how physical space is used (e.g., Is it an area open to residents and staff or staff only?), the symbolic meanings of places (e.g., nursing homes as places of fear), the physical layout of place (e.g., walls, tables, personal items), the function of structural and decorative features within an environment (e.g., Do they serve as barriers, facilitators, or identity markers?), and the precarity or level of insecurity associated with being in a particular place.

To further consider positioning in LTC, we present an illustrative case example of Rosie (a pseudonym), an 86-year-old widow who resided in a 20-bed nursing home unit for people living with dementia. Specific interactions related to positioning between Rosie and a staff member and other residents were documented through observational notes and interviews. By considering positioning in light of Rosie's

K. de Medeiros (✉)
Department of Sociology and Gerontology, Miami University, Oxford, OH, USA
e-mail: demedekb@miamiOH.edu

F. Ferdous, E. Roberts (eds.), *(Re)designing the Continuum of Care for Older Adults*, https://doi.org/10.1007/978-3-031-20970-3_10

experiences, we consider ways in which LTC settings can move beyond the over-sight needs of the staff to foster more equitable communicative possibilities for residents within the care environment.

## 1.1 Communication and Dementia

Changes in communicative abilities that occur with advancing dementia can cause challenges for staff and residents in LTC settings (Adams & Gardiner, 2005; Saunders et al., 2011; Savundranayagam & Moore-Nielsen, 2015). Many challenges are not related to language changes, but instead are shaped by social perceptions, stereotypes, and assumptions about the communicative abilities of people living with dementia. The literature on speech accommodation suggests negative stereotypes associated with conditions like dementia can cause a speaker make over-accommodations when speaking to someone living with dementia regardless of that person's actual language abilities (Coupland et al., 1988; Giles, 2016; Savundranayagam & Moore-Nielsen, 2015). For instance, a speaker may talk to a person living with dementia as if they were a child because of stereotypes that suggest they are childlike (Kemper, 1994; Williams et al., 2009).

Furthermore, people living with dementia have been depicted as akin to selfless "zombies" (Behuniak, 2011); as "tragic, weak, and completely incapable" (Bartlett & O'Connor, 2010, p. 98); and as "no longer people" (Bruens, 2013, p. 84). These and other damaging stereotypes create a type of separation between "us" (people not living with dementia) and "them" (those living with dementia) which contributes to stigmatization and social discreditation (Goffman, 2009; Gove et al., 2016; Young et al., 2011). Stereotypes like these reinforce the idea that people living with dementia have little or nothing to say of value since "they" are no longer like "us." This is especially true for people living with dementia who have been removed from the community and relocated to LTC, a particular type of place with negative associations, where they are unseen by the public.

It is also important to consider how power dynamics are negotiated, challenged, or reinforced through conversation. As mentioned briefly in the introduction, positioning theory has its roots in linguistics and social psychology. It broadly considers relationships and power as they are enacted through language, thoughts, and other communicative actions (e.g., gestures, facial expressions) (Harre & van Langenhove, 1999). Embedded in positioning theory is the notion that when engaging in conversational practices, people assume different roles which provide them with different rights and obligations (Adams & Gardiner, 2005). For example, a clinician may enact their role as expert by wearing a white coat and choosing technical words. In this way, the clinician positions themselves as having greater power in the conversation. As a conversation unfolds, participants may change their role in response to another's role, try to assume a more (or less) powerful position in the conversation, or enact other types of rights or obligations that they deem appropriate for the conversation. For example, the same clinician could position themselves as a "friendly expert" by dressing in layperson clothes and using nontechnical language as an attempt to achieve a more even power distribution in the conversation. If, however, the clinician over-accommodates and uses inappropriately simplistic language, they would be practicing a type of disabling speech or what Kitwood (1997) and Sabat and Lee (2011) have referred to as negative or malignant positioning.

Negative or malignant positioning describes a deficit view by one communicative partner toward another (Kitwood, 1997). It has been well documented in the research literature on communications between younger people and older people, regardless of dementia status (Young et al., 2011). Kemper (1994) coined the term "elderspeak" to describe the patronizing, childlike language often used by younger people when speaking to older people (Williams et al., 2003). Other types of over-accommodation that leads to negative positioning include using a high-pitched or exaggerated tone, choosing simple words, use of diminutives (e.g., "sweetie), interrupting, talking over the conversational partner, and disregarding the conversational partner altogether (Adams & Gardiner, 2005; Sabat, 2006; Savundranayagam & Moore-Nielsen, 2015; Young et al., 2011). Such over-accommodation not only reinforces unequal power dynamics between speaker and conversational partner, it also may contribute to withdrawal of the conversational partner from social interactions, thereby contributing to isolation.

As mentioned earlier, positions within a conversation are not one-sided or static. Building on the earlier example of a clinician using condescending talk, a person living with dementia may resist the clinician's position of "expert" and counter through conversational devices such as changing the subject, introducing humor, offering their own personal knowledge as a response, and so on. In these and other ways, power dynamics and roles in terms of one speaker's position to another unfold through discourse and other forms of communication (Harré & Van Langenhove, 1999). The clinician may practice enabling speech by recognizing that the person living with dementia is someone able to express input about their feelings and their care (Adams & Gardiner, 2005). In this way, the clinician would be positioning the person as someone worthy of talking with and listening to rather than talking at and disregarding (de Medeiros & Sabat, 2016).

Of course, language changes are likely to occur with advancing dementia which can present communication challenges for people living with dementia and their care providers. It is, however, important to note that language and communication changes differ according to dementia type and are not uniformly experienced. For example, around 36% of people in early stages and 100% of those in late stages of Alzheimer's disease are reported to have some form of aphasia or loss of ability to express or understand speech (Fraser et al., 2016). Other features of speech changes with Alzheimer's disease include difficulty with naming and word-finding and presence of "empty speech" or speech that lacks referential nouns, content words, and/or cohesion (Fraser et al., 2016; Klimova & Kuca, 2016; Mueller et al., 2018). Many of the speech changes associated with Alzheimer's disease are also experienced by people living with vascular dementia. In contrast, people living with Lewy body dementia or Parkinson's disease dementia are more likely to experience soft or non-articulated speech and lack of grammar cohesion which differ people living with Alzheimer's disease (Klimova & Kuca, 2016).

Overall, difficulties with language and communication can lead to frustration by people living with dementia and their caregivers, which in turn can lead to unpleasant interactions and social withdrawal (Savundranayagam & Moore-Nielsen, 2015). Consequently, improved communication is often identified as an important area in need of attention within dementia care broadly (Young et al., 2011). Stereotypical assumptions about communicative abilities have led many to erroneously assume that all people living with dementia experience similar types of language challenges and are unable to communicate in meaningful or insightful ways about their insights and experiences (Wang et al., 2019). Building on some of the ideas about communication and conversational positioning in this section, the next sections consider residential long-term care facilities (LTCFs) in terms of control through environmental positioning and communicative opportunities.

## 1.2 Residential Long-Term Care

Residential LTC dementia facilities such as nursing homes are what Goffman (1958) called "total institutions" – places where large groups of people are treated in similar ways; where sleep, play, and work occur in one location; and where the activities of the residents fall under one controlling authority charged with fulfilling the official aims of the institution (Agich, 2003; Eijkelenboom et al., 2017; van Hoof et al., 2016). Despite movements aimed at changing the nature of LTC, from total institutions to models that recognize and respect resident autonomy and personhood (White-Chu et al., 2009), residential long-term dementia care facilities are ultimately charged with providing appropriate medical and social care to people who are unable to care for themselves (Grubman, 2015). Consequently, such facilities are still institutions, even decades after culture change initiatives were introduced, and the staff still control daily schedules regardless of residents' preferences (Duan et al., 2020; Koren, 2010; Ward et al., 2008). Regardless of how "homelike" a facility might appear, institutions are a type of place but not a "home" (Kontos et al., 2021).

Home implies a private dwelling where one feels familiarity, belonging, safety, and comfort and can exercise choice and control (Eijkelenboom et al., 2017; Oswald & Wahl, 2005; Reed-Danahay, 2001; Rubinstein & de Medeiros, 2005). Place includes a particular physical location, locale or "the material setting for social relations" (Cresswell, 2009, p. 169), and the meanings associated with a particular place. Place identity describes how living in a particular community such as a nursing home influences a sense of identity associated with that community such that living elsewhere (e.g., in the community) would affect one's sense of identity (Andrews et al., 2007, 2017; Cuba & Hummon, 1993; Cutchin et al., 2003; Moore, 2014). In this way, understanding, or even questioning, who we are is related to where we are (Rubinstein & de Medeiros, 2003; Rubinstein & de Medeiros, 2005).

Unfortunately, as McParland et al. (2017) have observed, nursing homes are "the place where people with dementia must go when they have moved beyond manageable boundaries in our world … At their most cognitively impaired and thus most vulnerable, people with dementia are not regarded by the general public as 'of our world,' nor considered to be bound by the same rules, nor are their human or citizenship rights respected to the same extent as those without dementia" (p. 262). In addition, most LTC residents did not choose to leave their home in the community to live in the facility – a place. Once there, residents are constrained by the facility's rules and physical layout. They cannot leave without an escort, are restricted in access to other rooms and areas, and are dependent on others for care and social involvement (Ward et al., 2008). Regardless of the small choices that they may be given throughout the day (e.g., coffee or juice, participate in group singing activity or not), they have very little control over their living environment. Residents also will have had few of any opportunities to contribute to the design of a nursing home (van Hoof et al., 2016; Wang et al., 2019). When researchers do ask residents about their preferences within nursing homes, it is typically in relation to receiving care services or limited to their preferred interactions with staff rather than with regard to how residents would like to utilize space (Bangerter et al., 2016).

## 1.3 Environmental Positioning

Environmental positioning offers a way to further explore how LTCFs as places can become more like homes for residents by fostering communicative opportunities. As briefly mentioned earlier, environmental positioning describes "how the space and physical structures in an environment, as well as the sense of place that accompanies that environment, may enhance or limit a person's ability to express selfhood and identity and to engage socially with another person" (de Medeiros et al., 2013, p. 228). Environmental positioning considers how social roles are enforced through personal objects, how limits and opportunities are created through physical structures such as tables and walls, and the formal and informal "rules" that govern who has access to a physical or social space.

In addition, while the structural layout and décor of a given space can contribute to feelings of belonging or alienation (Chaudhury et al., 2018), they can also be sites of power. Staff exert tremendous control within nursing home spaces. They determine resident seating arrangements at meals, arrange furniture in particular ways for activities, and decide whether music is playing (and what type of music is played), all of which influence environmental positioning (Chaudhury et al., 2018; Doyle et al., 2012). For example, placing chairs too far apart could create a sense of distance rather than community (de Medeiros et al., 2009). Seating a noncommunicative resident next to one who enjoys conversation can silence both residents (de Medeiros et al., 2009). These and other acts of environmental positioning affect communicative opportunities and reflect one's superior (or inferior) social position within the environment, which in turn influences who gets to talk and whose talk is worth listening to.

Another important consideration of environmental positioning is the presence of precarity in a place. Nursing homes are typically viewed as terminal last stops – places where people go to die. Yet, living within a nursing home may also bring a high degree of precarity or uncertainty not related to death. Precarity has been described as "life worlds characterized by uncertainty and insecurity and as a concept that implies both a condition and rallying point for resistance" (Grenier et al., 2020, p. 2). People living with dementia may be positioned as failing socially as a result of negative positioning by caregivers, which in turn could lead to a precarious change in room assignment or relocation to a different facility altogether.

## 2   Research Objective

The research objective was to get an in-depth perspective on social and environmental positioning through the observed experiences of an LTC resident living with dementia. Of particular interest were the ways in which objects and structures in the environment were used by the resident, staff, and other residents to negotiate or challenge social positions.

## 3   Methods

An illustrative case study (Yin, 2017) of Rosie (a pseudonym), an 86-year-old woman living with dementia in a secured LTC facility, highlights several aspects of environmental positioning and communication via space and place. An illustrative case study describes the selection and use of a descriptive example which can provide unique insight into one or more key concepts (Yin, 2017). A key criterion when selecting a case example is having sufficient, rich material related to the phenomenon of interest (Flyvbjerg, 2006) or, in this chapter, environmental positioning. Rosie's case was identified through transcripts and observational field notes that provided clear examples of how space and place were experienced and sometimes contested by Rosie and staff. It is important to note that a case does not need to be linked to the study's original research question (Yin, 2011). In fact, case studies can provide needed insight into questions that were not asked by the original study since case studies are not bound by researcher preconceptions in the data-gathering phase of a study (Merriam, 1998).

Rosie was a participant in a 6-month ethnographic study designed to better understand friendships among residents living in a dementia care unit. Data were gathered through direct observations, resident chart reviews, and interviews with staff, family, and residents (de Medeiros et al., 2011). Rosie's unit, one of three 20-person assisted living units within a large (N = 167) dementia care facility, was selected since it was anecdotally known by staff as the "highest functioning" unit, although there were no data to corroborate this. All residents in the unit had a formal diagnosis of moderate to advanced dementia and were able to complete some activities of daily living (e.g., eating, dressing) on their own or with directed assistance. They also all had a legally authorized representatives (LARs) (e.g., relative, court-appointed guardian) who made care decisions on their behalf. LARs also provided written informed consent to participate in the research. Data were obtained through video and audio recordings of public spaces within the unit (e.g., dining room area, common hallways), detailed note-taking, and one-on-one interviews. Residents provided assent before each observation or interview. The original study was approved by the author's institutional review board. Pseudonyms are used throughout.

# 4 Results

## 4.1 The Notebook

Rosie had lived in the same assisted living unit for 3 years at the time of the research. She was widowed and did not have any children. Her LAR was her nephew who did not reside locally. Table 1. includes the transcript and notes from an interaction between Rosie and a staff member involving a notebook, an environmental artifact.

According to the observational notes, lunch had finished. Residents were being directed back into the dining room for an activity. Rosie entered the dining room area at 12: 09 p.m. She picked up a staff member's notebook from an empty table. The notebook contained brief biographical details and care notes for each resident. Lines 1 through 3 capture the start of communication, whereby the staff member positions Rosie as someone who is not worth her full attention when she responds to Rosie by saying "Mmmm Hmmm" (line 3). When Rosie tries to reassert her position by posing a question to the staff member (line 4), the staff member uses a disabling response (ignoring Rosie's question, lines 5–6) to negatively position her. When Rosie persists by looking at the notebook (line 7), the staff member first questions Rosie's action (line 8) and then dismisses Rosie's ability to find her own name (line 10). When Rosie affirms that her name is in the book, the staff person tells her that whatever Rosie might be looking at is not her name, even though it is (line14). In this way, the staff person discredits Rosie's statement as false, suggesting that Rosie lacks the ability to recognize her name in the book. The staff then positions herself as even more powerful than Rosie by asking her if she knows her (the staff person's) name. She holds her nametag up for Rosie to read. Rosie does not read the name (lines 18–20) for reasons that are unclear in the transcript.

Although the staff person again ignores Rosie and begins talking to another staff person, Rosie is undeterred. Rosie asks the staff person what she is doing (line 22). This is interesting since the dining room is theoretically Rosie's living space. Instead, the staff person again asserts her position by providing Rosie a confusing

**Table 1** Interaction between Rosie and a staff member

| 1 | Rosie: | [Looks at the binder and reads aloud the name of the unit that was printed |
| 2 | | on the notebook cover] |
| 3 | Staff1: | Mmm hmm. |
| 4 | Rosie: | What do you have in there about me? |
| 5 | Staff1: | I should not get the sheet out for nobody…I'm very upset. Don't ask |
| 6 | | me. I'm very, very upset. |
| 7 | Rosie: | [Looks at a paper in the binder] |
| 8 | Staff1: | What are you looking at? |
| 9 | Rosie: | My name. |
| 10 | Staff1: | Your name is not there. |
| 11 | Rosie: | Yes it is [Rosie says firmly.] |
| 12 | Staff1: | No. |
| 13 | Rosie: | Yes it is. |
| 14 | Staff1: | That's not your name. [Staff1 is not looking at the notebook.] |
| 15 | Rosie: | [Points at the paper]: Rosie Albertson. |
| 16 | Staff1 | [Starts speaking to another staff member, ignoring Rosie] |
| 17 | Rosie: | [While looking at the notebook] I think I might have been married. |
| 18 | Staff1: | [Speaking to Rosie] Do you know my name? |
| 19 | Rosie: | No, I don't know your name. |
| 20 | Staff1: | [Holds up her name tag for Rosie to read. Rosie tries to read it but is not able to.] |
| 21 | | Shirley. [Staff1 then talks to another staff person.] |
| 22 | Rosie: | What are you supposed to be doing? |
| 23 | Staff1: | A triple. |
| 24 | Rosie: | What is it? |
| 25 | Staff1: | Triple. |
| 26 | Rosie: | Well, triple doesn't tell me anything. |
| 27 | Staff1 | [Laughs]. A double. I am working 16 hours. |
| 28 | Rosie: | And how many days? |
| 29 | Staff1: | Just 1 day. |

response related to her work shift (lines 23–27). Rosie is once again able to reassert her own power within the conversation by following up with the question, "And how many days?" (line 28). In this way, Rosie demonstrates that she is interested and capable and does have some control over her environment: She can pick up and read the notebook.

With regard to environmental positioning in this example, the rules of place are at first in conflict. The staff member attempts to assert dominance only to be challenged by Rosie. The staff member's goal of providing care to the residents was in conflict with Rosie's desire to engage in a social interaction in a space that is supposed to provide Rosie with a sense of belonging. The staff member seemed to show no regard for Rosie's interest in the notebook possibly because she didn't think that Rosie was capable of or interested in reading the information. The staff member certainly did not seem to recognize that she, the staff member, was intruding on Rosie's living space rather than the other way around.

## 4.2   Where Am I?

A few days after the previous example, Rosie was guided back to the dining area by another staff member after having her hair done at the on-site beauty parlor:

> Staff 2 (to Rosie): Sit down. (Staff 2 then has another resident, Donna, sit next to Rosie.)
> Donna (to Rosie): Good afternoon.
> Rosie: I don't know. Where in the world am I?
> Donna: The same place I am.
> Rosie: Where's that?
> Donna: A nursing home. A very nice place. How did you get here?
> Rosie: I don't know. What's this place I'm in?
> Donna: I don't know,

In this excerpt, Rosie is directed into her place (her seat) next to a potential conversational partner, Donna. Donna and Rosie try to define where they are. Donna knows it's a nursing home, although Rosie is unsure where she is. A few days later, Rosie began setting the dining room tables with plates but was told by a staff member to stop, that the dining staff would bring the food on plates. Once again, Rosie was trying to be actively involved in her living space but was prevented from doing so by staff.

## 4.3   The Easter Card

Later in the month, Rosie was again unsure of where she was:

> [Rosie has an Easter card that says it's from her sister, but Rosie insists that she doesn't have a sister. She does not according to her files. Rosie reads the card aloud, but the other residents and staff aren't listening.]
> Rosie: Can someone tell me where we are? Don't all speak at once.
> A few seconds later:
> Rosie: Can someone enlighten me as to where we are?
> Daniel (a resident): I don't know the name of the place.

In this example, it is unclear whether Rosie may have picked up someone else's Easter's card, since she did not have a sister, or if staff gave her the wrong card, but the staff did not respond to her question. As in the previous example with Donna, Daniel does not know the name of the place. Whereas the staff could have provided him with the name and more of an explanation of where they were, they did not, making it difficult for Rosie to make sense of her space and place.

## *4.4   The Kitchen Remodel*

Approximately 3 months into the study, the kitchen area in the assisted living unit was remodeled. The kitchen and surrounding dining room were the center point between two corridors of resident rooms. The kitchen area functioned as a thoroughfare for residents to access a living room, located to the right of the kitchen area. Prior to the remodel, the kitchen featured an open design, whereby residents could pass from one side of the kitchen to the other in several spots. A counter-height, half-wall enabled residents to see across the dining room to the living.

Part of the kitchen remodel involved raising the height and depth of the half-wall and closing the shortcut through the kitchen. These changes closed off residents' access to the kitchen area and created a barrier between the two corridors of resident room hallways. Residents who lived to the right of the kitchen could still access the living room. However, residents on the left side were no longer able to see the living room and therefore were not able navigate across the kitchen area. This reduced their physical space and their social world. Seating arrangements during meals also changed following the remodel. The ten residents from hallway A now exclusively ate together at one side of the kitchen, while the ten residents from hallway B sat at the opposite side. The care facility's official reason for the change was to reduce the spread of germs and make it easier to locate residents for medications. In practice, the remodel reduced the residents' access to other residents with whom to socialize, from 20 residents to 10 residents.

Four months after the kitchen remodel, Rosie began a relationship with a male resident, Robert, one of the nine other people from her side of the hallway. In one observed conversation, Rosie sat by Robert, held up a leaf that was used in an earlier activity, and asked him, "Does this belong to you?"

"No," Robert said. "It belongs on the tree," to which Rosie laughed and responded, "Well run out there and put it on the tree."

Over the course of the next several weeks, Rosie and Robert spent much of their time together, sitting next to each other at meals, during facility-led activities, and nonscheduled free time. Through this relationship, Rosie seemed to have gained some control over her own space by spending time with a resident of her choice. Despite there being no objections to the relationship by Rosie's and Robert's family members, staff became uncomfortable. They said that the relationship interfered with their ability to perform caregiving tasks, especially at night when staff needed to prepare residents for bedtime. They often separated Rosie and Robert for reasons that were not made clear.

## 4.5 Rosie Is Transferred

Around 1 month after the kitchen remodel (3 weeks after meeting Robert), Rosie was transferred without notice to another assisted living unit within the facility. At first, Rosie's care chart provided no official reason for the transfer. When asked, nursing staff said that Rosie was relocated because her dementia had worsened. This seemed unlikely to the researchers since they had not recorded any cognitive changes in a recent series of assessments with her. Later, however, a staff member confided to one of the researchers that Rosie was relocated to make room for a new person whose family wanted him to live in the "highest functioning" unit. When the researcher suggested that Charles, a nonverbal and nonmobile resident, would have seemed to have been the more appropriate person to move given due to his functional abilities compared to Rosie's, the staff member explained that it was easier to get Rosie's nephew to agree to a move than Charles' daughter.

After a week of being in the new unit, Rosie was documented in her care chart as being "isolative during adjustment period" and that "there has been a decrease in her eating and weight recently." A few weeks later, another care provider noted that Rosie was "more depressed, isolative, less activity participation since moving," that she had lost 5.5 pounds, and that she remained in her room much of the time. Unfortunately, Rosie was ultimately positioned as less important than Charles because of potential advocacy of a family member rather than ability. Since Rosie had no way of finding or accessing her former living unit within the larger facility, her relationship with Robert was terminated by environmental and social barriers enforced by staff. Despite resisting being treated as "other" within her "home" on several occasions, the final move to a new unit where most of the residents were in advanced stages of dementia and unable to communicate positioned her in a way that she could not effectively counter. The precarity of her living situation which resulted in her being removed from her familiar surroundings led to her rapid decline.

## 5 Discussion

The chapter has argued that a key aspect of place involves communication; communication is an important way that power and social positions are negotiated, challenged, and resisted. One way to understand how speakers communicate power to their conversational partners is through positioning theory, which considers how speech practices (e.g., word choice, tone) assert one's identity in relation to another. For example, a nursing home employee who addresses a resident as "sweetie" is positioning the resident as childlike: endearing but in need of help. Subsequently, the resident's response can be to challenge the staff member's position (e.g., "Don't call me 'sweetie.' My name is Mary.") or to support it by not responding. How residents living with dementia in LTCFs are positioned within conversations is often overlooked. However, even the smallest acts of conversation can provide insight into the social standing of residents and staff within LTCFs.

In addition to understanding more about power construction through conversational practice, it is also important to consider how environmental features contribute to conversations and ultimately to power. Environmental positioning considers the ways that structures can facilitate or hinder what types of communication are possible. It considers space and place with regard to social positions. For example, on the one hand, nursing homes are places of employment; nursing home staff are charged with ensuring the safety and care of the residents. Staff can come and go at will. They decide when residents eat, what activities will take place, who will sit by whom, who will be relocated to a different room, and so on. On the other hand, nursing homes are a particular type of place with homelike spaces where residents live. Home implies a sense of familiarity, belonging, safety, comfort, choice, and personal control (Eijkelenboom et al., 2017; van Hoof et al., 2016). Residents like Rosie who ask other residents "Where in the world am I?" might receive an answer such as "The same place … A nursing home" or "I don't know the name of the place." As these conversations illustrate, the nursing home is a place but not a home where residents feel a sense of belonging or familiarity. This reinforcement of place rather than home could also be seen in the description of Rosie being told by staff to stop setting the table. In this example, Rosie was trying to exercise some control over her environment by participating in a familiar task – setting the table – but was reminded that she had little control over her space. Since residents don't have much control over their space, it begs the question of whether the goal of a creating a home environment within nursing homes is appropriate or if another environmental strategy would be better suited. More specifically, given that a person visiting (or living at) a hotel expects to be waited upon by staff, a resort model, rather than one based on an unrealistic idea of home, might be more satisfying and more desirable to residents. Environmentally, it might do a better job of communicating position within space than the illusion of home.

Consider some of the other examples of staff challenging Rosie's actions within her "home" such as the notebook left by staff on a dining room table. The staff member negatively positions Rosie through her responses and does not seem to appreciate that the notebook was placed in an area that was supposed to be Rosie's (and other residents') dining room. To the staff member, the dining room was one of many workspaces that she was responsible for. Despite the staff member's conversational rebuffs, Rosie resists the negative positioning and asserts herself as a capable person in the environment. As mentioned earlier, the tension between spaces within nursing homes functioning as work versus home can be seen in the staff/resident interaction within the environment. A worktable to a staff person is a dining table to a resident.

The kitchen remodel is a good example of how a change to the physical space created change in social opportunities for residents. Because of the raised wall (which was formerly counter-height) and the sealed access to the kitchen, residents experienced a profound truncation of their physical and social world. Although there was still a small walkway from one side of the dining room to the other and to living room, many residents could not spatially navigate the change. In this way, the environmental features of the newly remodeled kitchen negatively positioned them while positively positioning staff. Staff could now secure the kitchen, which could potentially lead to better protection of the residents against harm such as germ exposure. However, resident safety came at a social cost and further reinforced the notion of institution versus home. It is therefore important to strike a balance between ensuring the safety of residents while also providing social spaces. Considerations may include creating spaces with lower barrier walls that could serve as compartmental meeting areas for residents while also providing staff with the ability to monitor residents' safety. Such smaller social spaces could also help families and visitors experience a sense of having more privacy (Van Hoof et al., 2016).

The sense of precarity embedded within the institutional structure is another aspect to consider with regard to LTCFs. Despite often being challenged or ignored by staff, Rosie did develop friendships and relationships with others in the care unit. Unfortunately, she was ultimately moved without warning to make room for someone new. Although staff used the language of expert opinion (i.e., declining cognition) to justify the move, their reason was actually based on convenience since Rosie's nephew was not actively involved in her care. Such disregard for Rosie's wishes and her place within the environment underscores the unconscious bias that institution hold, reinforcing the message, explicitly or implicitly, that residents are not really people in a full moral sense but rather bodies living that can be controlled for their "own good."

A bold approach to creating environments that could address the social needs for residents through space would be to have architects, designers, and staff member spend a day living like a resident – being restricted to same spaces, having to rely on another for food, being guided on where to sit, and having to look at all the cues of place that reinforce position. While this would certainly be a fabricated situation and differs in myriad ways from an actual resident's experience, it may provide insight into the importance of place and space in communicative interactions. It would also give nonresidents the opportunity to communicate with residents outside of providing care-related tasks, which may also provide a deeper sense of empathy and understanding of the lived environment.

Another approach is to include people living with dementia who are living in LTCFs in the co-design of physical and social spaces. As stated earlier, most people who live in nursing homes did not choose to do so. Most people who are not living with dementia cannot imagine what their lives would be like with dementia or the challenges that they may face in LTCFs. Living with dementia in an LTCF is an experience that only truly be understood by people who are living it. In addition, although some people living with dementia experience some challenges with language, language change alone should not be a reason for excluding their perspectives. As noted earlier in the chapter, language abilities, and loss in communicative abilities, differ among individuals and by types of dementia. As the case example of Rosie illustrated, she was able to communicate quite effectively even though staff did not acknowledge her abilities and insight. Imagine if the staff member would have asked Rosie what she thought of the dining room, if she felt like she belonged, or what would make her environment more comfortable or satisfying for her.

Overall, LTC settings must move beyond rigidly controlled, oversight models that emphasize on controlled safety and interactions and policies that restrict communicative and social possibilities for residents. With its emphasis on detailed observations aimed at better understanding how social worlds evolve within the environmental confines of institutional settings, ethnographic-type research allow investigator to rely less on staff input and more so on ways place and space impact interactions, power, and well-being of these residents. To be successful, this approach involves partnerships between architects, designers, stakeholders (i.e., administrators, staff, residents, families, and future potential residents) who can sit back, observe, and design environments that equalize power differences, allowing one party (e.g., staff, administrators) to consider the in-depth needs of others.

## 6 Conclusion

How place is communicated to and by people within nursing homes is greatly affected by what is contained within spaces. Overall, if we truly are going to rethink how to move forward in considering LTC environments, we need to reconsider the "person" as an active participant in their environment, not as an object to be cared for or objects of activities we provide or move. By recognizing how dialogues are shaped by space and power within space, we can better consider how the built environment directly influences the lived environment. This means inviting residents to be co-creators in their space and in their social interactions. It also means challenging nonresidents involved in decision-making about space to become residents, even for a short time, to truly appreciate what it means to live in a particular place like a nursing home.

**Acknowledgments** This research was funded by the Alzheimer's Association, NIRG-08-91765.

## References

Adams, T., & Gardiner, P. (2005). Communication and interaction within dementia care triads: Developing a theory for relationship-centred care. *Dementia, 4*(2), 185–205. https://doi.org/10.1177/1471301205051092

Agich, G. (2003). *Dependence and autonomy in old age: An ethical framework for long-term care.* Cambridge University Press. https://doi.org/10.1177/1471301205051092

Andrews, G. J., Cutchin, M., McCracken, K., Phillips, D. R., & Wiles, J. (2007). Geographical gerontology: The constitution of a discipline. *Social Science & Medicine, 65*(1), 151–168. https://doi.org/10.1016/j.socscimed.2007.02.047

Andrews, G. J., Cutchin, M. P., & Skinner, M. W. (2017). Space and place in geographical gerontology: Theoretical traditions, formations of hope. In M. W. Skinner, G. J. Andrews,

& M. P. Cutchin (Eds.), *Geographical gerontology: Perspectives, concepts, approaches* (pp. 11–28). Routledge. https://doi.org/10.4324/9781315281216-2

Bangerter, L. R., Van Haitsma, K., Heid, A. R., & Abbott, K. (2016). Make me feel at ease and at home: Differential care preferences of nursing home residents. *The Gerontologist, 56*(4), 702–713. https://doi.org/10.1093/geront/gnv026

Bartlett, R., & O'Connor, D. (2010). *Broadening the dementia debate: Towards social citizenship.* Policy Press. https://doi.org/10.2307/j.ctt9qgmrg

Behuniak, S. M. (2011). The living dead? The construction of people with Alzheimer's disease as zombies. Ageing & Society, *31*(1), 70–92. https://doi.org/10.1017/S0144686X10000693.

Bruens, M. T. (2013). Dementia beyond structures of medicalisation and cultural neglect. In J. Baars & J. Dohmen (Eds.), *Ageing, meaning and social structure. Connecting critical and humanistic gerontology* (pp. 81–96). Policy Press. https://doi.org/10.1332/policypress/9781447300908.003.0005

Chaudhury, H., Cooke, H. A., Cowie, H., & Razaghi, L. (2018). The influence of the physical environment on residents with dementia in long-term care settings: A review of the empirical literature. *The Gerontologist, 58*(5), e325–e337. https://doi.org/10.1093/geront/gnw259

Coupland, N., Coupland, J., Giles, H., & Henwood, K. (1988). Accommodating the elderly: Invoking and extending a theory 1. *Language in Society, 17*(1), 1–41. https://doi.org/10.1017/S0047404500012574

Cresswell, T. (2009). *Place International encyclopedia of human geography* (Vol. 8, pp. 169–177). Elsevier.

Cuba, L., & Hummon, D. M. (1993). A place to call home: Identification with dwelling, community, and region. *Sociological Quarterly, 34*(1), 111–131. https://doi.org/10.1111/j.1533-8525.1993.tb00133.x

Cutchin, M. P., Owen, S. V., & Chang, P.-F. J. (2003). Becoming "at home" in assisted living residences: Exploring place integration processes. *The Journals of Gerontology Series B: Psychological Sciences and Social Sciences, 58*(4), S234–S243. https://doi.org/10.1093/geronb/58.4.S234

de Medeiros, K., & Sabat, S. (2016). Understanding the person with Alzheimer's disease from a cause and consequence perspective. In F. Moghaddam & R. Harré (Eds.), *Questioning causality: Explorations and causes and consequences across contexts* (pp. 221–236). ABC-CLIO.

de Medeiros, K., Beall, E., Vozzella, S., & Brandt, J. (2009). Television viewing and people with dementia living in long-term care: A pilot study. *Journal of Applied Gerontology, 28*(5), 638–648. https://doi.org/10.1177/0733464808330964

de Medeiros, K., Saunders, P. A., Doyle, P. J., Mosby, A., & Haitsma, K. V. (2011, September 20). Friendships among people with dementia in long-term care. *Dementia*. https://doi.org/10.1177/1471301211421186

de Medeiros, K., Rubinstein, R. L., & Doyle, P. (2013). A place of one's own: Reinterpreting the meaning of home among childless older women. In G. Rowles & M. Bernard (Eds.), *Environmental gerontology: Making meaning places in old age* (pp. 79–104). Springer.

Doyle, P. J., de Medeiros, K., & Saunders, P. A. (2012). Nested social groups within the social environment of a dementia care assisted living setting. *Dementia, 11*(3), 383–399. https://doi.org/10.1177/1471301211421188

Duan, Y., Mueller, C. A., Yu, F., & Talley, K. M. (2020). The effects of nursing home culture change on resident quality of life in US nursing homes: An integrative review. *Research in Gerontological Nursing, 13*(4), 210–224. https://doi.org/10.3928/19404921-20200115-02

Eijkelenboom, A., Verbeek, H., Felix, E., & van Hoof, J. (2017). Architectural factors influencing the sense of home in nursing homes: An operationalization for practice. *Frontiers of Architectural Research, 6*(2), 111–122. https://doi.org/10.1016/j.foar.2017.02.004

Flyvbjerg, B. (2006). Five misunderstandings about case-study research. *Qualitative Inquiry, 12*(2), 219–245.

Fraser, K. C., Meltzer, J. A., & Rudzicz, F. (2016). Linguistic features identify Alzheimer's disease in narrative speech. *Journal of Alzheimer's Disease, 49*(2), 407–422. https://doi.org/10.3233/JAD-150520

Giles, H. (2016). *Communication accommodation theory: Negotiating personal relationships and social identities across contexts.* Cambridge University Press. https://doi.org/10.1017/CBO9781316226537

Goffman, E. (1958). Characteristics of total institutions. *Symposium on preventive and social psychiatry.* The National Academies Press. https://doi.org/10.17226/20228.

Goffman, E. (2009). *Stigma: Notes on the management of spoiled identity.* Simon and Schuster.

Gove, D., Downs, M., Vernooij-Dassen, M., & Small, N. (2016). Stigma and GPs' perceptions of dementia. *Aging & Mental Health, 20*(4), 391–400. https://doi.org/10.1080/13607863.2015.1015962

Grenier, A., Phillipson, C., & Setterston, R., Jr. (2020). *Precarity and ageing: Understanding insecurity and risk in later life.* Bristol University Press. https://doi.org/10.1332/policypress/9781447340850.001.0001

Grubman, J. F. (2015). Methods for managing risk and promoting resident-centered care in nursing homes. *Columbia Journal of Law & Social Problems, 49*, 217–249.

Harre, R., & van Langenhove, L. (1999). *Positioning theory: Moral contexts of intentional action.* Blackwell Publishers.

Harré, R., & Van Langenhove, L. (1999). Positioning theory. *The Discursive Turn in Social Psychology*, 129–136.

Kemper, S. (1994). Elderspeak: Speech accommodations to older adults. *Aging and Cognition, 1*(1), 17–28. https://doi.org/10.1080/09289919408251447

Kitwood, T. (1997). *Dementia care reconsidered: The person comes first.* Open University Press.

Klimova, B., & Kuca, K. (2016). Speech and language impairments in dementia. *Journal of Applied Biomedicine, 14*(2), 97–103. https://doi.org/10.1016/j.jab.2016.02.002

Kontos, P., Radnofsky, M. L., Fehr, P., Belleville, M. R., Bottenberg, F., Fridley, M., Massad, S., Grigorovich, A., Carson, J., & Rogenski, K. (2021). Separate and unequal: A time to reimagine dementia. *Journal of Alzheimer's Disease, 80*(4), 1395–1399. https://doi.org/10.3233/JAD-210057

Koren, M. J. (2010). Person-centered care for nursing home residents: The culture-change movement. *Health Affairs, 29*(2), 312–317. https://doi.org/10.1377/hlthaff.2009.0966

McParland, P., Kelly, F., & Innes, A. (2017). Dichotomising dementia: Is there another way? *Sociology of Health & Illness, 39*(2), 258–269. https://doi.org/10.1111/1467-9566.12438

Merriam, S. B. (1998). Qualitative research and case study applications in education. In *Case study research in education.* Wiley.

Moore, K. D. (2014). An ecological framework of place: Situating environmental gerontology within a life course perspective. *The International Journal of Aging and Human Development, 79*(3), 183–209. https://doi.org/10.2190/AG.79.3.a

Mueller, K. D., Hermann, B., Mecollari, J., & Turkstra, L. S. (2018). Connected speech and language in mild cognitive impairment and Alzheimer's disease: A review of picture description tasks. *Journal of Clinical and Experimental Neuropsychology, 40*(9), 917–939. https://doi.org/10.1080/13803395.2018.1446513

Oswald, F., & Wahl, H.-W. (2005). Dimensions of the meaning of home in later life. In *Home and identity in late life: International perspectives* (pp. 21–45). Springer.

Reed-Danahay, D. (2001). 'This is your home now!': Conceptualizing location and dislocation in a dementia unit. *Qualitative Research, 1*(1), 47–63. https://doi.org/10.1177/146879410100100103

Rubinstein, R. L., & de Medeiros, K. (2003). Ecology and the aging self. In H.-W. Wahl, R. J. Schiedt, & P. G. Windely (Eds.), *Annual review of gerontology and geriatrics* (Vol. 23, pp. 59–82). Springer.

Rubinstein, R. L., & de Medeiros, K. (2005). Home, self, and identity. In G. D. Rowles & H. Chaudhury (Eds.), *Home and identity in late life international perspectives* (pp. 47–62). Springer.

Sabat, S. R. (2006). Mind, meaning, and personhood in dementia: The effects of positioning. In J. Hughes, S. Louw, & S. Sabat (Eds.), *Dementia: Mind, meaning, and the person* (pp. 287–301). Oxford University Press. https://doi.org/10.1093/med/9780198566151.003.0018

Sabat, S. R., & Lee, J. M. (2011, September 20, 2011). Relatedness among people diagnosed with dementia: Social cognition and the possibility of friendship. *Dementia*. https://doi.org/10.1177/1471301211421069.

Sabat, S. R., Johnson, A., Swarbrick, C., & Keady, J. (2011). The 'demented other' or simply 'a person'? Extending the philosophical discourse of Naue and Kroll through the situated self. *Nursing Philosophy, 12*(4), 282–292. http://onlinelibrary.wiley.com/doi/10.1111/j.1466-769X.2011.00485.x/abstract

Saunders, P. A., de Medeiros, K., Doyle, P., & Mosby, A. (2011). The discourse of friendship: Mediators of communication among dementia residents in long-term care. *Dementia, 11*(3), 347–361. https://doi.org/10.1177/1471301211421187

Savundranayagam, M. Y., & Moore-Nielsen, K. (2015). Language-based communication strategies that support person-centered communication with persons with dementia. *International Psychogeriatrics, 27*(10), 1707–1718. https://doi.org/10.1017/S1041610215000903

van Hoof, J., Verbeek, H., Janssen, B. M., et al. (2016). A three perspective study of the sense of home of nursing home residents: The views of residents, care professionals and relatives. *BMC Geriatrics, 16*, 16. https://doi.org/10.1186/s12877-016-0344-9

Wang, G., Marradi, C., Albayrak, A., & van der Cammen, T. J. (2019). Co-designing with people with dementia: A scoping review of involving people with dementia in design research. *Maturitas, 127*, 55–63. https://doi.org/10.1016/j.maturitas.2019.06.003

Ward, R., Vass, A. A., Aggarwal, N., Garfield, C., & Cybyk, B. (2008). A different story: Exploring patterns of communication in residential dementia care. *Ageing & Society, 28*(5), 629–651. https://doi.org/10.1017/S0144686X07006927

White-Chu, E. F., Graves, W. J., Godfrey, S. M., Bonner, A., & Sloane, P. (2009). Beyond the medical model: The culture change revolution in long-term care. *Journal of the American Medical Directors Association, 10*(6), 370–378. https://doi.org/10.1016/j.jamda.2009.04.004

Williams, K., Kemper, S., & Hummert, M. L. (2003). Improving nursing home communication: An intervention to reduce elderspeak. *The Gerontologist, 43*(2), 242–247. https://doi.org/10.1093/geront/43.2.242

Williams, K. N., Herman, R., Gajewski, B., & Wilson, K. (2009). Elderspeak communication: Impact on dementia care. *American Journal of Alzheimer's Disease & Other Dementias, 24*(1), 11–20.

Yin, R. K. (2011). *Applications of case study research*. Sage.

Yin, R. K. (2017). *Case study research and applications: Design and methods*. Sage.

Young, T. J., Manthorp, C., Howells, D., & Tullo, E. (2011). Developing a carer communication intervention to support personhood and quality of life in dementia. *Ageing & Society, 31*(6), 1003–1025. https://doi.org/10.1017/S0144686X10001182

# Adaptive Reuse of Closed Malls for Dementia Programs and Services: Community Focus Group Feedback

Emily Roberts and Heather Carlile Carter

## 1 Introduction

It is estimated that 5.4 million Americans have some form of dementia, and these numbers are expected to rise in the coming decades, leading to an unprecedented demand for memory care housing and services (Alzheimer's Association, 2020). In biomedical terms, dementia is not a disease, but a syndrome produced in large part by diseases such as Alzheimer's, Parkinson's, and vascular disease, with a cluster of symptoms and signs linked to the deterioration of cognitive abilities as a person ages (Haeusermann, 2018). The double societal hit of dementia and infectious disease outbreaks like the COVID-19 pandemic have raised a convergence of concerns for the future of care settings for people living with dementia (Wang et al., 2020).

People living with dementia need help with their daily activities in order to enable them to live safely and with dignity; therefore central to the ethics of dementia care is enhancing well-being and making the most of the strengths that are still present within the person (Rabig, 2009).

Yet often those living with dementia may be institutionalized, frequently with negative outcomes, as the individual with dementia becomes further disconnected from home, family, community, and activities with daily meaning (Black et al., 2013). These institutional environments are confining in design and size, with little access to outdoor spaces and other amenities (Roberts & Pulay, 2018). While it is

Part of this chapter is published in Roberts, E., & Carter, H. C. (2020). Making the Case for Centralized Dementia Care Through Adaptive Reuse in the Time of COVID-19. *INQUIRY: a journal of medical care organization, provision and financing, 57*, 46958020969305. https://doi.org/10.1177/0046958020969305. Used with permission of SAGE.

E. Roberts (✉) · H. C. Carter
Oklahoma State University, Stillwater, OK, USA
e-mail: emily.roberts12@okstate.edu

© The Author(s), under exclusive license to Springer Nature Switzerland AG 2023
F. Ferdous, E. Roberts (eds.), *(Re)designing the Continuum of Care for Older Adults*, https://doi.org/10.1007/978-3-031-20970-3_11

imperative that vulnerable populations are provided care settings which allow for support of their physical and mental health, dementia care settings more often are known to increase resident isolation and depression (Roberts, 2018). Through focus group feedback from architects and developers, this chapter describes the potential for adaptive reuse of closed malls for dementia programs and services to support innovation in memory care settings.

## 1.1   Supporting Autonomy in Dementia Care

In light of  images in the media of older adults in care settings confined to a single or shared room, autonomy is starting to be seen as an overarching problem in care settings, not only because institutions limit freedom, but because of the existential conditions that create the need for care rail against the autonomy of independent self-sufficiency (Agich, 2003). Barrett et al. (2019) describe a holistic approach to dementia care in which the impact of multiple dimensions are individually targeted in specific environments, and one innovative example of a holistic approach is the European dementia village model.

### 1.1.1   The Netherlands Dementia Village

The first dementia village (DV) opened in Holland in 2009, offering a new care model providing medical and psychosocial care in a community setting without the hospital façade. Several other European countries have since adopted this model (Chrysikou et al., 2018). The DV model allows for autonomy and continuation of patterns of daily living through housing integrated with large exterior walkways and gardens, restaurants, a grocery store, pub, and theater. The Dutch DV is home to 150 residents and encompasses 4 acres in familiar and normal surroundings, with multiple households of 8–10 individuals (Archer, 2012). DV residents live in a secure setting having access to the medical attention they may need while continuing to receive the daily stimulation from exercising outside and attending classes and clubs (Glass, 2014). This is an important distinction between the traditional care facilities we find in the United States which do not provide these broader amenities, particularly for residents with dementia who are often living in locked buildings without opportunities for indoor/outdoor experiences.

To date, there have been no other developments at the scale of the DV model in the United States, as care providers may not have the appropriately sized property to offer multiple activities and advanced medical services for residents, nor the funding to develop them. Providers are also concerned about the bottom-line costs associated with new construction for a care setting of this scope. One potential solution, therefore, may relate directly to the perennial challenge of care providers, planners, and designers: *how do we design with what we have?*

# 2  Adaptive Reuse for Community Healthcare Needs

In the healthcare industry, when patient volume outstrips capacity, the need for expansion initiatives carries significant costs. Adaptive reuse—the practice of identifying, acquiring, renovating, and placing back into service a building or similar structure for a purpose different than that for which it was originally designed—offers great potential for addressing the spatial expansion needs of healthcare establishments in a unique and mutually beneficial manner (Conejos et al., 2011; Elrod & Fortenberry, 2017).

Significant discussions have come out of the COVID-19 pandemic throughout the healthcare industry and governmental agencies about the conversion of existing hotels, community centers, convention centers, and other large unoccupied commercial buildings into quarantine or general patient care spaces. If the built space does not require significant structural reconstruction, rehabilitation may be timelier and less expensive than razing the building and rebuilding with ground-up construction (Amlani et al., 2020). In addition, recycling materials, reusing structural elements, and reducing demolition waste support material conservation, environmental sustainability, and a circular economy (Tan et al., 2020). Similarly, adaptive reuse of commercial properties may prove to be a viable option for the large sites required for developments similar to the DV. In particular, reuse of vacant urban malls may provide sites and space for mixed-use developments which include programs, medical services, and attached housing (CommONEnergy, 2017).

## 2.1  Mall Adaptations

Malls are buildings or complexes of buildings designed and built to contain many interconnected activities in different areas (CommONEnergy, 2017). These sites have a meaningful urban and social impact. Yet due to the 2008 economic downturn and online shopping, current forecasts suggest 10% of the nation's 1500 enclosed malls will have permanently closed by 2022 (Corroto & Richardson, 2019). In addition, the economic fallout from COVID-19 is also affecting those retailers that were already in dire circumstances before the current pandemic hit, possibly resulting in higher rates of closures than previously forecasted (Bodamer, 2020).

The regulatory and financing structures for vacant urban malls are evolving in a way that should allow more of these properties to be repurposed in a productive way (Dunham-Jones & Williamson, 2011). Mall demolition is costly, and demolition waste in landfills is environmentally unsustainable. In 2017, 569 million tons of total demolition debris were generated in the United States (EPA, 2019).

Consequently, property owners and developers are looking for other options for closed malls (Guimaraes & Porfirio, 2019), yet converting malls into different place types, which are not automatic referents to their previous built lives, is challenging for designers (Voien, 2017). In addition to structural issues, physical attributes influence the decision to convert malls into different occupancy types. Considerations include building type, aesthetic appeal, dimensional flexibility, physical footprint, and floor plan size. Even in the face of these challenges, repurposed, closed mall sites are currently thriving as medical centers, data centers, churches, colleges, apartments, office spaces, and mixed-use developments (Peterson, 2015). From the vantage point of land-use, vacated malls are full of adaptive possibilities (Burtch, 2017), and with extensive parking lots, malls are situated on large land parcels at easily accessible locations (Garreau, 2008).

## 2.2   Example Mall Conversion Sites

Several existing case studies demonstrate the environmental and social benefits that make adaptive reuse attractive to a variety of stakeholders (Burtch, 2017; Kohlstedt, 2016; Matchar, 2017; Peterson, 2015). For example, Vanderbilt University Medical Center expanded its size—approximately 440,000 square feet—by converting mall space into an additional campus with outpatient facilities, offices, an employee childcare center, and a fitness center (Burtch, 2017). Other malls are being redeveloped into mixed-use (hotels, gyms, apartment complexes, and grocery stores) lifestyle centers (Burtch, 2017).

## 3   The Dementia-Friendly City Center

The current challenge for our nation's long-term care system is to provide care settings which ensure autonomy for individuals to continue with preferred activities while at the same to supporting infection control (Zimmerman et al., 2016). The confined living arrangements and group activities of traditional dementia care, combined with understaffing and failure to comply with infection-control guidelines, are associated with high infection and disease transfer rates (Amlani et al., 2020; Glass, 2014).

### 3.1   A Convergence of Factors

In looking for innovative solutions to current issues around dementia care, there are a convergence of factors that are indicative of the societal needs moving forward. These factors include the growing numbers of older adults with dementia that will need care, the need for sustainable building practices as the impact of global climate change continues to impact our planet, and growing numbers of closed mall properties that will either need to be repurposed or torn down (Fig. 1).

This convergence of factors had led the research team to propose that malls may become sustainable **dementia-friendly city centers (DFCC),** as the internal

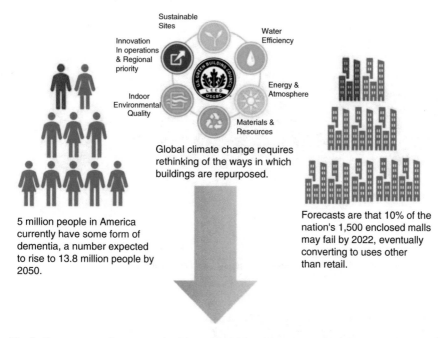

Sustainable Sites

Water Efficiency

Innovation In operations & Regional priority

Indoor Environmental Quality

Energy & Atmosphere

Materials & Resources

Global climate change requires rethinking of the ways in which buildings are repurposed.

5 million people in America currently have some form of dementia, a number expected to rise to 13.8 million people by 2050.

Forecasts are that 10% of the nation's 1,500 enclosed malls may fail by 2022, eventually converting to uses other than retail.

**Fig. 1** Convergence of current societal factors requiring innovative solutions

infrastructure is in place in existing mall structures for lighting, heating, and cooling systems, with varied spatial configuration of public spaces. Programming such as art and music venues, indoor/outdoor garden spaces, theaters, dining areas, and attached housing can link with core services, integrating into the larger DFCC (Fig. 2).

With adaptive reuse of malls for the DFCC model, there is also ample space for on-site core medical services as well as a quarantine center enabling staff to make decisions that address testing, isolation, and infection control on-site on an integrated campus. These and other medical services may be provided by a local healthcare network, and other site programming may be funded by local, state, and federal funds, similar to those available for the national Program for All Inclusive Care for the Elderly (PACE). The need for an integrated health and wellness model to address infection control represents the final piece in the convergence of factors leading to the planning of the DFCC model of care (Fig. 3).

## 3.2  The DFCC Case Study Site

Research into the DFCC model began with the development of architectural plans and renderings for a 800,000 square foot mall located in a mid-size Midwestern city. This mall site originally opened in 1974 and ceased operation in 2017 after several failed attempts at re-branding. The DFCC case study designs include an integrated

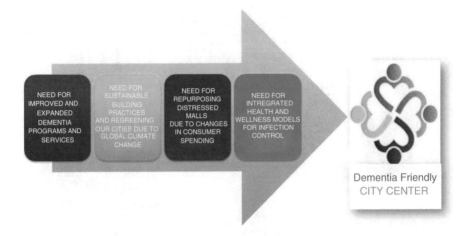

**Fig. 2** Factors embedded in the dementia-friendly city center model

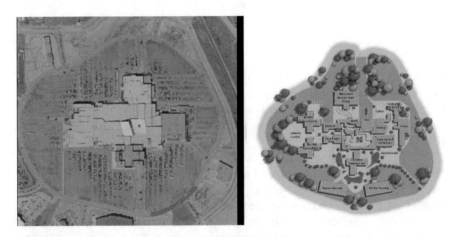

**Fig. 3** Existing closed mall site and conceptual site plan for the DFCC model of care

medical complex which will provide general medical care, as well as a specialized medical and quarantine unit. Also included in the design are a supermarket, library, full-service restaurant, and several outdoor areas for eating and socializing. Pedestrian streetscapes with secure entrances connect adjacent housing, and the removal of several sections of the existing roof provides large secure courtyards (Fig. 4). Three stages of purpose-built memory care housing are proposed, including independent living apartments for caregiver/care recipient dyads, assisted living, and 24/7 memory care. All are connected to the city center amenities through pedestrian walkways.

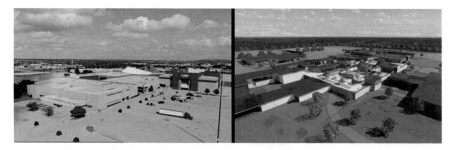

**Fig. 4** Birdseye view of closed mall site and the case study DFCC

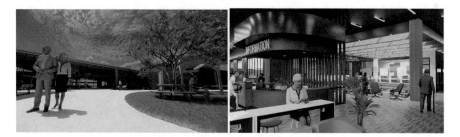

**Fig. 5** DFCC site opportunities for indoor/outdoor engagement

# 4 Methods

Following the development of DFCC case study plans and renderings, a community dementia care workshop was held with 65 attendees from several stakeholder groups including (1) medical providers, (2) independent living retirement home residents, (3) architects and developers, (4) dementia program and service providers, and (5) family caregivers. During the workshop the attendees were introduced to the DFCC concept and in the weeks following the workshop, attendees were sent a follow-up email requesting their participation in a focus group relating to their area of interest in smaller more directed conversations. Interested individuals received written information sheets about the research and consent forms to sign if they wished to participate. Those participants were then assigned a specific focus group relating to their area of interest, and the researchers chose to analyze focus groups separately due to the different content and focus in the questions. This chapter specifically focusses on the outcomes from the architect/developer focus group discussion involving the benefits and barriers to adaptive reuse of commercial properties to support vulnerable populations through the lens of building professionals. Previous focus group outcomes have been reported with the medical provider themes which include the spectrum of programming, on-site medical care, and applicability of the DFCC concept to the medical profession (Roberts et al., 2020) and independent living, service provider and family caregivers themes which include maintaining family connections, community education and acceptance, staffing, and resident adaptation (Roberts & Shehadeh, 2021) (Fig. 5).

The research questions which align with the architect/developer perspectives on adaptive reuse of malls for dementia programs and services include:

1. What are the key opportunities in creating a sustainable city center solution for residents living with dementia using the adaptive reuse of a mall structure?
2. What are the key barriers in creating a sustainable city center solution for residents living with dementia using the adaptive reuse of a mall structure?
3. What are the types of innovative community public/private partnerships which can be created for mixed-use developments?

## 4.1 Architect/Developer Focus Group

Focus group research is characterized by homogeneity, but with sufficient variation among participants to allow for contrasting opinions (Stewart & Shamdasni, 2014). The intent of focus groups is not to infer but to understand and provide insights about how people in groups perceive a situation appropriate to the purpose of the research. The architect/developer focus group was comprised of two male architects (A1, A2) and two male senior living developers (D1, D2) all who had attended the previously held community workshop. The focus group was conducted by a member of the research team at a community conference center and lasted 1 hour. Each participant had an opportunity to answer all of the ten protocol questions which were approved by the University Institutional Review Board with follow-up questions when a specific topic needed further investigation or detail (see Table 1).

**Table 1** Architect/developer focus group protocol

| Number | Question |
|--------|----------|
| 1 | Can you please share your initial reaction to the dementia-friendly city center concept? |
| 2 | Please share any experiences that you have with a family member with dementia. |
| 3 | Please share your experiences in retrofitting large commercial sites including enclosed malls. |
| 4 | What are the opportunities which you see in retrofitting existing enclosed malls for projects such as the dementia-friendly city center? |
| 5 | What are the barriers which you see in retrofitting existing enclosed malls for projects such as the dementia-friendly city center? |
| 6 | Using the case study mall site in the images on the easels, what are your initial ideas on the scalability of a site such as this for cost control? |
| 7 | What opportunities do you see for sustainable practices such as energy use, rain capture systems, and repurposing the existing infrastructure? |
| 8 | What barriers do you see for sustainable practices? |
| 9 | Do you have any suggestions on existing projects or sites that would be good points of references for a project of this scale? |
| 10 | Would you like to be a part of further research and design for this and future dementia centers? |

The questions and answers were audio recorded and then transcribed verbatim. Pseudonyms were then assigned to participants to ensure their confidentiality. An inductive content analysis was then used (Stewart & Shamdasni, 2014), with words, sentences, or strings of words that conveyed the same meaning assigned to essence-capture the codes. This allowed new themes to be identified from the transcription. Strategies used to enhance the trustworthiness of the findings included all researchers participating in coding and categorizing the findings. Disagreements in these processes were solved by discussions and consensus between the researchers. Quotes from participants were used to illustrate the themes and to keep the interpretation closely linked to the original data. Codes were presented based on the frequency of their use during the focus group session. The analysis and cross-analysis of the information gathered in the focus groups were then used to develop five themes which included: mixed-use precedents, sustainable building practices, linking the old to the new, financial implications, and development partnerships (Table 2).

**Table 2** Architect/developer focus group themes

| Theme | Definition | Example |
|---|---|---|
| | *Discussion of the barriers and opportunities for adaptive reuse for the dementia-friendly city center (DFCC) model of care* | |
| Mixed-use precedents | Discussion relating to precedents for adaptive reuse of malls for the DFCC mixed-use development | Mixed-use adaptive reuse is happening in mall sites, particularly those that are looking to build multi-family housing. Being able to convert the spaces into uses that would be appropriate for those individuals with dementia is an opportunity but it's also a challenge. |
| Sustainable building practices | Discussion relating to sustainable building practices in an adaptive reuse of a mall for the DFCC model of care | The biggest sustainable advantage that you have is you're not tearing down the building and putting all of that demolition debris in a landfill. You're saving that building and saving the energy cost of producing new bricks or new steel. There is an opportunity to replace old heating systems by introducing a ground source heat pump, because you have huge areas of parking lots that those wells could go in to. |
| Linking the old with the new | Discussion relating to linking the old and new construction in an adaptive reuse of a mall for the DFCC model of care | Shopping mall infrastructure is all there, you have the big box structure that can have a grid that allows the interior to be very flexible. You can take it away and put it back any way that you want. What I can see are mainly the MEP issues that make the new connectivity difficult. That gets very expensive and involves a lot of engineering. |

(continued)

**Table 2** (continued)

| Theme | Definition | Example |
|---|---|---|
| Financial implications | Discussion relating to the financial implications of the development of the DFCC model of care | A simple equation as a way to look at this is that the distressed mall property can be purchased at X % under market value for the cost of land/purchase of the property. You then will see a 25–30% bonus for the infrastructure, structure, and underground work that's on-site; probably 80% of your structure is already there. Finally, you can get state, local, and federal incentives. |
| Development partnerships | Discussion relating to the public/private partnerships necessary for the DFCC model of care | Public/private partnerships will make this kind of development fiscally viable. The partnership can create income from amenities, and then each of the care providers will develop their own purpose- built care facility. You could find a corporation or group of owners to take on the adaptive reuse of the mall and rent the converted space to a medical provider, adult day center, and/or public institutions like libraries, community workshops, or education centers. |

# 5   Results

## 5.1   Mixed-Use Precedents

Design factors such as the infrastructure, structural integrity, building's physical attributes, and roofing system must be considered as stakeholders evaluate new program types to determine which are best suited to taking maximum advantage of closed mall infrastructure, parking lots, and buildings. Mall sites have invested infrastructure, with embedded energy, which remains after retailers vacate the site and create strong conversion incentives (Bullen & Love, 2011). There was consensus within the focus group participants that malls are usually centrally located and surrounded by a substantial sized population that can be drawn on. One of the attractions of large malls is the fact that there is space and access for walking or exercise courses. A1 mentioned that malls in his community are currently used for walking and exercise for older adults:

> I know the malls close to where I live, they open up early in the morning for seniors to simply walk around in the mall to get their exercise. In fact, they have the course laid out in distances. But from a personal perspective I think being inside all of the time is not necessarily good, so pulling off a portion of the roof and exchanging it for open courtyards like you have done in the renderings could be beneficial.

The participants agreed that the layout of the case study site using a large open area at the center of the structure will be beneficial in fulfilling DFCC user needs. Most malls have wide areas of passage for circulation, and there are bearing walls at these zones that allow for opening of the space with full or partial roof removal. A2 sees the DFCC case study site to be similar to other sites around the country that are currently being renovated for mixed-use development:

> Mixed-use adaptive reuse is happening in mall sites, particularly those with tenants that are leaving like Sears and J.C. Penny that are looking to build multi-family housing around those malls to use the vacant spaces. Obviously, you've seen the examples of big box stores that have been turned into medical or urgent care centers. Some other things I've seen are large restaurants turned into entertainment centers that include multi-family housing. This model is certainly an extension of these mixed-use solutions, so viable precedents are there.

### 5.1.1 Mixed-Use Development for Dementia Programs and Services

While it is beneficial to look at existing mixed-use precedents, the participants also discussed the medical component of the DFCC. A2 was aware of adaptive reuse of malls in the cities that he has worked in, but as he explained, the development of a mixed-use site for vulnerable populations was something he had not heard or thought of previously:

> You're talking about a model that I had not heard of before. Quite frankly, the fact that these malls are typically substantial in size lends itself to that kind of thing, but there is a medical aspect to this project and anything to do with medical has a lot of code applications that come in to play. The challenge is how you make it work, how you fit all of those pieces together, it's very complex. That's probably why it hasn't been pursued before.

As D1 described it, "The DFCC concept is creating a little city with living environments and all of the amenities for those living with dementia. You are creating a mixed-use palate for better quality of life for residents with inside outside/spaces for feeling the weather." After looking at the site plan again, he commented on the benefits and barriers to opening up the city center:

> I think it's really interesting how we are looking at carving out the building, using space that's currently enclosed and opening it to the sky. From a healthcare perspective, it's pretty cool to have secure spaces that residents can wander and explore in. In traditional memory care environments that's always an issue. I do see a host of issues with the opened-up City Center that will need to be dealt with like accessibility and safety. Fall prevention will be particularly important for this population.

D1 also had organizational questions about how DFCC residents would intermix with the general public in places like the grocery store and library. He asked, "Is that OK and at what point is it not OK, I'm wondering how the staff would manage these safety and security issues." He also went on to point out that bringing providers into a new model such as the DFCC may prove to be difficult:

> Malls are generally large and it's a big undertaking. What uses can you put in there expeditiously and economically become key. Being able to convert the spaces into uses that would be appropriate for those individuals with dementia is an opportunity but it's also a challenge to find providers who would provide those kinds of senior services.

The participants agreed that the DFCC concept could be applied in other communities with closed mall properties relatively easily. D2 spoke of the adaptability of the large mall properties:

> I think this idea is scalable, or maybe adaptable is a better term. The approach that is taken with the DFCC is transferrable to other locations that could be larger or smaller than this case study site. I think there is enough flexibility in the concept that it has validity in that respect across the country.

D1 agreed and added:

> Its funny most of the projects that I work on have some kind of mixed use, and the retail component is usually the hardest thing to sell just because of the how much people are now shopping online. Transforming malls for senior care with our aging population makes a lot of sense and I think is great that you're pinning down what this is and what this isn't ahead of time. That way, you can hand the idea off to other developers saying, 'This is an idea, make it work in your community. These are the things that we've thought about and these are the things that you'd probably want to address.'

While mall sites are usually in areas with a large population to draw on, A2 pointed out that the geographical location of the site will impact the design decisions for indoor/outdoor spaces. "If you are in North Dakota for example, you may not want to pull off all of the roof due to the outside issues in the winter, while those looking at sites in Florida you would be dealing with heat or rain issues."

## 5.2    Sustainable Building Practices

Structural steel components (e.g., columns, plates, beams, decks) have a high potential for reuse at the end of their primary life because they are both durable and flexible. When suitably deconstructed, both non-structural and structural timber elements also have high reuse potential. Generalizing concrete's potential for reuse is less distinct because of the variety of material components (Iacovidou & Purnell, 2016).

Both architect participants have expertise in sustainable building practices and are credentialed in the Leadership in Energy and Environment Design (LEED) green building program. Both architects agreed that adaptive reuse of malls for the DFCC model can benefit the environment through the reduction of demolition debris going into landfills. A1 explained:

> The biggest sustainable advantage that you have is you're not tearing down the building and putting all of that demolition debris in a landfill. You're saving that building and saving the energy cost of producing new bricks or new steel. The flip side to that is that the building is already constructed and the infrastructure is already in place.

With that said, he did point out some potential barriers regarding reuse of existing heating, ventilating, and air conditioning (HVAC) systems, "If you reuse the existing HVAC system they probably would not be as efficient as new ones would be."

A2 suggested using a new heat pump system rather than reusing the older HVAC components as well as other sustainable building practices:

> There is an opportunity to replace old heating systems by introducing a ground source heat pump, because you have huge areas of parking lots that those wells could go in to. You can also develop sun harvesting grids and a substantial rain water harvesting system with your open courtyards and water retention ponds. So yes, there are definitely green building benefits in this proposal, but I think the biggest one is that you're reusing the building, that's sustainable in it of itself. If the mall infrastructure were scraped off completely, the demolition and waste disposal would be a major cost. The sustainability benefit of this scenario is that there is very little debris going into the land fill.

## 5.3   Linking the Old with the New

Adaptive reuse is an important conservation intervention to recycle the resources of the past and to transform them into experiences in and for the present (Hong & Chen, 2016). Older buildings, which are out of compliance with current regulations (e.g., life safety, seismic, tornado/hurricane safe room codes, ADA standards, etc.), may require structural changes or additional protective measures. A2 pointed out the challenges in linking the old and the new construction on large adaptive reuse projects:

> Adaptive reuse can be very challenging, particularly on large hospitality venues where much of the existing facility will be torn down while other sections are left as is. Then the combined original and newly built sections of the facility will be switched over to a new central energy plant. This is costly and wrought with a lot of unknowns that crop up and create more cost impact. The repurposing of the shopping malls is not as complex as that, you have the big box infrastructure that can have a grid that allows the interior to be very flexible. You can take it away and put it back any way that you want.

The connection of the structural elements is not as complex as the mechanical, electrical, and plumbing (MEP) components. As A1 points out, plugging in new energy supplies and infrastructure sources to the old building can be very costly at this scale:

> What I can see are mainly the MEP issues that make the new connectivity difficult. The central energy plant has boilers for the hydronic and a lot of these malls are going to have heat pump systems, that's the way they are typically done. That gets very expensive and involves a lot of engineering. You're taking something that was fairly straight forward, you're going from simple to more complex, that's a big challenge,

A1 added that when mechanical systems are redesigned for heating and cooling in a larger space, much of the system must be disposed up except for some of the ducting. Because of the rezoning, all of the mechanical aspects need to be balanced. As he explained it:

> You will have to start from scratch with the MEP. So what benefits you do get is your sanitary sewer and your structure, which is the big deal. You have that structure that is a big grid that gives you enormous flexibility, that's probably the easiest element to manipulate. Also the electrical services are probably very robust.

Participants also pointed out that reusing sections of the building after roof removal would require reengineering of the spaces now exposed to the elements. Roofs on closed malls have always been susceptible to weather deterioration, which denigrates its structural system and eventually creates problems within the built spaces below. From a design standpoint, while altering the existing roof provides opportunities for more compelling design schemes that break free from the box mall aesthetic (Hein & Houck, 2008), water and drainage, snow loads, and any new paving and planting will be added cost issues. In addition, maintenance of the newly developed outdoor courtyards will require gated vehicular access or storage for manageable, practical grounds and infrastructure maintenance.

## 5.4   Financial Implications

In addressing adaptive reuse, comparing the cost of retrofitting an existing structure vs. the cost of starting over with ground up construction are dynamics frequently faced. While from a sustainability perspective, it is optimal to keep materials in place, in a market-driven field of real estate development, finances drive the decision-making, often creating tough decisions and challenges. As D1 points out, the key concern is how to keep as much of the building elements of the mall walls, roof, and HVAC, while at the same to creating a forward-thinking functional design that has a high-yield return on investment (ROI):

> The benefits are economic. The shell is built, the structure is there. It's a matter of modifying it to suit the needs of the programs. That is very beneficial financially because you don't have to spend the money on building a new building. I guess the flip side to that are there are expenses involved in converting the space. But having the shell in place is a huge benefit.

For D2, the easiest way to look at the financial aspects of a DFCC development is to break them down into the cost saving factors:

> A simple equation as a way to look at this is that number one, the distressed mall property can be purchased at X % under market value for the cost of land/purchase of the property. Second, you then will see a 25–30% bonus for the infrastructure, structure and underground work that's on site, probably 80% of your structure is already there. You can get state, local and federal incentives as you are bringing back a distressed property for programs and housing for a vulnerable population. The end- user needs and regulatory issues involved add more complexity, but the gains are there on the outset, you have built in ROI.

This points to the fact that within the DFCC model, life cycle costs and waste are significantly reduced, and building functionality is improved, potentially improving value in a sustainable fashion across the lifespan of the development.

## 5.5   Development Partnerships

While holding many benefits, adaptive reuse can pose unique challenges including potential regulatory modifications. D2 sees the development of a business partnership plan for the DFCC as important as in any development scenario, if not more so.

Property owners who are holding on to closed mall properties at this point still have to pay property taxes as well as general property upkeep. They are ready to move on and get these properties either sold or into a new viable income stream opportunity. At the same time, the city and county agencies want to revitalize these closed commercial properties to bring back higher tax revenues, so a public/private partnership may be something that makes sense. D2 articulated the need for these types of partnerships:

> The way that nursing homes are regulated is the reason why this hasn't been done before. Reimbursement depends on the daily number of people in their beds. No provider at this time, with the current system, is going to independently spend the money to buy this size property and include all of those programs and services. Instead public/private partnerships will make this kind of development fiscally viable. The partnership can create income from the City Center amenities and then each of the care providers can develop their own purpose-built care facility. There will need to be a policy shift, the regulatory agencies like the Centers for Medicare and Medicaid (CMS) are going to have to write the policy to support it.

He also makes the point that the mixed-use format of the development can bring in established tenants which will have benefits to all of the stakeholders:

> I think there are a number of ways that you can approach this. If you take the simple model of the mall itself, it's generally a corporation or group of owners with tenants that rent the space from them. You could utilize this model if you could find a corporation or group of owners to take on the adaptive reuse and rent the converted space to a medical provider, adult day center, and/or public institutions like libraries, community workshops or education centers.

A1 and D2 discussed the probability that cities may grant property tax abatement for several years if the reused space is developed into senior living programs and services. It is in the interest of the city for the vibrancy of the area and the property tax income to be amenable to some of these property tax abatements and would pay off for all of the stakeholders in the long run. D1 went on to describe the fair market component that he has witnessed through his work in senior living development:

> What I've learned is each of these senior living providers has a unique take on what they're providing and what segment of the market they are trying to hit. The operators of senior living guide the market very powerfully and it would be important to figure out what profile or what developer/owner fit this might take. There are certainly really well known players in this market, it has consolidated quite a lot so you've got really big players and then the niche market or higher end market and everything in between.

The focus group participants also looked at the option of putting together a package of similar programs and services in every DFCC development, similar to the standardized tenant packages that many commercial properties use when they lease to the same restaurant, retail, and big box store chains. In the DFCC model, the formula for the best array of services and amenities would be streamlined to an aging population with special needs (i.e., pharmacy, bank, wellness center, etc.). This would create less risk as each DFCC would be developed with several similar amenities, and this business model of public/private partnerships would encourage the local municipality to allow for incentives because they are able to see the market precedents in other communities. Care center operators would also be interested in this business model as there would be programs, amenities, and services available on-site that the operator would not need to pay for but could use to market and drive clients to live in their facility.

# 6 Discussion

Now more than ever, adaptive reuse of commercial mall properties is being looked at to address bottom-line building costs and issues relating sustainable building practices in large-scale development projects. Therefore, the social and economic factors of this current moment in time could be a significant driver for innovative change in the provision of dementia care in the United States. Malls around the country are struggling, and all of the evidence points to this trend continuing as the economic consequences from COVID-19 shutdowns linger. Mall owners are at a point where creative ideas are being looked at with a more directed lens. Input from the architect/developer focus group covered a broad set of topics relating to adaptive reuse of malls for the DFCC model. While all participants were positive about the concept, some were less sure about its implementation.

When looking at research questions 1 and 2 focused on opportunities and barriers to adaptive reuse of malls for the DFCC project, the financing and development costs were seen as both an opportunity and a barrier by the focus group participants. Creating a reasonable cost analysis balance and ROI for a development group looking for a new way to provide care is imperative. This in turn leads to topics in research question 3 regarding public/private partnerships. The various stakeholders will all have an interest in finding the right make-up of the mixed-use amenities, programs, and services. This will be key to the model's success, in terms of economic feasibility, as well as acceptance and use by individuals living with dementia and their family members.

As the participants reported and the literature review highlighted, there are precedents for adaptive reuse of malls for mixed-use developments around the country. Connecting the dementia care piece is the outlier element to the DFCC proposed model. Conceptually three different levels of care would be brought in to develop the attached housing in the DFCC (independent living, assisted living, memory care), and the focus group participants stressed the importance of exploring how local and state tax incentives could benefit all stakeholders throughout the development process.

The focus group data also makes clear that future developments in the field of mall retrofits require considering sustainability, energy efficiency, and architectural qualities at the same time. The key to practices which encourage sustainable adaptive reuse of malls is the determination of the amount of the current building materials that can be retained and the types of MEP systems which can maintain the best energy efficiency on these large sites. Buildings should be adaptable and spaces flexible both in terms of usage and energy uses. However, functionality and technology should not be allowed to dominate at the cost of architectural quality (CommONEnergy, 2017).

Other areas of discussion revolved around the impact of specific design factors in the reused malls. The benefits of flexibility of the mall structural grid were discussed at length in terms of the ability to connect old and new sections of the building seamlessly. All participants agreed the MEP systems would create the greatest unknowns and potential cost upticks. This is where a complete cost analysis is critical in order to have a relatively well-thought out price per square foot budget to share with potential stakeholders.

Defining the potential impact of the DFCC model will be an iterative process, and there is a need for adjustments and detailed calculations to model satisfying energy and cost savings. Therefore, future research and evaluation of the model will address the therapeutic qualities of the spaces, as well as the economic indicators. Other questions that need to be addressed in future research include how the care facility operators and their residents will use the City Center amenities and spaces and what governing bodies will regulate those areas.

A known limitation of this study was the small architect/developer focus group size. While the questions and outcomes of the various focus group stakeholders are defined by differing areas of interest (i.e., medical provider discussions about integrated healthcare), a future cross-case analysis will be published looking at common themes between all of the focus groups. In addition, the findings from the focus group data analysis will be used to develop an online survey for a larger sample size of stakeholders. This survey will include more global questions about sustainable building practices, re-greening urban landscapes, and the economic impact of revitalization of urban centers. In addition, the research team will continue to focus on the opportunities to overcome the current regulatory and resource constraints and provision of resources for policy makers to help develop the public health infrastructure and public-private partnerships for this model. Despite these larger questions, this architect/developer focus group research has laid the groundwork for future conversations, helping to delineate the complexities from the built environment perspective of adaptive reuse of closed mall properties for dementia programs and services.

# 7 Conclusion

A convergence of societal factors has led to the development of the DFCC case study model including the growing population of individuals living with dementia, the need for sustainable building practices due to global climate change, the growing number of closed mall properties, and the need for integrated medical systems to strengthen infection control. While advancing the DFCC model can be seen as an investment not only for older adults now, but for ourselves in the future, it is clear there will be hurdles encountered throughout the development process.

Often it is problematic to introduce a new and innovative idea without a tangible precedent or prototype. On the whole, personal ownership of the issues around designing for an aging population may not be immediately obvious to the general community. Therefore, educating future stakeholders about the potential value of DFCC model of care will be critical in transforming current barriers into future opportunities.

In particular, as a society changed forever by the implications of the COVID-19 outbreak, awareness of the need for integrated health centers in all levels of care has been at a high point. While no one knows the ultimate toll of COVID-19 on the health of the US population and economy, integrated care models similar to the DFCC realized potentially provide a connected health and wellness community system which can be further evaluated through the lens of economic renewal, sustainable building practices, and infectious disease control. Identification of opportunities and barriers in new models of care becomes critical as we continue to strive to create real community within care communities. The focus group findings from architects and developers may well help to provide important information to professionals in the design and development fields regarding the opportunities created by adaptive reuse of closed malls for individuals living with dementia. It is hoped that continued design and research on this new place-type will allow for the rethinking of the way that building reuse and blended urban landscapes support vulnerable populations.

# References

Agich, G. (2003). *Dependence and autonomy in old age: An ethical framework for long-term care.* Cambridge University Press.

Alzheimer's Association. (2020). Alzheimer's disease facts and figures. *Alzheimer's Dementia, 16*(3), 392–460.

Amlani, T., Chamber, P., Hankin, J., & King, D. (2020). *Solutions for pandemic-related health-care capacity issues, health care design* https://www.healthcaredesignmagazine.com/trends/perspectives/solutions-for-pandemic-related-healthcare-capacity. Retrieved April 18, 2020.

Archer, D. (2012). *Stepping out in time: Help for Alzheimer's.* Retrieved from https://www.psychologytoday.com/us/blog/reading-between-the-headlines/201204/stepping-back-in-time-help-alzheimers. Retrieved May 2, 2020.

Barrett, P., Sharma, M., & Zeisel, J. (2019). Optimal spaces for those living with dementia: Principles and evidence. *Building Research & Information., 47*(6), 734–746.

Black, B. S., Johnston, D., Rabins, P. V., Morrison, A., Lykestos, C., & Samus, Q. (2013). Unmet needs of community residing person with dementia and their informal caregiver: Findings from the maximizing independence at home study. *Journal American Geriatric Society, 61*(12), 2087–2095.

Bodamer, D. (2020). *What commercial real estate will look like as America reopens national real estate investor* https://www.nreionline.com/industrial/what-cre-will-look-america-reopens/gallery?slide=8

Bullen, P. A., & Love, P. (2011). Factors influencing the adaptive re-use of buildings. *Journal of Engineering, Design and Technology, 9*(1), 32–46.

Burtch, A. (2017, July 3). *What to do with dead malls: A look at declining retail spaces and how to revitalize them from a land-use perspective.* Renaissance Planning. http://www.citiesthatwork.com/blog-renaissance/dead-malls

Chrysikou, E., Tziraki, C., & Buhalis, D. (2018). Architectural hybrids for living across the lifespan: Lessons from dementia. *Service Industry Journal, 38*(1–2), 4–26.

CommOnEnergy. (2017). *Guidelines on retrofitting of shopping malls. Deliverable 7.12.* European Commission DG Research and Innovation.

Conejos, S., Langston, C., & Smith, J. (2011). *Improving the implementation of adaptive reuse strategies for historic buildings.* Bond University ePublications @bond, Mirvac School of Sustainable Development Institute of Sustainable Development and Architecture.

Corroto, C., & Richardson, L. (2019). We have seen it all. At the mall. *Qualitative Inquiry, 25*(9–10), 1078–1084.

Dunham-Jones, E., & Williamson, J. (2011). *Retrofitting suburbia: Urban design solutions for redesigning suburbs.* John Wiley & Sons.

Elrod, J. K., & Fortenberry, J. L. (2017). Advancing indigent healthcare services through adaptive reuse: Repurposing abandoned buildings as medical clinics for disadvantaged. *BMC Health Services Research, 17*(4), 805.

EPA. (2019). *Construction and demolition: material-specific data. Facts and figures about materials, waste and recycling.* https://www.epa.gov/facts-and-figures-about-materials-waste-and-recycling. Retrieved May 29, 2020.

Garreau, J. (2008 November 16). *Don't trash big boxes, Repackage them!* The Washington Post Company. https://www.washingtonpost.com/wp-srv/artsandliving/style/2008/1116/bigbox/gallery.html.

Glass, A. P. (2014). Innovative seniors housing and care models: What we can learn from the Netherlands. *Senior Housing and Care Journal, 22*(1), 74–81.

Guimaraes, C., & Porfirio, P. (2019). Shopping centers in decline: Analysis of demalling in Lisbon. *Cities, 87,* 21–29.

Haeusermann, T. (2018). Professionalized intimacy: How dementia care workers navigate between domestic intimacy and institutional detachment. *Sociology of Health and Illness, 40*(5), 907–923.

Hein, M., & Houck, K. (2008). Construction challenges of adaptive reuse of historical buildings in Europe. *International Journal of Construction Education and Research, 4*(2), 115–131.

Hong, Y., & Chen, F. (2016). Evaluating the adaptive reuse potential of buildings in conservation areas. *Facilities, 35*(3/4), 202–219.

Iacovidou, E., & Purnell, P. (2016). Mining the physical infrastructure: Opportunities, barriers and interventions in promoting structural components reuse. *Science of the Total Environment, 557,* 791–807.

Kohlstedt, K. (2016, June 27). *Ghost boxes: Reusing abandoned big-box superstores across America.* 99% Invisible. https://99percentinvisible.org/article/ghost-boxes-reusing-abandoned-big-box-superstores-across-america/

Matchar, E. (2017, September 12). *The transformation of the American shopping mall.* Smithsonian Magazine https://www.smithsonianmag.com/innovation/transformation-american-shopping-mall-180964837/

Peterson, S. (2015, March 18). *Forget ruin porn: 5 awesome adapted spaces that used to be dead malls.* Vox Media, LLC. https://www.curbed.com/2015/3/18/9982614/things-that-used-to-be-malls

Rabig, J. (2009). Home again, small houses for individuals with cognitive impairment. *Journal of Gerontological Nursing, 35*(8), 10–15.

Roberts, E. (2018). Voices from down home: Family caregiver perspectives on navigating care transitions with individuals with dementia in Nova, Scotia, Canada. In W. Baily & A. Harrist (Eds.), *Family caregiving: Emerging issues in family and individual resilience.* Springer.

Roberts, E., & Pulay, A. (2018). Examining the nursing home physical environment though policy-driven culture change. *Journal of Housing for the Elderly, 32*(1), 1–22.

Roberts, E., & Shehadeh, A. (2021). Community visioning for innovation in integrated dementia care: Stakeholder focus group outcomes. *Journal of Primary Care & Community Health.* https://doi.org/10.1177/215013272110427911-9

Roberts, E., Kleszynski, K., Shehadeh, A., & Carter, H. (2020). Thinking outside of the box: Medical provider perspectives on adaptive reuse of closed mall sites for mixed-use dementia programs and services. *Journal of Aging and the Environment.* https://doi.org/10.1080/2689261 8.2020.18567531-22

Stewart, D., & Shamdasni, P. (2014). *Focus groups: Theory and practice.* Sage.

Tan, C. M., Pallaske, G., & Bassi, A. (2020). *Sustainable asset valuation tool: Materials management infrastructure.* IISD. https://www.iisd.org/sites/default/files/publications/sustainable-asset-valuation-tool-materials-management.pdf

Voien, G. (2017, August 20). *What should be done with America's abandoned malls?* Condé Nast. https://www.architecturaldigest.com/story/abandoned-malls

Wang, H., Li, T., Barbarino, P., Gauthier, S., Brodaty, H., Molinuevo, J. L., Xie, H., Sun, Y., Yu, E., Tang, Y., Weidner, W., & Yu, X. (2020). Dementia care during COVID-19. *Lancet, 395,* 1190–1191.

Zimmerman, S., Bowers, B., Cohen, L., Grabowski, D., Horn, S., & Kemper, P. (2016). New evidence on the Green House model of nursing home care: Synthesis of findings and implications for policy, practice and research. *BMC Health Services Research, 51*(1), 475–496.

# Extending the Continuum of Care for People with Dementia: Building Resilience

Gesine Marquardt and Kathrin Bueter

## 1 Dementia-Friendly Architecture

It is the constant wish of the vast majority of older adults to remain in their current home environment as they grow older. However, most of them are aware that this wish may remain unfulfilled (Binette & Vasold, 2018). Even when home-care networks are available and home modifications to accommodate age-related functional and cognitive decline are implemented, transition to long-term care (LTC) may become necessary, especially for people living with dementia (Holup et al., 2017). Consequently, dementia is present in approximately half of the residents in nursing homes.

An increase in nursing home residents in general and of people living with dementia among them is expected in the future (Liu et al., 2020). However, home and LTC settings are not the only places where it is necessary to consider the needs of people living with dementia. In recent years, hospitals have especially come into focus as the probability of hospitalization increases with age. Currently, approximately half of the patients in hospitals are older than 65 years (World Health Organization, 2020), and the prevalence of dementia symptoms in older patients ranges between 20% and 40% (Bickel et al., 2018; Briggs et al., 2017). To accommodate the needs of a growing number of people with dementia in health-care settings, strategies are necessary to deliver a continuum of care where individuals can move from one place to another without encountering any disruption that may lead to a deterioration of their abilities.

G. Marquardt (✉) · K. Bueter
Social and Health Care Buildings and Design Faculty of Architecture,
Technische Universitaet Dresden, Dresden, Germany
e-mail: gesine.marquardt@tu-dresden.de; kathrin.bueter@tu-dresden.de

It has been widely acknowledged that the architectural design of spaces influences human behavior and well-being. Established theories of human-environment research posit that the well-being and behavior of people depend on the interaction of environmental factors and their individual coping skills (Lawton & Nahemow, 1973). People living with dementia are particularly susceptible to their surroundings, as they do not experience them in the same way as healthy older people (Smith et al., 2004). Building on these findings, more than 30 years ago, the first design guidance and buildings accommodating the needs of people living with dementia emerged (Calkins, 1988; Cohen & Weisman, 1991). Currently, numerous researchers worldwide explore ways to design environments that are supportive and therapeutic for persons living with dementia (Calkins, 2018; Fleming et al., 2020a).

In this chapter, first, we summarize the research evidence on supportive, dementia-friendly architectural design and postulate ten evidence-based design criteria. Then we discuss the current state of dementia-friendly architectural design in LTC settings. Afterward, we transfer these findings into the design of hospitals and elucidate ways to implement the ten design criteria in acute care settings. Further, the results of a quasi-experimental study, which evaluated the influence of a redesigned hospital ward on patients with dementia outcomes, are presented. Finally, we argue that our design criteria help to build a continuum of care that brings dementia-friendly care to hospital environments and, ultimately, will even contribute to building resilient health-care settings for the future.

## 1.1   Research Findings on Supportive Nursing Care Environments

Research on dementia-friendly environments has produced a range of findings on how architecture can have a positive influence on alleviating the symptoms and progression of dementia and helps to make individuals living with dementia feel at home in nursing care settings.

The layout and interior design of nursing care settings have been investigated extensively. Small-scale nursing care settings, which house up to 15 people per unit, have shown many advantages for residents. The fact that small-scale units can create opportunities for individualized care and attention to residents' personal needs contributes to a better quality of life and greater well-being (Dyer et al., 2018). Furthermore, fewer hospitalizations, lower use of medication, and better orientation are associated with small-scale settings (de Boer et al., 2018; Harrison et al., 2018; Marquardt, 2011). Less decline in global cognitive functioning compared to that of residents in larger care settings has even been reported (Kok et al., 2016). Most importantly, small-scale settings are conducive to the emergence of a homelike milieu, which is one of the recurring elements of design guidance for people living with dementia.

The architectural layout is a major influencing factor on the abilities and care outcomes of residents. Supporting orientation and way-finding abilities, which deteriorate with the progression of dementia, is an important goal to pursue with the design of the initial floor plan. In small-scale settings, open plan environments allow for better visual access to support orientation, while in larger units, straight corridors with meaningful spatial reference points have been found to be supportive. A live-in kitchen constitutes an excellent spatial reference point, and its design can further facilitate increased resident independence, autonomy, and social interaction (Chaudhury et al., 2017; Davis & Weisbeck, 2016; de Boer et al., 2018; Marquardt & Schmieg, 2009). Spending time outside, maybe even engaging in gardening activities, has also been shown to have a positive influence on people living with dementia (Whear et al., 2014). Therefore, the connection between indoor and outdoor spaces should be planned carefully to allow for residents' independent transition.

The appearance of the interior design of care settings is determined mainly through furniture and fixtures, colors, signs, and pictures. Their design can create a homelike atmosphere that is beneficial for residents' daily life, as it promotes greater engagement in activities and social interaction (de Boer et al., 2017, 2018). Their deliberate design further enables them to serve as cues for orientation to time, place, and situation (Davis & Weisbeck, 2016; Marquardt, 2011). Finally, the interior design needs to provide sensory stimulation that can lead to varied levels of natural environmental signals that lessen boredom, a sense of isolation, and improve the residents' quality of life (Strøm et al., 2016).

## 1.2   Dementia-Friendly Design Criteria to Transfer Research Results into Architectural Practice

At present, we can state that a coherent body of research on dementia-friendly architectural design measures has evolved (Fleming et al., 2020a; Chaudhury et al., 2018; Calkins, 2018). Building on these research findings, extensive design guidance specifically aimed at informing architects, health-care providers, and operators has been published. It covers a wide range of environments (Fung, 2015; Fleming et al., 2020b), such as home care environments (Grey et al., 2015), daycares (Moore et al., 2006), nursing homes (Cunningham et al., 2011), hospitals (Bueter & Marquardt, 2020), outdoor spaces (Pollock & Cunningham, 2018), and public buildings (Fleming et al., 2020b).

Based on the research evidence presented in the previous section of this chapter, we developed ten key criteria for designing dementia-friendly care environments. These design criteria are not all-encompassing, but they specifically provide design strategies that we consider practicing architects and designers should adapt and develop further for their specific projects. These criteria pertain not only to nursing care settings but also to all settings that people living with dementia may encounter.

### 1.2.1   Floor Plan Structure

Simple, clearly defined building structures and room layouts are the basis for dementia-friendly architecture. They have a significant impact on spatial orientation and, as a result, the activities of individuals living with dementia. In addition, they facilitate workflow efficiency. Properties of a supportive floor plan structure are small unit sizes, architectural typologies with a straight design of horizontal circulation areas, and the provision of spatial anchor points, which are meaningful and highly recognizable places.

### 1.2.2   Floor Space Requirements

Due to limited mobility, disorientation, or insecurity in unfamiliar environments, many people living with dementia are unable to move beyond their immediate environment. They may even put themselves in danger, so it is not advisable for some people living with dementia to walk away unaccompanied. As dementia can also lead to an increase in restlessness, there must be sufficient room for them to move about and suitable places for them to spend time within a protective framework. Due to their age-related impairments, many people with dementia require mobility aids, which also necessitate more space.

### 1.2.3   Safety

Safe and protected spaces for moving about are necessary for individuals living with dementia. This does not imply closed environments, however, but rather easily accessible, clearly laid out and high-quality spaces, which promote individuals' mobility and autonomy. Implementing barrier-free design standards as mandated by building regulations is an important prerequisite.

### 1.2.4   Orientation

Dementia-related difficulties with spatial, temporal, and situational orientation manifest in different ways. Design that supports way-finding not only facilitates direct navigation but can also help with temporal orientation (times of the day and durations) and support situational comprehension of their own presence in the environment and, thus, how others expect them to behave in certain situations and in the overall setting.

### 1.2.5  Guidance and Orientation Systems

Guidance and orientation systems help people living with dementia find their way around buildings. Such systems incorporate clearly legible signage and easily interpretable symbols as well as address different senses by including visual, tactile, auditory, and olfactory cues. Guidance and orientation systems must always be developed following a holistic approach by implementing a clearly defined floor plan structure.

### 1.2.6  Lighting

Light intensity and lighting design are key aspects of a dementia-friendly environment. Basic room lighting should be bright and glare-free, which supports the perception of the surrounding space. Natural light is conducive to well-being and controlling the sleep-wake rhythm. Furthermore, lighting concepts can support spatial orientation.

### 1.2.7  Colors and Contrast

The perception of colors changes with age, resulting in the need for stronger contrasts to compensate for age-related visual impairments. Spatial elements that are of importance to the individual can be emphasized by stark contrasts, and nonrelevant elements can be camouflaged by low contrast. Colors create mood and atmosphere, although there is no scientific evidence on how individual colors affect individuals living with dementia.

### 1.2.8  Atmosphere

Transitioning to an unfamiliar environment is challenging for individuals living with dementia. In addition to a calming and aesthetically pleasing interior design, a spatial structure that facilitates and instigates communication, social interaction, and participation is vital. The combined spatial and social environment can create an ambiance that emanates security and orientation, making individuals feel welcome and appreciated.

### 1.2.9  Activation Concepts

Having a purpose and assigned tasks maintains self-confidence and prevents functional and cognitive decline. It also helps to prevent challenging behaviors due to under-stimulation and boredom. In all care settings, spaces for activity, a stimulating design that induces self-sufficient informal activity, and structured programs that keep individuals active are necessary.

### 1.2.10 Stimulus Densities

Dementia limits the ability to adequately filter, process, and interpret environmental information, hampering an appropriate response. Both sensory overload and the absence of sensory stimulation must be avoided. The degree of stimulation needed varies among individuals. Therefore, offering variable stimulus densities to respond to the different needs of individuals is essential.

## 2 Current State of Dementia-Friendly Architectural Design in Long-Term Care Settings

There is widespread consensus among architects in practice and nursing home operators that the implementation of dementia-friendly design measures is possible and useful. To date, there are several publications available that present case studies from LTC with successful designs. The buildings included can be found in various countries around the world and incorporate very different climatic, societal, and economic situations (Feddersen & Luedtke, 2014; Fleming et al., 2020b; Palmer et al., 2021; Regnier, 2018; Tsekleves, & Keady, 2021). Reviewing the designs presented, we realize that many research findings on dementia-friendly design were incorporated. Of course, to varying degrees and with shifting focus, many other factors (such as building regulations and costs) are also to be taken into account in the design of a building. Nevertheless, we find the dementia-friendly design criteria we postulated to be valid in architectural practice.

In light of the extensive information available on dementia-friendly design, the question of why there are still so many facilities that do not adhere to these design criteria inevitably arises. The lack of awareness can be ruled out as a reason since the design guidance has been widely proliferated not only in academic books and journals but also in many outlets directed at the operators of care facilities and architects who are commissioned with the design of refurbishments or new construction of facilities. Even a quick Internet search will yield many results and raise awareness of this topic.

Neither do we find any indication that dementia-friendly design raises costs to the extent that overstrained budgets result in neglecting these design aspects against better knowledge. As a result of these deliberations, we can only assume that care providers and operators that do not implement dementia-friendly design features are unaware of their importance and the benefits both for residents and staff. Additionally, they appear to be fearful of the costs of such measures, which they tend to overestimate (Heiss et al., 2010). To overcome this predicament, we urge architects in practice to familiarize themselves with dementia-friendly design measures, encourage their implementation, and, most importantly, evaluate their impact on construction costs. Researchers, on the other hand, need to provide design guidance that can efficiently be incorporated into the planning process by architects in practice.

## 3   Continuing Dementia-Friendly Care in Hospital Environments

Dementia-friendly design is not only feasible for LTC settings. People living with dementia will encounter other health-care settings and will need to find dementia-friendly design measures to extend there. Often, the carefully balanced situation of older adults living with dementia in a care setting is suddenly disrupted through the urgent need for hospital admission.

Dementia, itself, is rarely the reason for hospitalization. Others, often age-related conditions, including orthopedic, respiratory, and urologic factors, as well as multi-morbidity, polypharmacy, and lower functional ability, come into play. Many patients display multiple conditions concurrently (Toot et al., 2013; Shepherd et al., 2019). When older adults are admitted to the hospital, dementia is often only a secondary diagnosis, if it is known at all (Rao et al., 2016). Nevertheless, 40% of inpatients over the age of 65 exhibit cognitive impairments, and one-fifth show symptoms of dementia (Bickel et al., 2018).

Being admitted to a hospital with dementia can have a significant impact on the outcome of treatment and therapy. Hospital processes are designed primarily for patients who understand the purpose of their stay and are accepting and cooperative in their treatments. However, people living with dementia are at odds with standardized, workflow-oriented processes; they may not understand where they are and what condition brought them into the hospital and, thus, have little or no understanding of the necessity for treatment and care procedures. This often results in adverse outcomes for people living with dementia, such as higher complications and mortality rates, increased length of stay, and increased use of psychotropic medication (Moellers et al., 2019).

Patients with dementia are also at particular risk of further cognitive and functional decline because of the passive, "sedentary behavior" that is commonly expected from patients in hospital routines. However, with dementia, self-care abilities quickly atrophy if they are not used, and reduced mobility results in a dramatic loss of muscle mass and aerobic capacity (Sourdet et al., 2015).

In LTC settings, people living with dementia are kept active and maintain their self-care abilities by being encouraged to participate in everyday tasks, such as socializing, sharing meals, cooking, cleaning, and gardening. These activities cannot easily continue in the hospital environment. First and foremost, patients may be too sick to move about and take care of themselves, but even if they could do so, individual activities are often at odds with hospitals' care routines. Most importantly, spatial prerequisites for activities (such as common rooms, therapeutic kitchens, or garden access) are scarce and typically not available on hospital wards at all. Therefore, extending dementia-friendly care to the hospital context relies on specific modifications to the environments encountered there (Belala et al., 2019; Xidous et al., 2020).

## 3.1 Architectural Properties of Dementia-Friendly Hospitals

The disadvantageous situation of people living with dementia in hospitals has become the focus of multiple stakeholders during the past decade. Among others, the King's Fund[1] from the United Kingdom and the Robert Bosch Foundation[2] from Germany have been driving forces to identify ways to redesign hospital wards to accommodate the needs of people with dementia. Both organizations encouraged and funded several model projects and disseminated the results, including design guidance on dementia-friendly hospital environments (Kings Fund, 2014; Kirchen-Peters & Krupp, 2019; Bueter & Marquardt, 2020; Waller et al., 2017). Furthermore, the topic has increasingly gained attention from researchers investigating the relationship between dementia-friendly hospital design and the outcomes of patients with dementia to derive design guidance (Grey et al., 2019; Parke et al., 2017). An empirical study has shown that most dementia-friendly hospital design measures are associated with significant improvement in patients' self-care abilities (Kirch & Marquardt, 2021).

In a dementia-friendly hospital, the goal of all design considerations is to create an environment that has a positive influence on patients' well-being and recovery. Additionally, their family, caregivers, and visitors need space to play their part. At the same time, hospitals are workplaces that must facilitate optimum performance of treatment and care processes. Other framework conditions for architectural design are economic factors and the fulfillment of medical, technical, and hygienic requirements. There can be no trade-offs between these aspects; moreover, they must be integrated into an overall concept.

Specifically, we propose that effective dementia-friendly hospital environments include additional aspects beyond the physical characteristics. Design measures must be embedded in an overall concept to cater to individuals living with dementia, considering organizational and human resources. An architecture presumed to be dementia-friendly should not be based on a stigmatizing design that perpetuates outdated notions of the design preferences of "elderly people."

Rather, hospital designs should mirror the sample principles applied for home care and LTC settings. Specifically, these designs should (1) foster patient independence and encourage mobility and activity to preserve patients' cognitive capabilities and physical functions; (2) give patients emotional security, stability, and orientation; (3) help medical staff work to the best of their ability; (4) make relatives, caregivers, and visitors feel welcome and involved; and (5) combine functionality, hygiene, and aesthetics, offering all users an environment of dignity and respect. Ultimately, hospital architecture must balance requirements such as economy, efficiency, hygiene, and use of technology with the desire to design spaces that promote convalescence. The designs should feature high-quality and contemporary aesthetics that emanate dignity and respect, avoiding the stigmatization of a group of patients. In Table 1, we present ways to easily implement our ten design criteria in hospital environments.

---

[1] https://www.kingsfund.org.uk/projects/enhancing-healing-environment/ehe-design-dementia

[2] https://www.bosch-stiftung.de/en/project/people-dementia-hospitals

**Table 1**  Implementing dementia-friendly design criteria in the hospital context

| Design criterion | Architectural implementation |
|---|---|
| Floor plan structure | Clear and legible corridors and a central nursing station serve as spatial reference points that support spatial orientation |
| Floor space requirements | Common rooms are large enough to accommodate groups for shared meals. Wall recesses and storage spaces are available for mobility and care aids |
| Safety | Barrier-free design accommodates age-related physical and sensory impairments |
| Orientation | Multisensory information on time, situation, and place is given. Room functions can easily be interpreted |
| Guidance and orientation systems | Simple signs and multiple cues that appeal to different senses are used |
| Lighting | Bright, even and glare-free room lighting supports the perception of ward environments, while individually adjustable lights are available in patients' rooms |
| Colors and contrast | Areas relevant to patients' independent movement are highlighted, while the hospital's functional sections are concealed |
| Atmosphere | Requirements of clinical functionality and a non-institutional ambiance that appeals to a wide range of patients are well balanced |
| Activation concepts | Informal occupational activities are offered in seating niches, and supervised activities are scheduled in common areas |
| Stimulus densities | Secluded seating niches offer privacy to spend time alone or with visitors. Sitting areas near the central nursing station provide distraction |

## 3.2   Quasi-Experimental Study: Results of a Dementia-Friendly Redesign of a Hospital Ward

The following example of redesigning a hospital ward shows how dementia-friendly architecture can be implemented. The project was planned by the authors and executed at the standard care Diakonissenkrankenhaus Hospital in Dresden, Germany. The internal medicine ward was chosen for a redesign because it was found to have the highest percentage of older patients living with dementia within the hospital. It has a total of 22 beds and includes a patient common room. The nursing station, personnel, and storage rooms, as well as the therapeutic bath, were centrally located. There was a focused phase of concept development before the planning process. It was based on a comprehensive status quo analysis to systematically observe how patients used the space. Employee and patient surveys were also conducted. As a result, three major spatial deficits that prevented needs-driven care of patients living with dementia were identified: (1) a lack of common areas and activity options, (2) confusing way-finding systems, and (3) inadequate equipment of patient rooms. Based on this analysis and taking into account the latest findings on dementia-friendly architecture, a design concept was developed and coordinated with the ward's nursing staff, nursing management, and the hospital's construction department.

In the following section, we show how the identified spatial deficits were addressed by implementing different dementia-friendly design criteria:

**Floorplan Structure** A new common area was created at a central location on the ward corridor. It was built as a nook by reorganizing secondary rooms and remodeling walls and ceilings. The nook is opposite the nursing station, offering a direct line of sight between the two areas.

**Activation Concepts and Stimulus Densities** The new common area offers seating, a table with clearance for wheelchair users, and various activities and occupations for patients, which can be pursued without significantly increasing the workload on the nursing staff. For example, a flush-mounted screen emulates an aquarium, an audio station lets patients listen to music and short stories, and there are books, photo books, and magazines for reading (Fig. 1).

**Guidance and Orientation Systems** An orientation system was added to the ward corridor to support way-finding and orientation. Based on a pilot study (Motzek et al., 2017), all patient room doors were fitted with signage consisting of large-format room numbers and a regional image. The ward corridor was also given a bright coat of paint, the patient room doors were highlighted through colors, and writing and symbols were added to patient-relevant rooms. The letter was hung in patients' field of vision, and a highly legible size and font were chosen. Doors to patient-relevant rooms, such as the patient common area or the nurses' station, were given larger letters than doors to storage and function rooms (Fig. 2).

**Atmosphere and Orientation** Patient rooms were given a new, dementia-friendly design. A new floor covering in warm and dark colors promotes clear spatial orien-

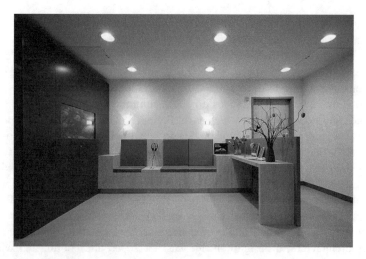

**Fig. 1** The new common area offers seating and several activities for patients. Diakonissenkrankenhaus Hospital in Dresden

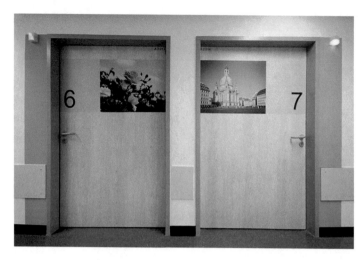

**Fig. 2** The patient room signage is made up of the room number and a regional image. Diakonissenkrankenhaus Hospital in Dresden

tation and creates a non-institutional atmosphere. Medical and media equipment was concealed behind a wall clad with a wood finish to be less prominent. Personal areas such as beds and coat racks are color-coded. This color is repeated in the patient bathrooms to mark personal shelves and towel rails. New signage was also added to the bathroom door, consisting of a large-format bathtub symbol and the word "Bathroom" in large letters. A light strip was installed in the skirting board along the wall opposite the beds and above the bathroom door to help patients find the bathroom at night. The light is switched on from a call bell control panel that can be operated from the bed. An analog clock and a wall mural were also added on the wall opposite the beds to support temporal and situational orientation. The wall mural features the hospital logo, the room number, and the same regional image as on the door. In the en suite bathrooms, the original white fittings, such as handles, toilet seats, shelves, and towel hooks, were replaced with high-contrast fittings to increase visibility and, therefore, facilitate independent use (Fig. 3).

To assess the effectiveness of the architectural redesign measures, a quasi-experimental study was conducted. A pre-post design was chosen, and data were collected over 5 weeks at an interval of roughly 1 year. Ninety-four hours of observation were recorded per data collection period, and the hours of observation were distributed evenly. The key objective was to identify structural and design factors that influence the mobilization and activation of individuals living with dementia in acute care hospitals. Behavior mapping, a method of systematically observing the behavior of persons in relation to their spatial environment (Ng, 2016), was the primary data surveying instrument. Due to their symptoms, asking individuals living with dementia directly is either impossible or of limited value. Therefore, behavioral observation is a suitable alternative to measure the influence of the spatial environment on persons living with dementia. The type, time, duration, and

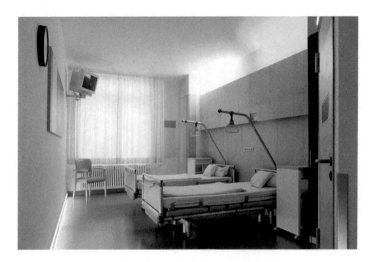

**Fig. 3** Warm colors and materials make the patient rooms more homelike. Individual areas are color-coded. Diakonissenkrankenhaus Hospital in Dresden

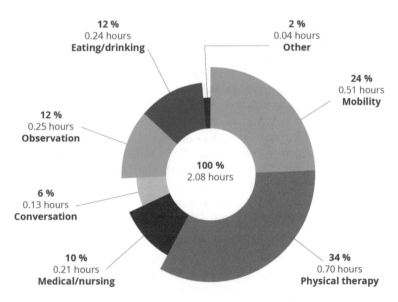

**Fig. 4** Patients' activities before the redesign

location of behaviors are noted on a data survey form. As part of the study, patients were observed in the public areas of the hospital ward—the ward corridor and common area. No observations were conducted in the patient rooms due to patient privacy reasons.

The diagram shows how patients with dementia spent their time during their hospital stay. Before the redesign (Fig. 4), patients with dementia were primarily

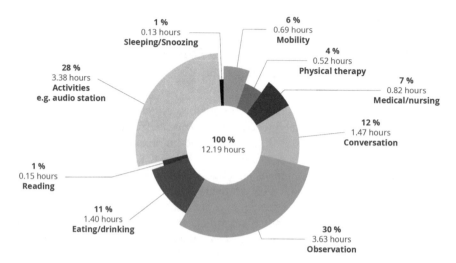

**Fig. 5** Patients' activities after the redesign

involved in mobility-related activities (24.4%) and physical therapy activities (33.3%). The third most common activities were medical and nursing activities, which took up 19.2% of their active time, followed by the categories of observation (12%) and eating/drinking (11.6%). Significant changes can be observed after the redesign (Fig. 5). The patients are now involved in more diverse activities. The primary activities are now observation (29.8%) and using the new audio stations (27.8%). They were also seen conversing (12%) and eating/drinking (11.5%). The absolute duration of mobility and physiotherapy remained virtually unchanged between the two survey periods. However, due to the higher overall duration of observations, these activities took up proportionately less time.

The dementia-friendly redesign of the ward was found to have positive effects on the nursing staff. The results of the staff survey reveal a lower perceived level of stress and load on the part of the nursing staff. Improvements were reported in almost all areas surveyed. Both the orientation problems of patients with dementia and the risk of their leaving the ward unnoticed were considered less of a strain. Increased job satisfaction among the nursing staff was also reported after the interventions. Nurses also indicated improvements in nurse-patient interactions. They expressed greater satisfaction with the standard of care for patients with dementia in their ward. They also described looking after patients as a more enjoyable experience and stated that they had a good relationship with them. This can be interpreted as a better standard of care for patients with dementia in the ward.

Concluding this example of a dementia-friendly redesign of a hospital ward has shown that the dementia-friendly design criteria that are valid in LTC can be extended to the hospital context, thus expanding the continuum of care for people living with dementia.

# 4   Discussion

## 4.1   Dementia-Friendly Design as a Driver for Human-Centered Design

Dementia-friendly design not only benefits a group of individuals with a very specific condition. Moreover, the properties of a dementia-friendly environment are deeply rooted in design efforts that center on the fulfillment of very basic human needs. As such, we could see people living with dementia as seismographs for the design quality of the built environment. It needs to be made clear that environments for people with dementia do not have a fundamentally different appearance from other environments. It is not necessary to apply a specific style of furnishing or to make use of a certain set of wall colors, which may lead to the stigmatization of people in this specific environment. In this way, the architectural design would even work against the human need for social inclusion. However, to further promote the implementation of dementia-friendly design, some barriers need to be broken down. First, a modern and individualized image of aging, which reflects the actual diversity of our aging society, should be advanced. Second, the perception that the primary way to design for dementia entails old-fashioned, stereotypical architecture needs to be overcome. Architects and designers must show that dementia-friendly design is a creative challenge, which implies high aesthetic quality and designers' knowledgeability and sensibility. Thus, the entire setting of health-care facilities should become as supportive as possible to benefit all the people they serve. By incorporating the available evidence on dementia-friendly design into the principles of inclusive design, a better health-care environment for everyone, including visitors and staff, will emerge. For example, spacious, safe, and barrier-free architecture is needed not only by wheelchair users but also by young parents with strollers. Intuitive cues for orientation to place, time, and situation not only help to compensate for cognitive decline due to dementia but are also helpful for anyone affected by fear and stress during hospital admission. Guidance and orientation systems make visitors feel welcome. Finally, supporting the maintenance of self-care abilities is necessary for anyone recovering in a hospital. In light of these findings, we can hypothesize that a stronger orientation toward vulnerable people and their needs might lead to increased sensitivity by architects and designers, resulting in an increase in human-centered designs.

Therefore, the challenge of a growing number of individuals with dementia in health-care facilities holds great potential to inspire health-care providers, operators, architects, and designers to reimagine health-care buildings and design them with human beings and their needs in mind, resulting in positive outcomes for all patients, visitors, and staff. The dementia-friendly design criteria introduced in previous chapters can serve as helpful guidance toward a more friendly architecture that meets the needs of all people. Against the background of increasing life expectancy and the correspondingly growing number of people living with dementia, implementing appropriate design measures can become a driving force toward the further proliferation of human-centered design efforts in many aspects of our built environment, especially in health-care settings.

## 4.2 Potential of Dementia-Friendly Design in Building Resilient Structures in the Future

The architectural designs of newly built (health) care facilities will need to serve their purpose for many years, often decades. However, when integrating the available scientific evidence into design, it remains uncertain whether our existing principles and evidence will help to envision structures that accommodate the challenges and changes that lay ahead. We assert that buildings that perform well in the future must be resilient, capable of standing up to disasters, disruptions, and adverse events. Some future developments are already visible now, and they need to be incorporated into today's designs:

**Demographic Change**  A growing number of older adults will require care, and many of them will have dementia. At the same time, the number of younger people is shrinking and thus reducing the pool of available caregivers, nurses, and doctors (United Nations, 2019).

**Climate Change**  For older adults and people in (health) care facilities, heat waves increase the risk of mortality. This effect is even higher for people living with dementia (Fritze, 2020). Furthermore, heat stresses nursing professionals, adding additional strain to those required to wear personal protective equipment (Jegodka et al., 2021). Both exacerbation and acceleration of recurring events, such as regional droughts, floods, and storms, also need to be accommodated in building designs.

**Pandemics**  COVID-19 has developed into a pandemic that affects human societies worldwide, and we must assume that this virus will become endemic in humans (Philips, 2021). Even if living with COVID-19 will become feasible in the future, epidemics that infect the world's population to a significant degree are expected every 10 to 20 years (Dodds, 2019). The rise of bacteria resistant to antibiotics further increases the need to avoid the transmission of infections through hygiene measures integrated into building design (Gradmann, 2018). (Health) care facilities were largely unprepared for the rapid spread of COVID-19, resulting in numerous deaths among residents in long-term care facilities (AARP, 2021). Structural unpreparedness, not only with regard to the availability of personal protective equipment and tests but also to the quick adaptation of the care processes, contributed to this.

Clearly, the future of dementia-friendly designs will need to consider the application of design principles that will facilitate resident safety while providing care during staff shortages and natural disasters. At this point, we would like to elucidate whether dementia-friendly design can contribute to building resilient structures in the future. To do so, in Table 2, we once again draw on the design criteria we have postulated, this time in light of resilience toward future crises.

**Table 2** Potential of dementia-friendly design criteria in light of building resilience toward future crisis

| Design criterion | Architectural implementation |
|---|---|
| Floor plan structure | Circulation systems that feature short paths reduce encounters between visitors, staff, and patients/residents and avoid the transmission of germs. Small unit sizes can operate independently to contain infections and can form clusters for the daily lives of patients/ residents |
| Floor space requirements | Sufficient space allows for an ad hoc adaptation of care routines, e.g. built temporarily sluice rooms and add additional technical devices such as air cleaning, heating, or cooling. Furthermore, buffer zones can be created where people may be queuing, waiting or safely passing each other in hallways |
| Safety | Critical information can be shared immediately through communications technology. Sensors detecting unusual heat, cold, water, viral or bacterial load alert staff and facility management |
| Orientation | Contingency plans for adverse events can be incorporated into guidance systems. If frequent contact and communication with the world outside the ward or facility are cut off, necessary information can be conveyed through environmental cues |
| Guidance and orientation systems | Short-notice and emergency assistance by individuals not familiar with the environment are facilitated. Strong way-finding measures help avoid wandering and unnecessary encounters |
| Lighting | Ample natural light permeating the building sustains daytime lighting during power outages. Windows not only let light into the building but also air, allowing for energy-neutral cooling and heating concepts for interior spaces as well as dilution of contaminated air |
| Colors and contrast | Stark contrast highlights objects and places that are relevant in emergencies, such as evacuation or firefighting. Low contrasts camouflage objects and places that may be dangerous to patients or residents |
| Atmosphere | Encouraging frequent social interaction builds trust among patients or residents, staff, and visitors, thus building community and promoting a sense of belonging |
| Activation concepts | Individuals who maintain their self-sufficiency and self-care abilities are less reliant on the availability of care and support. Outdoor spaces can encourage exercise, and the risk of infection transmission is lower outdoors. Communication technology not only allows access to information but also a chance to reduce isolation |
| Stimulus densities | In unstable situations, quickly increasing or reducing stimuli may become necessary to deescalate. Variable stimuli can be interchanged (e.g., use tactile material discontinued when contamination likely) |

## 5   Conclusion

Concepts of dementia-friendly design have been well researched over the past decades, and a coherent body of scientific evidence has evolved. As dementia-friendly designs have been implemented in many countries worldwide, the translation of these research results into practice has proven feasible. Nevertheless, the extension of corresponding design efforts to the hospital context is still emerging.

Even though hospitals operate differently from LTC settings in many ways, we identified design criteria that pertain to both environments. We argue that architects, hospital operators, and health-care providers need to be open to incorporating successful design strategies from LTC. We would also like to stress that dementia-friendly design does not imply the creation of environments that are perceived as different from others. We argue that dementia-friendly design is an integral part of any human-centered design, leading to inclusive designs that are conducive to everyone's well-being and best performance. Our reassessment of our criteria for dementia-friendly design in the face of staff shortages and natural disasters also points to the need to challenge current principles to design resilient structures that accommodate crises that inevitably will challenge us in the future. In this respect, dementia-friendly design not only benefits all stakeholders of today but also contributes to building structures that are resilient to future developments.

**Acknowledgments** The authors gratefully acknowledge funding of their work by the German Research Foundation, DFG (Gz. MA 5384/1-1), and the Robert Bosch Foundation Stuttgart, Germany. Further, they would like to extend their thanks to the hospital staff and patients who supported the quasi-experimental study at the Diakonissenkrankenhaus in Dresden, Germany.

# References

AARP. (2021). *AARP nursing home COVID-19 dashboard.* https://www.aarp.org/ppi/issues/caregiving/info-2020/nursing-home-covid-dashboard.html

Belala, N., Maier, C., Heldmann, P., Schwenk, M., & Becker, C. (2019). A pilot observational study to analyze (in)activity and reasons for sedentary behavior of cognitively impaired geriatric acute inpatients. *Z Gerontol Geriat, 52,* 273–281. https://doi.org/10.1007/s00391-019-01644-x

Bickel, H., Hendlmeier, I., Heßler, J. B., Junge, M. N., Leonhardt-Achilles, S., Weber, J., & Schäufele, M. (2018). The prevalence of dementia and cognitive impairment in hospitals: Results from the general hospital study (GHoSt). *Deutsches Ärzteblatt International, 115*(44), 733.

Binette, J., & Vasold, K. (2018). Home and community preferences: A national survey of adults age 18-plus. *AARP Research.* https://doi.org/10.26419/res.00231.001

Briggs, R., Dyer, A., Nabeel, S., Collins, R., Doherty, J., Coughlan, T., O'Neill, D., & Kennelly, S. P. (2017). Dementia in the acute hospital: The prevalence and clinical outcomes of acutely unwell patients with dementia. *QJM: Monthly Journal of the Association of Physicians, 110*(1), 33–37. https://doi.org/10.1093/qjmed/hcw114

Bueter, K., & Marquardt, G. (2020). *Dementia-friendly hospital building. Construction and design manual.* DOM Publishers.

Calkins, M. P. (1988). *Design for dementia: Planning environments for the elderly and the confused.* National Health Publishing.

Calkins, M. P. (2018). From research to application: Supportive and therapeutic environments for people living with dementia. *The Gerontologist, 58*(Suppl 1), S114–S128. https://doi.org/10.1093/geront/gnx146

Chaudhury, H., Hung, L., Rust, T., & Wu, S. (2017). Do physical environmental changes make a difference? Supporting person-centered care at mealtimes in nursing homes. *Dementia, 16*(7), 878–896. https://doi.org/10.1177/2F1471301215622839

Chaudhury, H., Cooke, H. A., Cowie, H., & Razaghi, L. (2018). The influence of the physical environment on residents with dementia in long-term care settings: A review of the empirical literature. *The Gerontologist, 58*(5), e325–e337. https://doi.org/10.1093/geront/gnw259

Cohen, U., & Weisman, J. (1991). *Holding on to home: Designing environments for people with dementia.* Johns Hopkins University Press.

Cunningham, C., Galbraith, J., Marshall, M., McClenaghan, C., McManus, M., McNair, D., & Dincarslan, O. (2011). *Dementia design audit tool.* University of Stirling.

Davis, R., & Weisbeck, C. (2016). Creating a supportive environment using cues for way-finding in dementia. *Journal of Gerontological Nursing, 42*(3), 36–44. https://doi.org/10.3928/00989134-20160212-07

de Boer, B., Hamers, J. P., Zwakhalen, S. M., Tan, F. E., Beerens, H. C., & Verbeek, H. (2017). Green care farms as innovative nursing homes, promoting activities and social interaction for people with dementia. *Journal of the American Medical Directors Association, 18*(1), 40–46. https://doi.org/10.1016/j.jamda.2016.10.013

de Boer, B., Beerens, H. C., Katterbach, M. A., Viduka, M., Willemse, B. M., & Verbeek, H. (2018). The physical environment of nursing homes for people with dementia: Traditional nursing homes, small-scale living facilities, and green care farms. *Healthcare, 6*(4), 137. https://doi.org/10.3390/healthcare6040137

Dodds, W. (2019). Disease now and potential future pandemics. In W. Dodds (Ed.), *The world's worst problems* (pp. 31–44). Springer. https://doi.org/10.1007/978-3-030-30410-2_4

Dyer, S. M., Liu, E., Gnanamanickam, E. S., Milte, R., Easton, T., Harrison, S. L., Bradley, C. E., Ratcliffe, J., & Crotty, M. (2018). Clustered domestic residential aged care in Australia: Fewer hospitalisations and better quality of life. *Medical Journal of Australia, 208*(10), 433–438. https://doi.org/10.5694/mja17.00861

Feddersen, E. & Luedtke, I. (2014). *Lost in Space. Architecture and Dementia.* Birkhaeuser.

Fleming, R., Zeisel, J., & Bennett, K. (2020a). *World Alzheimer report 2020: Design dignity dementia: Dementia-related design and the built environment* (Vol. 1). Alzheimer's Disease International. https://www.alzint.org/u/WorldAlzheimerReport2020Vol1.pdf

Fleming, R., Zeisel, J., & Bennett, K. (2020b). *World Alzheimer report 2020: Design dignity dementia: Dementia-related design and the built environment* (Vol. 2). Alzheimer's Disease International. https://www.alzint.org/u/WorldAlzheimerReport2020Vol2.pdf

Fritze, T. (2020). The effect of heat and cold waves on the mortality of persons with dementia in Germany. *Sustainability, 12*(9), 3664. https://doi.org/10.3390/su12093664

Fung, J. C. (2015). *Dementia design sourcebook. Design guide + design elements.* Centre for Advanced Studies in Architecture (CASA), Department of Architecture, National University of Singapore.

Gradmann, C. (2018). From lighthouse to hothouse: Hospital hygiene, antibiotics and the evolution of infectious disease, 1950–1990. *History and Philosophy of the Life Sciences, 40*(1), 1–25. https://doi.org/10.1007/s40656-017-0176-8

Grey, T., Pierce, M., Cahill, S., & Dyer, M. (2015). *Universal design guidelines dementia friendly dwellings for people with dementia, their families and carers.* Centre for Excellence in Universal Design. http://universaldesign.ie/Web-Content-/UD_Guidelines-Dementia_Friendly_Dwellings-2015-full-doc.pdf

Grey, T., Fleming, R., Goodenough, B. J., Xidous, D., Moehler, R., & O'Neill, D. (2019). Hospital design for older people with cognitive impairment including dementia and delirium: Supporting inpatients and accompanying persons. *Cochrane Database of Systematic Reviews, 11.* https://doi.org/10.1002/14651858.CD013482

Harrison, S. L., O'Donnell, L. K., Milte, R., Dyer, S. M., Gnanamanickam, E. S., Bradley, C., Liu, E., Hilmer, S. N., & Crotty, M. (2018). Costs of potentially inappropriate medication use in residential aged care facilities. *BMC Geriatrics, 18*(1), 1–10. https://doi.org/10.1186/s12877-018-0704-8

Heiss, O., Degenhart, C., & Ebe, J. (2010). *Barrier-free design: Principles, planning, examples.* Birkhäuser.

Holup, A. A., Hyer, K., Meng, H., & Volicer, L. (2017). Profile of nursing home residents admitted directly from home. *Journal of the American Medical Directors Association, 18*(2), 131–137. https://doi.org/10.1016/j.jamda.2016.08.017

Jegodka, Y., Lagally, L., Mertes, H., Deering, K., Schoierer, J., Buchberger, B., & Bose-O'Reilly, S. (2021). Hot days and Covid 19-unusual heat stress for nursing professions in Germany. *Med Rxiv.* https://doi.org/10.1101/2021.01.29.21250592

King's Fund. (2014). *Is your ward dementia friendly? EHE environmental assessment tool.* The King's Fund. https://www.kingsfund.org.uk/sites/default/files/EHE-dementia-assessment-tool.pdf.

Kirch, J., & Marquardt, G. (2021). Towards human-centred general hospitals: The potential of dementia-friendly design. *Architectural Science Review, 1–9.* https://doi.org/10.1080/0003862 8.2021.1933889

Kirchen-Peters, S., & Krupp, E. (2019). *Praxisleitfaden zum Aufbau demenzsensibler Krankenhäuser.* Robert Bosch Stiftung.

Kok, S. J., Heuvelen, M. J. G., Berg, I. J., & Scherder, E. J. A. (2016). Small scale homelike special care units and traditional special care units: Effects on cognition in dementia: A longitudinal controlled intervention study. *BMC Geriatrics, 16*(1), 1–8. https://doi.org/10.1186/s12877-016-0222-5

Lawton, M. P., & Nahemow, L. (1973). Ecology and the aging process. In C. Eisdorfer & M. P. Lawton (Eds.), *The psychology of adult development and aging* (pp. 619–674). American Psychological Association.

Liu, J., Hlávka, J., Hillestad, R. J., & Mattke, S. (2020). 2020 Alzheimer's disease facts and figures. *Alzheimer's Dement, 16,* 391–460. https://doi.org/10.1002/alz.12068

Marquardt, G. (2011). Wayfinding for people with dementia: A review of the role of architectural design. *HERD: Health Environments Research & Design Journal, 4*(2), 75–90. https://doi.org/10.1177/2F193758671100400207

Marquardt, G., & Schmieg, P. (2009). Dementia-friendly architecture: Environments that facilitate wayfinding in nursing homes. *American Journal of Alzheimer's Disease & Other Dementias, 24*(4), 333–340. https://doi.org/10.1177/2F1533317509334959

Moellers, T., Stocker, H., Wei, W., Perna, L., & Brenner, H. (2019). Length of hospital stay and dementia: A systematic review of observational studies. *International Journal of Geriatric Psychiatry, 34*(1), 8–21. https://doi.org/10.1002/gps.4993

Moore, K. D., Geboy, L. D., & Weisman, G. D. (2006). *Designing a better day: Guidelines for adult and dementia day services centers.* JHU Press.

Motzek, T., Bueter, K., & Marquardt, G. (2017). Investigation of eligible picture categories for use as environmental cues in dementia-friendly environments. *HERD: Health Environments Research & Design Journal, 10*(4), 64–73. https://doi.org/10.1177/2F1937586716679403

Palmer, L., Wallace, K., & Hutchinson, L. (2021). *Architecture for dementia. Stirling gold: 2008–2020.* University of Stirling.

Parke, B., Boltz, M., Hunter, K. F., Chambers, T., Wolf-Ostermann, K., Adi, M. N., Feldman, F., & Gutman, G. (2017). A scoping literature review of dementia-friendly hospital design. *The Gerontologist, 57*(4), e62–e74. https://doi.org/10.1093/geront/gnw128

Phillips, N. (2021). The coronavirus is here to stay-here's what that means. *Nature, 590*(7846), 382–384. https://doi.org/10.1038/d41586-021-00396-2

Pollock, A., & Cunningham, C. (2018). *The room outside. Designing outdoor living for older people and people with dementia.* HammondCare Media.

Rao, A., Suliman, A., Vuik, S., Aylin, P., & Darzi, A. (2016). Outcomes of dementia: Systematic review and meta-analysis of hospital administrative database studies. *Archives of Gerontology and Geriatrics, 66,* 198–204. https://doi.org/10.1016/j.archger.2016.06.008

Regnier, V. (2018). *Housing design for an increasingly older population: Redefining assisted living for the mentally and physically frail.* John Wiley & Sons.

Shepherd, H., Livingston, G., Chan, J., & Sommerlad, A. (2019). Hospitalisation rates and predictors in people with dementia: A systematic review and meta-analysis. *BMC Medicine, 17*(1), 1–13. https://doi.org/10.1186/s12916-019-1369-7

Smith, M., Gerdner, L. A., Hall, G. R., & Buckwalter, K. C. (2004). History, development, and future of the progressively lowered stress threshold: A conceptual model for dementia care. *Journal of the American Geriatrics Society, 52*(10), 1755–1760. https://doi.org/10.1111/j.1532-5415.2004.52473.x

Sourdet, S., Lafont, C., Rolland, Y., Nourhashemi, F., Andrieu, S., & Vellas, B. (2015). Preventable iatrogenic disability in elderly patients during hospitalization. *Journal of the American Medical Directors Association, 16*(8), 674–681. https://doi.org/10.1016/j.jamda.2015.03.011

Strøm, B. S., Ytrehus, S., & Grov, E. K. (2016). Sensory stimulation for persons with dementia: A review of the literature. *Journal of Clinical Nursing, 25*(13–14), 1805–1834. https://doi.org/10.1111/jocn.13169

Toot, S., Devine, M., Akporobaro, A., & Orrell, M. (2013). Causes of hospital admission for people with dementia: A systematic review and meta-analysis. *Journal of the American Medical Directors Association, 14*(7), 463–470. https://doi.org/10.1016/j.jamda.2013.01.011

Tsekleves, E., & Keady, J. (2021). *Design for People Living with dementia: Interactions and innovations*. Routledge.

United Nations. (2019). *World population prospects 2019: Highlights*. https://population.un.org/wpp/Publications/Files/WPP2019_10KeyFindings.pdf

Waller, S., Masterson, A., & Evans, S. C. (2017). The development of environmental assessment tools to support the creation of dementia friendly care environments: Innovative practice. *Dementia, 16*(2), 226–232. https://doi.org/10.1177/2F1471301216635829

Whear, R., Coon, J. T., Bethel, A., Abbott, R., Stein, K., & Garside, R. (2014). What is the impact of using outdoor spaces such as gardens on the physical and mental well-being of those with dementia? A systematic review of quantitative and qualitative evidence. *Journal of the American Medical Directors Association, 15*(10), 697–705. https://doi.org/10.1016/j.jamda.2014.05.013

World Health Organization (2020). The top 10 causes of death. Factsheet. https://www.who.int/news-room/fact-sheets/detail/the-top-10-causesof-death

Xidous, D., Grey, T., Kennelly, S. P., McHale, C., & O'Neill, D. (2020). Dementia friendly hospital design: Key issues for patients and accompanying persons in an Irish acute care public hospital. *HERD: Health Environments Research & Design Journal, 13*(1), 48–67. https://doi.org/10.1177/2F1937586719845120

# Designing the Post-Pandemic Hospice Environment: "The Last Place"

Sharmin Kader

## 1 Introduction

The German philosopher Martin Heidegger, in his famous analysis of death in *Being and Time*, wrote that "death is not an event but rather an existential phenomenon. (Heidegger, 1996). In these days, people die either in their home or in an end-of-life care facility, hospice. Hospice is a place to accommodate this phenomenon, death. It is a place to provide end-of-life care to individuals certified as "terminal" and their families (Government Printing Office, 2000 in Swenson, 2009, p. 9). End-of-life care is a multidisciplinary care and support (non-curative) system designed to address the physical, emotional, psychosocial, and spiritual concerns of terminal patients (NCP, 2004; and Medical Dictionary, 2012), which makes the hospice care model unlike other healthcare models (Siebold, 1992). Accordingly, the design of hospice settings differs from the design of other healthcare settings in important ways. In contemporary design philosophy, end-of-life care service has five basic types of models (Verderber & Refuerzo, 2006): in-hospital hospice or palliative care units (PCUs); home; nursing institutes with dedicated beds for hospice care; medical center-affiliated free-standing hospice; and nonhospital-affiliated autonomous hospice. This chapter discusses post-pandemic design considerations for the latter two categories: free-standing hospice facilities with or without hospital affiliation.

S. Kader (✉)
College of Architecture and Environmental Design, Kent State University, Kent, OH, USA
e-mail: sharminkader@yahoo.com; skader1@kent.edu

© The Author(s), under exclusive license to Springer Nature
Switzerland AG 2023
F. Ferdous, E. Roberts (eds.), *(Re)designing the Continuum of Care for Older Adults*, https://doi.org/10.1007/978-3-031-20970-3_13

## 2   The Hospice Environment

Hospice facility design has a significant impact on dying patients and their families because the place experience helps determine patient "quality of life" (Cohen et al., 2001) and the possibility of a "good death" as defined by Tong et al. (2003). The physical environment is a part of the entire care milieu which also includes personal, social, and organizational dimensions as suggested by Cohen and Weisman (1991) and shown in Fig. 1. The organizational component is conceptualized in terms of the policies and programs, the social component is represented by family and fellow residents, and the architectural component is defined in terms of the experiential qualities or attributes of the environment. The therapeutic goals serve as unifying intentions which can direct congruent decision-making in the organizational, social, and physical realms and thereby provide a useful foundation for planning and design (Cohen & Weisman, 1991) Fig. 1.

In 2015, one study by Kader and Diaz Moore identified eleven therapeutic goals for the hospice care environment that consider the dying experience for patients, their families, and caregivers. Employing a systematic and wide-ranging literature review with an approach developed by Hawker et al., 2002, this study conducted an extensive search including seven electronic databases (PubMed, PsyciNFO, Social Science Citation Index, Science Citation Index, ProQuest Dissertations & Thesis, Avery, and Cochrane Library), reference lists, literature recommended by relevant experts, and Google for books, reports, and guidelines. A total of 847 papers were identified and assessed based on inclusion and exclusion criteria, and 48 texts were

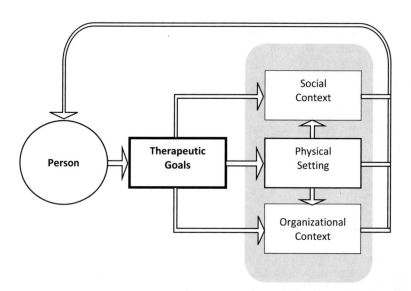

**Fig. 1** A conceptual framework for the organization of the person-environment system. (Adapted from Cohen & Weisman, 1991, figure 1.2)

**Table 1** Therapeutic goals of hospice environment

| | |
|---|---|
| Provide continuity of self | Environmental characteristics that help preserve or support patients' past activities, preferences, and awareness |
| Provide access to nature | Environmental characteristics that provide opportunities for visual and physical access to nature |
| Provide privacy | Environmental characteristics that facilitate patient choice in various levels of privacy through regulation of visual and auditory stimuli |
| Facilitate social interaction | Environmental characteristics that facilitate and enable meaningful interaction between patients and staff, their family, and other patients |
| Maximize safety and security | Environmental characteristics that maximize the safety and security of patients, their families, and staff |
| Provide autonomy | Environmental characteristics that enable patients to exercise choice and personal preference about their environment and everyday life |
| Regulate stimulation and support sensory therapies | Environmental characteristics that contribute to an appropriate quantity and quality of sensory experience and support palliative therapies |
| Provide support for spiritual care | Environmental characteristics that facilitate opportunities for patients' spiritual care, including religious, philosophical, existential, and personal beliefs, values, practices, and preferences |
| Provide family accommodation | Environmental characteristics that facilitate patient family accommodation and support control, functional independence, comfort, privacy, recreation, and spiritual care |
| Provide support after death | Environmental characteristics that support care and dignity for patients and their families from the moment of death through body removal, bereavement, and remembrance |
| Maximize support for staff | Environmental characteristics that support staff for better efficiency, communication, observation, satisfaction, and Well-being |

selected to develop the therapeutic goals of hospice care environment. Those goals and their definitions are presented in Table 1.

According to Lawton et al. (2000), the therapeutic goals reflect two characteristics: each expresses a basic or derived major patient needs and a potential environmental facilitator for the satisfaction of that need. The physical settings of hospice along with a carefully designed organizational environment can contribute to the realization of desired therapeutic goals and have a positive effect on the lives of dying patients. In 2016, Sharmin Kader published the design criteria to achieve these goals. This study used three methods to develop the evidence-based design considerations for each goal: a systematic literature review, interviews with an experts' panel using the Delphi method to obtain their opinions, and five case study surveys. Hospice design considerations to achieve each goal are discussed later.

## 3   COVID-19 and the Hospice Environment

The COVID-19 pandemic is an unprecedented situation that has created many challenges for healthcare facilities, including hospice or end-of-life care facilities
(Rogers et al., 2021). Generally, hospice facilities face unique challenges during
times of disasters as their patient populations are particularly vulnerable due to terminally ill conditions, decreased mobility, and dependence on medical technology
(Rogers et al., 2021). Additionally, hospice care facilities accommodate patient
families and provide spaces for social interaction, and the interdisciplinary care
model includes many volunteers and social workers, creating a risk of spreading
infection among patients, family members, and staff (Anderson et al., 2020). In
addition, restricted family visitations, constraints on social interaction, control over
shared activities (such as spiritual care), and the need for staff to wear personal
protective equipment all create an extra level of mental stress, increasing depression
and patient and staff dissatisfaction (Rogers et al., 2021; Gergerich et al., 2020).

After conducting a literature review, the author has identified six major design-
related challenges of post-pandemic hospice care facilities (Abbott et al., 2020;
Anderson et al., 2020; Bettini, 2020; ECDC, 2021; Etkind et al., 2020; Gergerich
et al., 2020; Ghosh, 2020; Gregory, 2021; Hughes & Vernon, 2021; Kader &
Gharaveis, 2020; Mercadante et al., 2020; Ness et al., 2021; Rogers et al., 2021; Sun
et al., 2020; Tay et al., 2021; Tomlin et al., 2020; and Tseng et al., 2020).

### 3.1   Improve Infection Control

It is difficult but vital to make all the necessary changes in a hospice facility to
improve infection control, such as changing finish materials for easier cleaning,
installing touch-free faucets or fixtures, and installing sneeze shields in reception or
nurse station areas.

### 3.2   Accommodate COVID-19 Patients Along
with Regular Patients

Although hospice facilities are generally designed with one or two isolation rooms
with negative pressure for infectious patients, it is challenging to accommodate
multiple infectious patients and isolate the regular patients and their families.

## 3.3    Accommodate Patients' Families in the Facilities

Accommodating overnight guests and providing them access to the regular amenities (kitchen, laundry, etc.) is difficult due to social distancing and cleaning protocols. Also, it is challenging to regulate the number of visitors and visitation hours for actively dying patients. Screening family members before they enter the facility is another critical function.

## 3.4    Create a Safe and Supportive Place for Healthcare Workers

All healthcare facilities including hospices have faced challenges to ensure staff safety and create a supportive environment for care providers. Studies have found that COVID-19 has created a mental health burden for healthcare workers and increased rates of psychological stress, depression, anxiety, and insomnia. Providing an environment that supports staff well-being is incredibly significant and challenging.

## 3.5    Provide Palliative Therapies and Spiritual or Grief Support

Hospice care provides psychological and spiritual support to patients, their families, and staff. The bereavement support for family continues for 13 months after patient's death. It is difficult to provide some palliative therapies and spiritual care while maintaining infection prevention guidelines.

## 3.6    Increase in-House Surge Capacity

There has been a growing demand for hospice care during the peak of the COVID-19 pandemic. Generally, a hospice facility has one or two isolation rooms with negative pressure. This is clearly insufficient to accommodate the influx of contagious patients and the required medical supplies and equipment.

## 4    Therapeutic Goals of Hospice Environments

This section defines and explains the significance of each therapeutic goal developed by Kader and Diaz Moore in 2015 and briefly discusses the key design considerations for each goal developed by Kader in 2016 through an intensive study. It also identifies any conflicts or challenges in incorporating COVID-19 design and pandemic resilience criteria.

## 4.1 Goal 1: Provide Continuity of Self

**Definition** Environmental characteristics that help preserve or support patients' past activities, preferences, and awareness:

> *I'd rather be home, of course, but they brought things from home and when I wake up, nice, cozy, then you don't have that longing.* (Hospice patient, as cited in Larkin et al., 2007, p. 74)

Dying patients experience complex emotions and a sense of instability and ephemerality. To avoid lack of familiarity and disorientation in hospice care, the creation of a "domestic" or "homelike" environment is a top priority. It is important to recreate meaningful surroundings for patients to ease the transition from home to institution.

**Design Considerations** Homelike environments can be achieved in two ways: by avoiding an institutional appearance and by enabling patients to personalize their spaces. Building size, scale, layout, exterior appearance, and landscape design should be residential in size and scale. Outdoor spaces should be integrated with indoor spaces to provide nice views from most areas. Patient units should mimic a residential setting with multiple bedrooms clustered around a living room. Long corridors and large central social spaces should be avoided. Instead, designs should create multiple small, intimate social spaces. The overall interior design needs careful attention to the use of color, selection of furniture, quality of light, selection of finishes, exploration of views, and artwork. Special consideration should be given to designing patient beds and headwalls to hide mechanical systems and thus create a non-institutional look. The overall design should promote orientation with space, time, and outside weather condition, such as having a window and a wall clock with visibility from the patient's bed head. Room design should also include wall shelves, picture hooks, and adequate space to accommodate patients' personal belongings, such as photos, paintings, a special chair or rug, and mementos.

**COVID-19 Challenges** The only issue is the selection of homelike finish materials and furniture (e.g., wood or stone, a curtain or a rug) which must be easily cleanable and withstand harsh cleaning chemicals. Patients' personal belongings may create difficulties in maintaining environmental hygiene.

## 4.2   Goal 2: Provide Access to Nature

**Definition**  Environmental characteristics that provide opportunities for physical and visual access to nature:

> *To be able to go out, to enjoy the trees and the air and the flowers and the colors, and to hear the birds singing, that's quality of life.* (Hospice patient as cited in Cohen & Leis, 2002, p. 5)

Having a physical and visual connection to nature provides significant benefits to patients, lifting spirits, increasing comfort, and improving quality of life in hospice care. As a dying patient tends to spend more and more time indoor and confined in a limited space, a view of natural landscape through windows can enhance positive feelings and reduce fear, anxiety, and pain.

**Design Considerations**  Maximize daylight, outdoor views, and fresh air through design. Building layout should consider outside views to landscape and organize accordingly. Try to provide maximum view to outside landscape and gardens from each patient's bed, social spaces, spiritual spaces, and staff break rooms. Provide natural daylight in most of the spaces. Have an operable window or door in patient rooms to allow fresh air. Provide transitional spaces (e.g., patio, veranda) between indoor and outside spaces. Create a large transitional space attached with social space to accommodate a large gathering or family event (barbeque party, birthday party, etc.). Provide bed accessibility to outdoor spaces and garden by designing wide pathways with appropriate finish materials. Create gardens with beautiful landscaping, flowers, plants, water features, bird feeders, sculptures, and multiple seating arrangements. Provide a visual interest and destination area with seating. Seating arrangements should allow for both group gatherings and individual solitude. In high-rise buildings, provide a roof garden. In cold weather areas, create small indoor gardens or use natural features inside the building.

**COVID-19 Challenges**  All of these design considerations are very supportive in a pandemic situation, but attention should be paid to selecting the natural materials and features (e.g., water fountains) to comply with the high level of infection prevention criteria in healthcare settings.

## 4.3   Goal 3: Provide Privacy

**Definition**  Environmental characteristics that facilitate patient choice in various levels of privacy through regulation of visual and auditory stimuli:

> *A good death is to give privacy to the family and the resident to work out there at the end.* (Hospice staff member as cited in Brazil et al., 2004, p.88)

Privacy is particularly salient to the dignity, independence, quality of life, and emotional well-being of patients and their families. Family and staff find privacy more important than patients. Lack of privacy due to the presence of a roommate may create discomfort and dissatisfaction. A dying patient and family should have privacy to spend time together, share feelings, and say goodbye.

**Design Considerations**  A single room with an attached bathroom provides better privacy for family accommodation, confidentiality of conversation, avoidance of distress from watching other patients' suffering, and private television watching or music playing than rooms with two or more patients. Design should avoid visibility of a patient's bed head from the circulation corridor. For rooms on the ground level, ensure visual privacy at night from outside gardens or paths. Improve acoustic privacy through the use of acoustic or absorbent materials in the ceilings, non-glossy surfaces in floors and walls, wood and fabric in the furniture, curtains in windows, and a building layout that creates a buffer zone (e.g., toilet) between patient rooms and corridors. Multiple small, intimate spaces provide better privacy for patients, families, and staff than one large central social space. Provide designated spaces for private communication between staff and families. Provide an outdoor social space with enough visual privacy for private family gatherings with patients.

**COVID-19 Challenges**  Select good acoustic-friendly finish materials and design features (e.g., cushions, curtains, carpets) to comply with infection control.

## 4.4   Goal 4: Facilitate Social Interaction

**Definition**  Environmental characteristics that facilitate and enable meaningful interaction between patients and staff, their families, and other patients:

> Very few people know what it feels like to know they are facing their last months of life. There can be a loneliness that is different from any other. It is a loneliness of the heart, even when you have people around you. (American Cancer Society, 2011)

Physical and emotional proximity to loved ones during the dying experience is one of the key themes of a good death. It improves patients' social life and lessens the feeling of loneliness. To facilitate patients' social interaction, accommodation of family and visitors and access to phone calls or letters has been emphasized in end-of-life care. Patients also benefit from interacting with other patients; it offers them self-reflection, mutual empathy, and companionship.

**Design Considerations**  With the decline of physical status, patients' desired level of socialization varies, and patients spend more time in and around their bed areas. A single room is preferable to have the opportunity of private interaction with family. Patient room should have enough space to accommodate many visitors to sit and to stand around bed. Provide a comfortable chair, recliner, or daybed for family members to relax and sleep. Provide opportunity for phone conversations and

Internet connection. In some cases, shared rooms are preferable. To have constant companionship and to witness a quiet, painless death of a roommate can help patients deal with their own end-of-life fears. Moveable partitions may provide better privacy than curtains during bathing and personal care in shared rooms. As privacy need increases as disease progresses, dying patients may move to a single room. Three beds rather than two in shared rooms can help soften the impact of the death of a roommate. Flexible rooms or trans-programmatic bedrooms can be easily convertible into single units when required. Make at least one room big enough to convert into a double bed or shared room to accommodate spouses, partners, or friends.

Social interactions also take place in hallways, living rooms, dayrooms, kitchen/café areas, and outdoor places or gardens. Design should incorporate a variety of cozy spaces to allow both group interaction and intimate discussion. Provide a residential look with comfortable furniture, a place for children to play freely under supervision, and outdoor landscape areas with shelter and sitting amenities. Having a large patio with visual privacy from other parts of the facility serves as a private family gathering space for patients to celebrate or take photos or to meet a pet (e.g., horse).

**COVID-19 Challenges** Maintaining social distancing in the social spaces.

## 4.5 Goal 5: Maximize Safety and Security

**Definition** Environmental characteristics that maximize the safety and security of patients, staff, and families:

*Hospice patients and their families experience emotional and other traumas, and are in need of safety, security, and refuge.* (Verderber & Refuerzo, 2006, p. 65)

Safety and security are among the most important issues of any healthcare facility (Ulrich et al., 2004), and there is a significant amount of research suggesting in-depth design considerations related to the safety and security of hospice care environments for patients, families, children, and staff. These considerations address accessibility, fire codes, theft and vandalism, fall prevention, infection control, and secure continuity of providing care.

**Design Considerations** Hospice care facilities must be fully barrier-free for disabled persons, should comply with regional fire safety codes and standards, and should be secured from theft and vandalism. Access and entrance points should be screened without sacrificing the overall openness and welcoming environment. Avoid patient falls by providing safety features inpatient beds (e.g., height adjustable beds) and a nurse call system. Provide grab bars in toilets and enough space in bathrooms so that at least two people can assist patients.

Considerations in the selection of furniture, fittings, and finishes include performance and clinical and infection control. Furniture must have stability, and corners on table benches and cupboards will preferably be rounded. Glass or clear plastic furniture should be avoided. Elements supportive of functional independence of patients and their families should be secured (stoves, kitchen utilities, microwaves, electronic appliances, etc.) and easy to monitor by staff. Covered porches should be provided for transferring patients during adverse weather.

The selection of furniture, fittings, and finishes should also consider infection control, and designs should provide handwashing sinks and sanitizing stations. Provide separate family toilets to avoid cross contamination from patient toilets. Provide one or two isolation rooms with appropriate standards. For disaster preparedness, facilities must be equipped with continuous power supply and necessary medical supplies, oxygen supply, a patient call system, and so on. Design should ensure security of the entire facility, including the parking area, from theft and vandalism.

**COVID-19 Challenges**  No conflict.

## 4.6   Goal 6: Provide Autonomy

**Definition**  Environmental characteristics that enable patients to exercise choice and personal preference about their environment and everyday life:

> *We are trying to give him everything he wants. From the special incense on his table, special drops in his water, his own pillow and slippers beside his bed, even if he is not able to walk.*
> (Hospice nurse technician as cited in Lindqvist et al., 2012, p. 4)

A dying patient should have a sense of control, and losing this can cause discomfort and dissatisfaction. Patients should have the opportunity to maintain as much control over their physical environment (e.g., furniture arrangements, personalization, temperature, noise, lighting, ventilation, smells) and their daily activities (e.g., bathing, eating, entertainment, and smoking) as possible. It is vital to understand a dying patient's wishes and allow them to exercise their choices as much as possible.

**Design Considerations**  Provide a sense of control in patient rooms and social spaces. Window design and location should consider the control of glare, climate, and ventilation. Dimmer switches and operable curtains provide greater control over lighting levels. Noise can be from different sources, such as televisions, phones, bells, loud staff conversations, and patients shouting, moaning, or groaning, which needs to be addressed by designing sound containment throughout the entire facility. A single room provides better control over the micro-environment. Provide operable windows and doors in patient rooms and in some social spaces to allow fresh air. Provide ceiling fans with dimmer switches in patient rooms. To avoid food smells from the kitchen, locate it a little further from patient rooms and use a high-quality exhaust fan. To provide control over physical settings, provide flexible furniture in patient room and a few movable chairs in indoor and outdoor social spaces to allow patients and families to create a desirable arrangement. To provide control over daily routine and activities (bathing, eating, smoking, watching television, etc.), provide a 24-hour family kitchenette for patient food preparation, Wi-Fi, and phone use. Provide designated indoor and outdoor smoking areas. More design considerations can be found in an article (Kader, 2017).

**COVID-19 Challenges**  No conflicts.

## 4.7  Goal 7: Regulate Stimulation and Support Sensory Therapies

**Definition**  Environmental characteristics that contribute to an appropriate quantity and quality of sensory experience and support sensory therapies (palliative therapies):

> You know, what is quality of life for someone lying in bed unable to do almost anything except breathe and open their mouth? That's about it. So, is it just doing those things, having that person in the fresh air or where there's stimulation of some sort? (A hospice patient's wife, as cited in Russell et al., 2008, p. 91)

Sensory stimulation offers therapeutic treatment for pain, depression, and many other symptoms, which are basic criteria of palliative care. Sensory stimulation may generate response in the patient—"a spark, a smile, a memory or a moment of lucidness" (NHPCO, 2007; p. 5). Different types of sensory therapies (music, aromatherapy, art, massage, horticulture, spa/hydro, multi-sensory, etc.) are increasingly used in hospice care to improve patient quality of life. Studies found environmental factors can influence patients' sensory experience (Ulrich et al., 2004). A meaningful view, for example, reduces stress and pain; color can affect mood; "exposure to daylight" reduces depression, eases pain, lessens agitation, and improves sleep and circadian rhythms (Joseph et al., 2006); and artwork (paintings, sculptures, water features, etc.) has multiple benefits for patients. Art representing nature in particular evokes a positive response in patients.

**Design Considerations**  Provide positive therapeutic stimuli through environmental design. Regulate levels of acoustic stimulation, visual stimulation, and olfactory stimulation (often the intrusion of noxious stimulation). In general, hospice facilities are known for their lack of tactile stimulation, which limit the need for regulation. Provide support for therapies (music therapy, aromatherapy, horticulture therapy, multi-sensory room design). Although there is little empirical research focusing on sensory environments for dying patients, designing for positive stimulation in the hospice environment means a peaceful, warm, and non-institutional interior design with the presence of natural light, attractive views, access to nature, and display of artworks. Also, designing for customization is important; personal photographs around the bed, a favorite perfume or scent, and comfortable cushions or pillows can also be highly therapeutic.

Some specific therapies require definite environmental characteristics. For example, spa therapy requires a quiet room free from noise and outside distraction. Horticultural therapy requires a raised platform for gardening or a greenhouse. Spaces for special therapies, such as a multi-sensory room or a spa/hydrotherapy room, have their own design criteria.

**COVID-19 Challenges** Attention should be paid to selecting the natural materials and features (e.g., water fountain) to comply with high level of infection prevention criteria.

## 4.8   Goal 8: Support for Spiritual Care

**Definition** Environmental characteristics that facilitate opportunities for patients' spiritual care, including religious, philosophical, and existential or personal beliefs, values, practices, and preferences:

> *Spirituality is the aspect of humanity that refers to the way individuals seek and express meaning and purpose and the way they experience their connectedness to the moment, to self, to others, to nature, and to the significant or sacred.* (Puchalski et al., 2009, p. 887)

Spiritual care is a fundamental component of hospice or palliative care, offering support for patients' personal striving for health, wholeness, comfort, and meaning at the end of life. According to National Consensus Project (NCP) Guidelines (2009), "the palliative care service facilitates religious or spiritual rituals or practices as desired by patient and family, especially at the time of death." As each person's definition of spirituality is individualized and may or may not include a religious preference, so spiritual care should be defined broadly and include practices such as meaning-oriented therapy, meditation, yoga, art therapy, etc.

**Design Considerations** Provide more than one spiritual care space. Provide formal spiritual care spaces: a sanctuary or chapel or meditation space to accommodate group prayers or rituals (for at least 10 to 12 people). Provide at least one quiet room or meditation space for small gatherings (3 to 5 people) for meditation, quiet reflection, or prayer; it might also work as a grieving room or consultancy room for chaplains, religious workers, or funeral directors. These indoor spiritual spaces should be accessible by wheelchair or bed, should consider good acoustic design to ensure a calm contemplative environment, and should have comfortable and flexible furnishings. Environmental aesthetics (paintings, pictures, décor, outside views) should encourage reflection and foster self-nurturing behaviors, and the spaces can be enriched with architectural delight (e.g., use of skylight, stained glass, nice view, water features). Patient rooms (private or shared) must have enough space around patient beds to perform bedside prayer, worship, or rituals. Have shelves or side tables to display patients' religious artifacts. Different moods of artificial light help create a contemplative environment. Garden or outdoor places can also be used for meditation or spiritual reflection. Provide an outdoor chapel or a designated outdoor space to perform rituals or a range of spiritual care practices.

**COVID-19 Challenges** Maintaining social distancing in the spiritual care spaces.

## 4.9 Goal 9: Provide Family Accommodation

**Definition** Environmental characteristics that facilitate patient family accommodation and support control, functional independence, comfort, privacy, recreation, and spiritual care:

> Family means those closest to the patient in knowledge, care and affection. This includes the biological family, the family of acquisition (related by marriage/contract) and the family of choice and friends (not related biologically or by marriage/contract). (Hospice Unit Generic Brief, 2000, p. 54)

The importance of "family presence" during the experience of death is well established in palliative care, and it has also been confirmed by studies in other related fields. Relatives need support in caring for a dying patient as well as in maintaining their own well-being.

**Design Considerations** The important design considerations include easy accessibility and clear directions or wayfinding for visitors; patient rooms large enough to accommodate overnight stays and a large number of visitors; a separate family bedroom in case the patient is in a shared room and actively dying; enough storage space for family use only; patient control over surrounding environments and daily activities, such as the ability to adjust temperature or move furniture; and amenities for functional independence, such as laundry, kitchen, and Wi-Fi. Provide different sizes of social spaces to accommodate visitors, from a large number to a few family members; a safe place for children to play under supervision; a place for pets that is "unobtrusive, hygienic, and yet close in proximity to patients"; a "family zone" or private break-out area for relaxation and recreation; an outdoor garden for socialization and individual solitude; a smoking area; appropriate space for spiritual care; and space for bereavement support.

**COVID-19 Challenges** As mentioned earlier, family overnight accommodation with regular amenities (kitchen, laundry, etc.) is difficult due to social distancing and cleaning protocol. Also, it is challenging to regulate the number of visitors for an actively dying patient and to screen visitors before they enter the facility.

## 4.10 Goal 10: Provide Support After Death

**Definition** Environmental characteristics that support care and dignity for patients and their families from the moment of death through body removal, bereavement, and remembrance:

> The room was filled with peace. They had put a white cloth on the bedside table and lit a candle. He was so beautiful in his best shirt, and everything was nice and clean. They had even laid a rose in his hand. (Kaarbo, 2011, p. 1129)

The event of death has some unique design and environmental considerations for hospice facilities. This time period starts right before the moment of death, continues through the transfer of the deceased and provision of bereavement support for families, and ends with the expression of remembrance. Patients may have some specific wishes about their death event, such as wanting to die in a garden, or families may have wishes such as wanting to perform bedside rituals.

**Design Considerations** Room size should be large enough to accommodate a large gathering around the patient bed during the event of death. Provide an operable opening (window or door) to support the belief in "allowing the soul to leave" during the moment of death. Provide a signage system outside the door to inform the staff and others that the deceased body is still inside. Provide individual temperature control systems in rooms that will allow lower temperatures to help keep the body for a few hours. Provide a small grieving or quiet room for families to gather after death (located near the inpatient area). Provide a discreet and sensitive route to transfer deceased patient bodies from bedroom to funeral car. The route must avoid service exits. Have a covered porch to transfer during adverse weather. Locate a bereavement suite or meeting room near the entrance to avoid a route through inpatient units. Provide storage space to keep patient belongings for a few months while waiting for family members to pick them up. Provide a flower room with a sink to organize flowers from the funeral hall. Provide dignified ways of expressing remembrance for the deceased. For example, have a designated remembrance wall (e.g., brink tile wall, donor wall, memory tree wall) or outdoor garden (with special memorial stones or landscape features).

**COVID-19 Challenges** There are a few strict guidelines for handling the body of a deceased COVID-19 patient. For transport and storage, the body must be placed and secured in a bag or other wrapping in a manner that prevents leakage. For viewing purposes, have a designated space, preferably a semi-outdoor or outdoor space (patio), for COVID patients. The body should be transferred through a separate exit and not cross the public route.

## 4.11   Goal 11: Maximize Support for Staff

**Definition**   Environmental characteristics that support staff for better communication, observation, efficiency, satisfaction, and well-being:

> *They are taking care of seriously ill people and need all the help they can get through efficient design, and pleasant work areas.* (Moorhouse, 2006, p.12)

Hospice staff take care of seriously ill people and their families and deal with death 24/7. At the same time, they are responsible for creating a comfortable, lively, quality environment. Patients value staff members with good dispositions and good communication skills. Staffs' satisfaction, productivity, and overall well-being are vital to the success of a hospice facility.

**Design Considerations**   Hospice design must provide an efficient, pleasant, and safe work environment for the staff. The environment should provide privacy and a comfortable work area; support socialization, relaxation, and recreation; support ease in observation and care; and maximize safety and security.

To ensure privacy, building layout should consider separate zoning for the staff area, a separate staff parking area, and separate staff entrance. It also helps to have travelling healthcare staff enter and exit the building without crossing the public route. To provide a comfortable work area, create intimate scale office spaces with a more residential look, have enough work area and storage space, have an efficient layout, have daylight and a nice view, and provide comfortable and flexible furnishings.

To support staff socialization, relaxation, and recreation, create at least one staff break area for inpatient and outside staff. Provide multiple intimate scale workspaces instead of one large space. Provide comfortable and flexible furnishings, daylight, a nice view to outside, visual and acoustic privacy, an attached outdoor area with seating opportunities, and recreational facilities (television, games, books, videos). Provide a quiet area besides the staff break area for individual solitude with a nice view to outside. Provide a small break area attached to the nurse station if the central break area is a long walking distance; it is convenient at night. Provide access to outdoor landscape for retreat or meditation. Provide at least one staff-only outdoor area with access to a walking trail or garden.

To ease the patient observation and care process, building layout should consider a short corridor run from nurse station to patient rooms and supply areas. Provide visual and acoustic privacy at the nurse station and the necessary equipment and mechanical systems (nurse calling system, patient lift systems, cameras, etc.). Provide staff zones in patient rooms with a supply closet so that at night the staff can enter easily and monitor patients without interrupting family. Provide adequate storage near the nurse station. Provide good surveillance of the building and parking lot to secure it from theft and vandalism.

**COVID-19 Challenges**   Number of occupancy rates (size of areas per worker) need to be reconsidered for dedensification purposes.

# 5 Prospective Design Considerations for COVID-19

Generally, hospice facilities are small and building layouts incorporate outdoor landscape to maximize access to nature. Rooms are designed with nice views to outside and mostly with private verandas, and there are multiple small-scale social spaces and outdoor seating arrangements. All these criteria are incredibly support-ive for accommodating the design considerations of the COVID-19 pandemic. Although current hospice design strategies are helpful, to incorporate increased lev-els of infection control measures and emergency preparedness, several prospective design concepts are explored in the following section based on the literature review and analysis (Anderson et al., 2020; Chen et al., 2020; ECDC, 2021; Fadaei, 2021; Gola et al., 2021; Gordon et al., 2021; Isha et al., 2020; Kader, 2016; Kader & Gharaveis, 2020; Liu et al., 2020; Naomi, 2020; Ronca et al., 2021; and Wang, 2021).

## 5.1 Planning and Programming

Planning and programming should incorporate infection prevention, increase the number of isolation rooms, increase in-house surge capacity, incorporate pandemic resiliency, and plan for alternative care sites. Due to intensive cleaning processes, the space allocation and utilization rate will change and should be considered dur-ing programming. Site planning should incorporate multiple points of access to the building, separate parking lots, separate patient entrances, and an area to triage people before they enter the building, which can be achieved by providing an oppor-tunity for temporary structures and waiting areas. Administrative offices can be in a separate structure with a separate entrance. Design should ensure security of the entire facility including the parking area and provide secure night entry to the inpa-tient units for staff and family.

## 5.2 Building Configurations

To reduce the number and density of patients, staff, and visitors in one single build-ing, the functions can be broken into small parts and joined through a circulation spine. Design patient units for a small number of patients, and have multiple bed-rooms clustered around a shared living room. COVID-19-positive or contagious patient units should have a separate entrance for patients, visitors, and staff, and there should be an option for a separate HVAC system. Anterooms or changing sta-tions should be incorporated in these units for staff to remove PPE without contami-nating other areas. Plan building layout to separate the staff area from inpatient units and social spaces. Provide a separate parking area and entrance to the staff area so that staff can enter without crossing public spaces. Building layout should also consider a night zone or 24-hour zone and a separate day zone (administrative area) to provide more limited and focused security at night. Building layout should consider outside views to landscape and organize accordingly. Try to provide maximum view to outside landscape and garden from each patient's bed, social spaces, spiritual spaces, and staff break rooms.

## 5.3   Overall Interior Design

One of the major objectives of post-pandemic interior design is maximizing infection prevention. Choose design features that can be easily cleaned and use finishes that withstand harsh chemicals. UV light or sterilizing mists can be used in high- to medium-risk areas. Low-risk areas also need more thorough cleaning protocols and room turnover processes. Select lightweight, kinetic, and flexible furniture, which is easily movable, rearrangeable, and sanitizable. Provide touchless technology and upgraded building mechanical systems with automatic doors with motion sensors or facial recognition, motion sensors for lights and faucets, and elevators and AV systems that can be controlled from a smartphone. Use self-cleaning materials for hot-spot surfaces which have the ability to remove any debris or bacteria from their surfaces in a variety of ways. All of this needs to be done without sacrificing the warmth and hospitality of today's designs.

## 5.4   Staff Area

Limit shared workspaces for staff by reconsidering room sizes and separating workstations. Eliminate the large break room or locker room, and provide multiple discrete, small spaces. Create workstations prioritizing physical distancing. As telemedicine increases, provide small virtual conference rooms with required technical support. Provide multiple small staff break areas or seating spaces prioritizing physical distancing. Use glass to separate these spaces for a sense of transparency and connectivity. Provide more storage areas, changing stations, and hand sanitizing stations. Use hands-free fixtures and appliances in bathrooms and kitchens. Limit the amount of surface areas that staff touch. Provide more private recreational spaces. The administrative department can be in a separate building or floor.

## 5.5   Patient Rooms

Previous research has found that private bedrooms with private bathrooms provide better infection control. It is easier to use these rooms to isolate confirmed or suspected COVID-19 patients and accommodate family members. Shared rooms for two or three can also accommodate COVID-19 patients without family or respite patients. Providing enough space around patient beds helps maintain social distance for visitors and therapists. Having access to a private veranda or patio from patient rooms improves the experience of patients, families, and staff, as shown in Fig. 2. The presence of an intermediate space or foyer between bedrooms and circulation areas can be used as an anteroom, as shown in Fig. 3. Handwashing sinks or hand sanitizer can be placed in those spaces. Providing built-in closets in those spaces that can be accessed from both sides can help staff load linens and supplies without entering patient rooms.

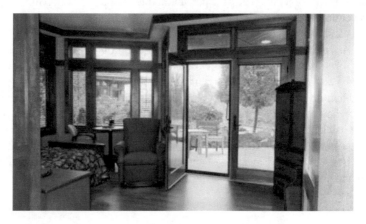

**Fig. 2** Patient room of one project is designed with a private patio and bed-accessible French doors and bay window. The patient's bed is placed to provide maximum view to outside. @ Sharmin Kader

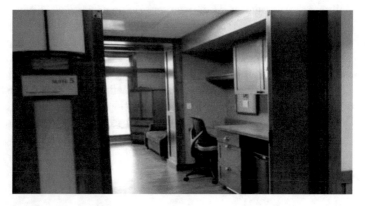

**Fig. 3** The foyer space between the corridor and patient's room provides privacy for the patient and the opportunity to use this space as an anteroom. @ Sharmin Kader

## 5.6    Social/Family Spaces

Instead of having one single large, central social space for the entire facility, distribute multiple small intimate spaces throughout the facility. Pod-style unit design with multiple bedrooms clustered around a living room provides better infection control. Change the layout of common spaces, waiting rooms, lobbies, dining facilities, kitchens, and spiritual care spaces to facilitate social distancing and appropriate queuing. Provide outdoor seating and exterior social areas for families and visitors. Provide separate bedrooms with bathrooms for actively dying patient families to stay overnight.

## 5.7    Outdoor Spaces and Gardens

Outdoor spaces play a vital role in the mental and physical health of staff, family members, and patients during a pandemic (Hobday & Cason, 2009.). Early research found outdoor hospital spaces had undetectable or incredibly low concentrations of the COVID-19 virus (Liu et al., 2020). Outdoor landscape and garden areas can be used for meditation or private family meetings and can create a separate entrance to the facility, as shown in Fig. 4. The transitional spaces (veranda, patio, etc.) and the seating spaces in gardens should be divided into three areas: only for staff, only for infectious patients, and for families. Outdoor pathways can also be used to create a separate entrance to the building, especially to the COVID-19 units.

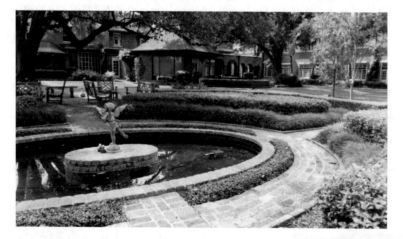

**Fig. 4** Garden view of one project. The garden with a small water pond at the center provides an opportunity for meditation and can be used as a private family meeting place. @ Sharmin Kader

## 6 Conclusions

In the era of an increasingly aging population, the need to design new hospice care facilities and expand and remodel existing facilities is no surprise. Additionally, this pandemic has forced hospice facilities to figure out how to make emergency changes with limited supplies and resources. In the coming years, hospice facilities need to adjust their operations for future pandemics and need to rewrite design guidelines to safely encounter these new situations. Further research is needed to develop evidence-based design guidelines which will improve a dying patient's quality of hospice care and ensure better resiliency and pandemic preparedness. This chapter plows new territory in attempting to identify the gaps and issues created by the COVID-19 pandemic to achieve the eleven salient therapeutic goals of hospice environments and, in so doing, challenges architects and society to create more enabling and inspiring environments to support a high-quality dying experience for all involved. This chapter has focused only on free-standing hospice facilities, not other settings, such as ICUs or nursing homes. Further research should be conducted regarding those environments. We must remember that there is no time at which we are more vulnerable and the environment more latent with meaning than in our last places. The right to a quality environment at the time of the dying experience is an inalienable right and needs no empirical justification.

## References

Abbott, J., Johnson, D., & Wynia, M. (2020). Ensuring adequate palliative and hospice care during COVID-19 surges. *Journal of the American Medical Association, 324*(14), 1393–1394. https://doi.org/10.1001/jama.2020.16843

American Cancer Society. (2011). *Your emotions or what you might feel.* Retrieved March 23, 2013, from American Cancer Society website: http://mstage.qa.cancer.org/treatment/nearingtheendoflife/nearingtheendoflife/nearing-the-end-of-life-emotions

Anderson, D. C., Grey, T., Kennelly, S., & O'Neill, D. (2020). Nursing home design and COVID-19: Balancing infection control, quality of life, and resilience. *Journal of the American Medical Directors Association, 21*(11), 1519–1524. https://doi.org/10.1016/j.jamda.2020.09.005

Bettini, E. A. (2020). COVID-19 pandemic restrictions and the use of Technology for Pediatric Palliative Care in the acute care setting. *Journal of hospice and palliative nursing: JHPN: the official journal of the Hospice and Palliative Nurses Association, 22*(6), 432–434. https://doi.org/10.1097/NJH.0000000000000694

Brazil, K., McAiney, C., Caron-O'Brien, M., et al. (2004). Quality end-of-life Care in Long-Term Care Facilities: Service Providers' perspective. *Journal of Palliative Care, 20*(2), 85–92.

Chen, Q., Liang, M., Li, Y., Guo, J., Fei, D., Wang, L., He, L. I., Sheng, C., Cai, Y., Li, X., & Wang, J. (2020). Mental health care for medical staff in China during the COVID-19 outbreak. *The Lancet Psychiatry, 7*(4), e15–e16.

Cohen, S. R., & Leis, A. (2002). What determines the quality of life of terminally ill cancer patients from their own perspective? *Journal of Palliative Care, 18*(1), 48.

Cohen, U., & Weisman, G. (1991). *Holding onto home: Designing environments for people with dementia.* John Hopkins University Press.

Cohen, S. R., Boston, P., Mount, B. M., & Porterfield, P. (2001). Changes in quality of life following admission to palliative care units. *Palliative Medicine, 15*(5), 363–371.

Etkind, S. N., Bone, A. E., Lovell, N., Cripps, R. L., Harding, R., Higginson, I. J., & Sleeman, K. E. (2020). The role and response of palliative care and hospice services in epidemics and pandemics: A rapid review to inform practice during the COVID-19 pandemic. *Journal of Pain and Symptom Management, 60*(1), e31–e40.

European Centre for Disease Prevention and Control. (2021, February 9). *Infection prevention and control and preparedness for COVID-19 in healthcare settings – Sixth update*. ECDC.

Fadaei, A. (2021). Ventilation systems and COVID-19 spread: Evidence from a systematic review study. *European Journal of Sustainable Development Research, 5*(2).

Gergerich, E., Mallonee, J., Gherardi, S., Kale-Cheever, M., & Duga, F. (2020). Strengths and struggles for families involved in hospice care during the COVID-19 pandemic. *Journal of Social Work in End-of-Life & Palliative Care*, 1–20.

Ghosh, D. (2020). End-of-life issues in the era of the COVID-19 pandemic. *The Korean Journal of Hospice and Palliative Care, 23*(3), 162–165.

Gola, M., Botta, M., D'Aniello, A. L., & Capolongo, S. (2021). Influence of nature at the time of the pandemic: An experience-based survey at the time of SARS-CoV-2 to demonstrate how even a short break in nature can reduce stress for healthcare staff. *HERD: Health Environments Research & Design Journal, 14*(2), 49–65. https://doi.org/10.1177/1937586721991113

Gordon, D., Ward, J., Yao, C. J., & Lee, J. (2021). Built environment airborne infection control strategies in pandemic alternative care sites. *HERD: Health Environments Research & Design Journal, 14*(2), 38–48.

Government Printing Office. (2000). *U.S. code of federal regulations 42CFR418.1*. Retrieved from http://www.access.gpo.gov/nara/cfr/waisidx_00/42cfr418_00.html

Gregory, D. (2021). Code lavender: Designing healthcare spaces to enhance caregiver wellness. *HERD: Health Environments Research & Design Journal, 14*(2), 13–15. https://doi.org/10.1177/1937586721993785

Hawker, S., Payne, S., Kerr, C., Hardey, M., & Powell, J. (2002). Appraising the evidence: Reviewing disparate data systematically. *Qualitative Health Research, 12*(9), 1284–1299.

Heidegger, M. (1996). *Being and time: A translation of sein und Zeit*. SUNY Press.

Hobday, R. A., & Cason, J. W. (2009). The open-air treatment of pandemic influenza. *American Journal of Public Health, 99*(S2), S236–S242.

Hospice Unit Generic Brief. (2000). The aged, Community and Mental Health Division, Melbourne, Australia: Victoria Government Department of Human Services.

Hughes, M. C., & Vernon, E. (2021). Hospice response to COVID-19: Promoting sustainable inclusion strategies for racial and ethnic minorities. *Journal of Gerontological Social Work, 64*(2), 101–105.

Isha, S. N., Ahmad, A., Kabir, R., & Apu, E. H. (2020). Dental clinic architecture prevents COVID-19-like infectious diseases. *HERD: Health Environments Research & Design Journal, 13*(4), 240–241.

Joseph, A., Zimring, C., Harris-Kojetin, L., & Kiefer, K. (2006). Presence and visibility of outdoor and indoor physical activity features and participation in physical activity among older adults in retirement communities. *Journal of Housing for the Elderly, 19*(3–4), 141–165.

Kaarbo, E. (2011). End-of-life care in two Norwegian nursing homes: Family perceptions. *Journal of Clinical Nursing, 20*(7–8), 1125–1132.

Kader, S. (2016). *Development of hospice environmental assessment protocol (HEAP): A post occupancy evaluation tool*. Doctoral dissertation, University of Kansas). http://hdl.handle.net/1808/21798

Kader, S., 2017. Environmental characteristics that enable dying patients to exercise choice and personal preference. *Proceedings of the EDRA48 Conference on Voices of Place* (pp. 116–126). https://cdn.ymaws.com/www.edra.org/resource/collection/8F43AFA7-151E-4AE2-8E3F-F71DF0ABF411/EDRA-Proceedings-2017.pdf

Kader, S. & Diaz Moore, K. (2015). Therapeutic dimensions of palliative care environment. *Proceedings of the ARCC Conference on Future of Architectural Research* (pp. 492–499). http://hdl.handle.net/1808/23329

Kader, S., & Gharaveis, A. (2020, September 7). *Transformation of hospital design after a 'disaster' or 'unforeseen event'* [Webinar]. [Online]. Academy of Architecture for Health. Available from: https://network.aia.org/viewdocument/transformation-of-hospital-design-a

Larkin, P. J., Bernadette Dierckx, D. C., & Schotsmans, P. (2007). Transition towards end of life in palliative care: An exploration of its meaning for advanced cancer patients in Europe. *Journal of Palliative Care, 23*(2), 69–79.

Lawton, M. P., Weisman, G. D., Sloane, P. D., Norris-Baker, C., Caulkins, M., & Zimmerman, S. I. (2000). Professional environment assessment procedure for special care units for elders with dementing illness and its relationship to the therapeutic environment schedule. *Alzheimer's Disease and Associated Disorders, 14*(1), 23–38.

Lindqvist, O., Tishelman, C., Hagelin, C. L., Clark, J. B., Daud, M. L., Dickman, A., et al. (2012). Complexity in non-pharmacological caregiving activities at the end of life: An international qualitative study. *PLoS Medicine, 9*(2), e1001173.

Liu, Y., Ning, Z., Chen, Y., Guo, M., Liu, Y., Gali, N. K., Sun, L., Duan, Y., Cai, J., Westerdahl, D., & Liu, X. (2020). Aerodynamic characteristics and RNA concentration of SARS-CoV-2 aerosol in Wuhan hospitals during COVID-19 outbreak. *Bio Rxiv, 8*, 2020.

Medical Dictionary for the Health Professions and Nursing © Farlex. 2012.

Mercadante, S., Adile, C., Ferrera, P., Giuliana, F., Terruso, L., & Piccione, T. (2020). Palliative care in the time of COVID-19. *Journal of Pain and Symptom Management, 60*(2), e79–e80.

Moorhouse, T. (2006). *Hospice design manual for in-patient facilities.* Hospice Education Institute.

Naomi, A. S. (2020). Access to nature has always been important; with COVID-19, it is essential. *HERD: Health Environments Research & Design Journal, 13*(4), 242–244. https://doi.org/10.1177/1937586720949792

NCP. (2004). National consensus project for quality palliative care: Clinical practice guidelines for quality palliative care, executive summary. *Journal of Palliative Medicine, 7*(5), 611–627.

Ness, M. M., Saylor, J., Di Fusco, L. A., & Evans, K. (2021). *Healthcare providers' challenges during the coronavirus disease (COVID-19) pandemic: A qualitative approach.* Nursing & Health Sciences.

NHPCO. (2007). *Caring for persons with Alzheimer's and other dementias guidelines for hospice providers.* National Hospice and Palliative Care Organization. Retrieved on March, 2013 from http://www.nhpco.org/sites/default/files/public/Dementia-Caring-Guide-final.pdf

Puchalski, C., Ferrell, B., Virani, R., Otis-Green, S., Baird, P., Bull, J., et al. (2009). Improving the quality of spiritual care as a dimension of palliative care: The report of the consensus conference. *Journal of Palliative Medicine, 12*(10), 885–904.

Rogers, J. E. B., Constantine, L. A., Thompson, J. M., Mupamombe, C. T., Vanin, J. M., & Navia, R. O. (2021). COVID-19 pandemic impacts on US hospice agencies: A national survey of hospice nurses and physicians. *American Journal of Hospice and Palliative Medicine®, 38*(5), 521–527.

Ronca, S. E., Sturdivant, R. X., Barr, K. L., & Harris, D. (2021). SARS-CoV-2 viability on 16 common indoor surface finish materials. *HERD: Health Environments Research & Design Journal*, 1937586721991535.

Russell, C., Middleton, H., & Shanley, C. (2008). Research: Dying with dementia: The views of family caregivers about quality of life. *Australasian Journal on Ageing, 27*(2), 89–92.

Siebold, C. (1992). *The hospice movement: Easing death's pains.* Twayne Publishers.

Sun, N., Wei, L., Shi, S., Jiao, D., Song, R., Ma, L., Wang, H., Wang, C., Wang, Z., You, Y., & Liu, S. (2020). A qualitative study on the psychological experience of caregivers of COVID-19 patients. *American Journal of Infection Control, 48*(6), 592–598.

Swenson, D. L. (2009). *Designated hospice rooms in nursing homes: A new model of end-of-life care.* Doctoral dissertation. Retrieved from Pro Quest Dissertations & Theses Global (Accession Order No. 3455510).

Tay, D. L., Thompson, C., Jones, M., Gettens, C., Cloyes, K. G., Reblin, M., Hebdon, M. C. T., Beck, A. C., Mooney, K., & Ellington, L. (2021). "I feel all alone out here": Analysis of audio diaries of bereaved hospice family caregivers during the COVID-19 pandemic. *Journal of Hospice and Palliative Nursing, 23*(4), 346–353. https://doi.org/10.1097/NJH.0000000000000763

Tomlin, J., Dalgleish-Warburton, B., & Lamph, G. (2020). Psychosocial support for healthcare workers during the COVID-19 pandemic. *Frontiers in Psychology, 11*, 1960.

Tong, E., McGraw, S. A., Dobihal, E., et al. (2003). What is a good death? Minority and non-minority perspectives. *Journal of Palliative Care, 19*(3), 168.

Tseng, T. G., Wu, H. L., Ku, H. C., & Tai, C. J. (2020). The impact of the COVID-19 pandemic on disabled and hospice home care patients. *The Journals of Gerontology: Series A, 75*, e128.

Ulrich, R., Zimring, C., Quan, X., Joseph, A., & Choudhary, R. (2004). *The role of the physical environment in the hospital of the 21st century*. Report sponsored by The Robert Wood Johnson Foundation and The Center for Health Design.

Verderber, S., & Refuerzo, B. J. (2006). *Innovations in hospice architecture*. Taylor & Francis.

Wang, Z. (2021). Use the environment to prevent and control COVID-19 in senior-living facilities: An analysis of the guidelines used in China. *HERD: Health Environments Research & Design Journal, 14*(1), 130–140. https://doi.org/10.1177/1937586720953519

# Part IV
# Evidence-Based Applied Projects and Next Steps

# Autonomy, Identity, and Design in the COVID-19 Era

Valerie Greer and Keith Diaz Moore

The novel coronavirus disease of 2019 (COVID-19) is responsible for what the World Health Organization identified as a global pandemic in March 2020 and continues to spread as of this writing. One of the first galvanizing events in the United States was an outbreak in a skilled nursing facility (SNF) resulting in 35 deaths in the State of Washington. Since that time, there has been significant concern about the dangers COVID-19 poses for older adults, particularly those with comorbidities (e.g., diabetes, heart disease, asthma) and especially those in congregate care settings. As Davidson and Szanton (2020: 2758) write, "The COVID-19 pandemic is providing us with many painful lessons particularly the vulnerability of individuals living with chronic conditions and the need for preparedness, coordination and monitoring."

This chapter examines the state of response and likely long-term implications across the housing continuum for older adults, specifically examining independent housing and skilled care with a focus on how physical settings and technological systems can empower autonomy and identity in response to vulnerabilities exposed by the COVID-19 pandemic. Building upon Chaudhury and Oswald's (2019) Integrative Framework of Person-Environment (P-E) Exchange, the chapter argues that autonomy and identity are critical developmental attributes for healthy aging and that environments serving older adults should facilitate the creation of such attributes. The chapter will first present the Framework of P-E Exchange, diving into the core concepts of autonomy and identity. It will then sequentially address the place types of independent housing and skilled care through a description of the place type, an exploration of COVID-19's impact on those place types, and finally a discussion of design opportunities illuminated by considering the attributes of

V. Greer (✉) · K. D. Moore
College of Architecture & Planning, University of Utah, Salt Lake City, UT, USA
e-mail: valerie.greer@utah.edu; diazmoore@utah.edu

F. Ferdous, E. Roberts (eds.), *(Re)designing the Continuum of Care for Older Adults*, https://doi.org/10.1007/978-3-031-20970-3_14

autonomy and identity. The chapter concludes with a call to radically reconceptualize the nature of these places as we turn toward the mid-twenty-first century.

## 1 Framework of Person-Environment Exchange

Chaudhury and Oswald (2019)'s Integrative Framework presents a logic model to understand P-E exchange in later life. This framework begins with four categories of contextual inputs which they call components of P-E interaction: individual characteristics, social factors, physical/built environments, and technological systems. These components constitute a milieu within which the P-E processes of agency and belonging occur. Chaudhury and Oswald (2019) take an environmental psychology perspective toward human experience, considering the "ABC's"—affect, behavior, cognition—as modalities of experience (Weisman et al., 2000). Agency is focused "on goal-directed behaviors related to making use of the objective physical-social environment" (Chaudhury & Oswald, 2019: 4), while belonging relates to both the affective ties to place and cognitive evaluations of a place. The model suggests that the recurring negotiation of those processes through myriad place experiences over time shapes the development-relevant outcomes of autonomy and identity (Fig. 1).

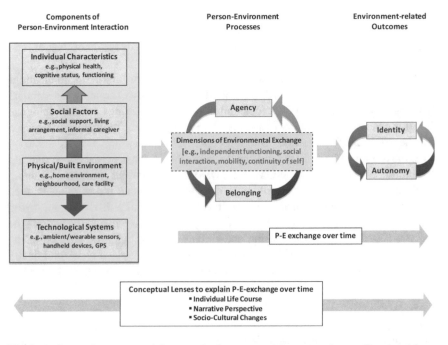

**Fig. 1** An integrative conceptual framework of person-environment exchange. (Reprinted from *Journal of Aging Studies, 51*, H. Chaudhury and F. Oswald, Advancing understanding of person-environment interaction in later life: One step further, p. 100821, Copyright 2019, with permission from Elsevier)

## *1.1 Autonomy, Identity, and the Integrated Development Model*

Both autonomy and identity are meta-constructs incorporating numerous developmentally salient attributes that merit further discussion. Scharlach and Leining (2015) present a model of six such attributes: compensation, control, challenge/comfort, continuity, connection, and contribution. The first three attributes are associated with the concept of autonomy as described by Chaudhury and Oswald (2019) and the subsequent three associated with the concept of identity. Here we will focus on the theoretical concepts of autonomy and identity most related to the built environment and technology.

**Autonomy** Chaudhury and Oswald (2019) emphasize that remaining independent for as long as possible is a fundamental development task as one ages. This includes traditional measures of independence found in the gerontological literature such as activities of daily living (ADLs) (performing personal hygiene, maintaining continence, dressing, eating, transferring) (Katz et al., 1970) and instrumental activities of daily living (IADLs) (meal preparation, shopping, housework, managing medications and finances) (Lawton & Brody, 1969), but they also highlight activities such as mobility and community participation. They reference both Lawton and Nahemow's (1973) competence-press model and Baltes' (1997) selective optimization with compensation (SOC) theory as relevant to the concept of autonomy in older adults.

The competence-press model asserts the level of comfort or challenge one finds in an environment is the result of the dynamic between the demand of that environment and the particular competence of the person in regard to a particular domain of functioning. SOC theory suggests older adults select domains of functioning particularly important to their own sense of autonomy and seek to optimize those domains, often involving compensatory strategies such as assistive devices, environmental modifications, or social support. A critical dimension of the SOC theory is the personal control one has in making those decisions. "Whereas compensation focuses on the need for support, control focuses on the actual and perceived ability to effect change" (Scharlach & Diaz Moore, 2016: 414). Parmalee and Lawton (1990: 465) highlight that the control dimension of autonomy is always in dialectic with security, "a state in which pursuit of life goals is linked to, limited by, and aided by dependable physical, social, and interpersonal resources."

This framework allows us to understand environmental challenges to autonomy in terms of misfit, or excessive challenge, perceived by the person in regard to the environment, the control one has to compensate for challenges, and the security one has in supports being available. During the COVID-19 pandemic, challenges to each of these aspects were exacerbated across the continuum of residential environments. The degree of control a person possessed to compensate for the situation resided in not only availability to systems of resources (e.g., telehealth with its requisite broadband Wi-Fi, laptop computers, appropriate computer applications (apps)) but the knowledge of those resources, the understanding of how to effectively utilize them, and the dependability of support systems.

**Identity** Identity is shaped through a negotiation between an individual's perceptions and behaviors in relation to the social structures of their context. Chaudhury
and Oswald (2019) connect identity to concepts such as "insideness" (Rowles,
1983) and "environmental mastery" (Golant, 2011). For our purposes, identity has
three associated constructs: continuity, connection, and contribution. Scharlach and
Diaz Moore (2016: 413) argue that "(m)aintaining continuity with regard to personal identity and self-construct is especially relevant in later life, in the face of a
variety of forces that threaten to undermine one's sense of self." Our environments
play four roles with continuity of self-identity: (1) history, referring to maintaining
links to the past such as through photographs; (2) habit, capturing the familiar routines that help maintain function; (3) heart, attempting to capture the meaning we
imbue to elements and settings; and (4) hearth, the role home has in relation to
ownership and belonging (Rowles & Watkins, 2003).

Social connectedness is usually considered essential to healthy aging, or aging
well. Being socially connected may well help encourage healthier lifestyles, but
also buffers stress through enhancing adaptive capacities of older adults through the
provision of emotional, informational, or tangible resources (Wong & Waite, 2016).
Antonucci et al. (2014) suggests these social relations constitute a "social convoy"
of support, which Smith and Ekerdt (2011) extended to possessions that support
daily life by arguing for a "material convoy." Diaz Moore et al. (2019: 104) assert
"that as much as individuals have both social and material convoys, they also have
environmental convoys that either constrict or facilitate potential social
connectedness."

Closely related to connection is the concept of contribution. Here the idea is that
people seek to be useful and helpful and to have a contributory orientation (Midlarsky
et al., 2015). Contributory activities include volunteerism, participation in civil
society, providing informal assistance to friends and/or neighbors, and providing
care for partners, pets, or family members.

This framework allows us to understand challenges to identity that older adults
experienced during the pandemic through the conceptualization of how interactions
with social structures are connected to individual senses of self. Recognizing the
dialectic between social connection, contribution, and continuity in the construction
of self-identity, we can better understand and characterize challenges that older
adults face in maintaining strong sense of identity due to the abrupt end to in-person
social activities. For residents in SNFs who experienced cancellation of social programming and communal gathering, as well as for independently living older adults
who relied on senior centers, libraries, and volunteer opportunities as social convoys
of support, the immediate disconnection to social structures poses a threat to continuity of identity.

## 2    The Continuum of Care: Independent Housing to Skilled Nursing

Environments for aging have been distinctly challenged by the COVID-19 pandemic as gaps and vulnerabilities in physical and technological environments have been exacerbated in response to the virus. Older adults have faced disproportionately dire consequences related to health outcomes and social connections. Industry experts in senior living widely agree that existing models of care settings must be reconsidered and redesigned (Inzitari et al., 2020), making it imperative to explore dimensions of P-E interactions across a continuum of care settings. To consider challenges and opportunities through the lens of two distinctly different place types, this text will focus on the dialectic between independent housing and skilled care, what Robinson (2004) refers to as "institution and home." We define and explore environments as being encompassing of physical and technological attributes as well as programs, activities, people, and change over time.

### 2.1    Independent Housing

Here, independent housing is meant to convey the concept of one residing in an environment under their own personal control. This may be through ownership or rental and therefore ranges from the traditional single-family home to condominiums, townhouses, and apartments. This is typically the type of setting where people discuss "aging-in-place," such as Greenfield (2012: 1), who defines aging in place as "being able to remain in one's *current residence* even when faced with increasing need for support because of life changes, such as declining health, widowhood, or loss of income" (p. 1, *emphasis added*).

#### 2.1.1    COVID Issues in Independent Housing

Let us begin by observing that the majority of older adults age 65+ live in community-based dwellings, and living independently represents a powerful source of autonomy and identity (Oswald & Rowles, 2006). Home confinement during the pandemic left people feeling constricted, disoriented, or displaced, with loneliness among older adults found to be greatest among women, lower-income individuals, individuals living alone, individuals with no children, and individuals unsatisfied with their contact with neighbors (Seifert & Hassler, 2020). Compensatory services such as meal delivery were disrupted, thus increasing the challenges of maintaining autonomy. Routines associated with IADL changed significantly as well, requiring more time and effort to complete tasks such as shopping or banking. Health and wellness resources, including exercise classes and physical therapy, shifted to being online. While COVID-19 and its related socioeconomic shutdown challenged everyone's sense of control, its impact was particularly felt by older adults with greater social isolation, enhanced economic risk, delayed medical treatment, and challenges to accessing resources (Miller, 2020). The disproportionate impact on disadvantaged and marginalized populations of community-dwelling older adults is increasingly straining access to financial, health, and social resources, compromising perceptions of safety, and creating a wide range of challenges to living independently (Wilder, 2021; Lee & Miller, 2020).

Autonomy and Independent Housing: Compensation, Control, Challenge

Home confinement during the pandemic has required adaptation and flexibility of domestic spaces in order to support work, communication, and recreation. The ability to reorganize domestic spaces to host activities that normally occur outside of the home—such as converting a spare bedroom into a home office—is an example of a compensatory strategy that supports autonomy. In addition to the need to adapt living spaces for programmatic flexibility, older adults often face a parallel challenge of making home modifications to support safety. In-home modifications such as installation of grab bars or slip-resistant flooring, as well as support for home maintenance, have been shown to significantly improve daily activity performance and be of benefit to older adults aging in place (Stark et al., 2009); however access has been particularly challenging during the pandemic due to increased costs of construction, increased demand for materials, and decreased availability of labor.

Supportive interventions put in place during COVID-19 rely heavily on digital technologies, such as Zoom and other apps to meet needs. Online access to healthcare, groceries, news, and group socialization has transformed rapidly during the pandemic, requiring a basic level of digital literacy and access to benefit from remote services. The pandemic made manifest the age-based "digital divide" which describes inequality in the access to and skills to make use of technology. This "gray" divide has been exacerbated by the pandemic, leaving older adults less able to benefit from digital measures put in place to help close the gap in isolation measures (Van Jaarsveld, 2020). Paradoxically, older adults who represent the population most negatively impacted by the pandemic may also least likely to be able to leverage compensatory benefits due to digital literacy.

Identity and Independent Housing: Connection, Continuity, Contribution

While barriers in physical and technological environments undermine autonomy, the issue of maintaining identity through connection, continuity, and contribution represents an equally dire challenge. There is no question that social isolation related to the pandemic disproportionately impacts community-dwelling older adults whose primary social contact is outside of the home, such as at senior centers or at places of worship (Armitage & Nellmus, 2020). Social isolation among older adults was recognized as a "serious public health concern" prior to the pandemic

(Gerst-Emmerson & Jayawardhana, 2015), elevating known risks to cardiovascular and autoimmune health, as well as to mental health conditions including anxiety, depression, and cognitive decline (Ganzer & Jacobs, 2021; Sachs-Ericsson et al., 2005). Even in the environment of neighborhoods, design factors such as the continuity of sidewalks and perceptions of safety and security may disproportionately impact the sense of isolation for older adults (Garcia & deLa Torre, 2019).

Additionally, social isolation experienced over a long period of time may well have begun to manifest aspects of the "partial institution," with older adults feeling deprived of social contact and an almost total loss of control to external factors. These real barriers to the outside world point to what Goffman refers to as "contaminative exposure" (Goffman, 1961: Salari & Rich, 2001). Early on in the COVID-19 pandemic, older adults were viewed as at high risk and encouraged to go into almost total lockdown. Images of grandparents waving to grandkids through their windows were devastatingly plentiful. Attachment is critical throughout the life course but takes increasing importance as we age (Wahl & Lang, 2004). Experiences of partial institution undermine attachment, which is theorized as connected to one's sense of self (Rubinstein & de Medeiros, 2004). This calls attention to the role of place attachment, or the emotional bond between people and place, as a strong source of support (Ramkissoon, 2020). The bonds that older adults have to their neighborhood, community, and history of places where they reside provide a sense of continuity, connection, and belonging which can be a buffer to stress and a contributor to maintaining self-identity (Scheidt & Norris-Baker, 2003).

Finally, within the discussion of independent housing, it should be noted the pandemic has exacerbated the phenomenon of homelessness among older adults (Canham et al., 2021) and questions the assumed baseline of "permanent" dwelling on which much aging-in-place work builds. This raises the prospect of architectural innovation in transitional housing for those recently homeless who are likely to have significant comorbid physical and mental conditions. From a policy standpoint, it suggests additional humanitarian rationale for programs such as Housing First along with supplementary service support (Humphries & Canham, 2021).

### 2.1.2   Design Opportunities in Independent Housing: Digital Technology

The pandemic has underscored the role of in-home technologies in order to bolster the sense of control, compensation, and connectivity in independent living. This calls attention to the opportunity to consider how digital environments are designed as age-friendly places and how digital environments are integrated with physical environments to create more responsive and resilient services, environments, and technologies (SETs) and promote autonomy. Questions arise such as how can an integration between technology and the physical environment be designed to be age-inclusive, intuitive, and affordable?

It strikes us that the inevitable linkage of environmental gerontology, geographical gerontology, and gerontechnology is now present and ought to reflect itself in such core issues as refining the definition of age-friendly communities to explicitly include the digital environment of such communities to affect their desired outcomes. Ambient assisted living is an emergent term referring to the use of integrated digital technologies such as smart devices, medical sensors, and wireless networks connecting data and analysis, for health monitoring (Rashidi & Mihalidis, 2013). Early versions focused on topics such as nutrition and physical activity, but now include more sophisticated monitoring of vitals, medication adherence, and enhanced mobility (Cicirelli et al., 2021). The COVID-19 pandemic has amplified the utility and accelerated the reliance upon both Internet-based technology (IBT) and mobile technologies (MT) yet simultaneously has raised significant issues ranging from HIPAA compliance to dependence (and therefore loss of control) for many older adults on caregivers to serve as technological support (Ganzer & Jacobs, 2021).

While ambient assistive living technologies can support control and compensation, online social platforms have the potential to further enhance connection and contribution. Designing online platforms as age-friendly places that provide social connections and access to community resources presents an avenue to support continuity of self-identity, particularly for older adults who rely upon places outside of the home for social connection (Poscia et al., 2018). Age-related changes such as those related to visual acuity, fine motor skills, audition, response time, and cognitive abilities must be considered with the design of virtual spaces (Mannheim et al., 2019). Protecting cyber security for older adults in digital environments is an additional dimension warranting attention (Morrison et al., 2020).

Finally, increasing the affordability and intuitive use of online platforms is a paramount design need as older adults face barriers related to material access as well as training opportunities (var Jaarsveld, 2020). As Chen (2020: 984) asserts, "COVID-19 is an alarm bell, reminding us that urgent attention should be paid to improve technology literacy among older people, as well as support caregivers and health professionals to use technological innovations as a complementary tool for delivering care services." Issues related to the digital divide—including broadband access, entry cost for smart phones and laptops, inclusive design of interfaces, digital skills—will prove paramount to enable both autonomy and identity attributes.

### 2.1.3 Design Opportunities in Independent Housing: Physical Environment

All of these digital interventions become impossible without broad-based, easily accessible Wi-Fi access. The response to COVID-19 has underscored how critical electric and broadband infrastructure is to maintaining autonomy in twenty-first-century living. Related to this, neighborhood infrastructure and age-friendly homes should consider the criticality of reliability of these systems and back-up electrical supply. Provision of community Wi-Fi hotspots for data access should be considered to promote dependability of resources (Beaunoyer et al., 2020).

Beyond physical infrastructure, social isolation associated with suburban settlement models has proven particularly problematic during COVID-19. There is a need for greater zoning flexibility in order to allow more inclusive models of dwelling and promote greater choice and control to older adults to find "their place." Such flexibility will enhance older adults' ability to age-in-place by providing them economic and lifestyle options (Forsyth et al., 2019). The rise of "zoom towns"— new destination communities affording attributes of livability but disassociated with the geography of employment allowed by digital technology such as Zoom (Florida & Ozimek, 2021)—during the pandemic may shift both older adults' priorities for retirement locale but also enable potential caregiving family members to live in their hometown locale with aging parents. Zoning codes that regulate the construction of accessory dwelling units (ADU) can further encourage alternatives for aging in place near or with loved ones.

Co-housing models, campus-affiliated communities, and senior cooperatives are other examples of alternative housing models that might be leveraged to allow older adults remain in residential environments. The Dutch Apartment for Life offers a model for promoting autonomy while having the tacit commitment to maintain older adults through the end of life through the provision of inclusive design, with a digitally supported care information system and home care-based service delivery (c.f. Regnier, 2018). Age-friendly community initiatives (c.f. Diaz Moore et.al, 2018) have piloted enhanced personal and healthcare delivery in the home while also making neighborhoods and communities more accessible and attractive for older adults.

Another critical need in the physical environment to support autonomy is the ability for older adults to make retrofits or modifications to home environments in an affordable and timely manner. A survey conducted by the Associated General Contractors of America in March 2021 indicates that, 1 year into the pandemic, over half of contractors are experiencing project delays or disruptions due to a shortage of materials, equipment, and parts; approximately a third of contractors are reporting delays due to shortage of labor, limiting the capacity for work and driving up construction costs (Yoders, 2021). Broadening financial assistance for older adults to perform in-home construction and maintenance related to upkeep is imperative to support independent living (Black & Oh, 2021).

This discussion highlights personal choice/control and the related concept of security stemming from the dependability of resources. We believe that trends will include an increase in the diversity of housing types and greater flexibility in settlement patterns that support healthy aging—all with the goal of optimizing/maintaining independence in one's own dwelling of choice. For designers, the implementation of inclusive principles regarding design at the full range of scales will prove an essential competence in the coming decades (Maisel et al., 2017).

## 2.2 Skilled Nursing Facilities

The history of SNFs is rooted in a backlash to the inhumane treatment of older persons in public poorhouses through the 1930s. On passage of the Social Security Act in 1935, Congress did not allow payments from this social safety net to be passed on to such poorhouses. There was growth in proprietary nursing homes up until a 1954 amendment to the Hill-Burton Act which provided "funds to nonprofit organizations for the construction of skilled nursing facilities that met certain definitions and hospital-like building standards" (Institute of Medicine, 1986). Still, there was a great diversity in such facilities necessitating the development of standards associated with the advent of Medicare and Medicaid in 1965. Even with that, states are highly divergent in how such standards are enforced.

What has brought a greater degree of architectural uniformity has been building codes. Currently, the International Building Code defines I-1 occupancies as facilities used by more than 16 people, not including staff, who reside on a 24-hour basis within a supervised environment and receive custodial care, while I-2 are buildings used for medical care on a 24-hour basis for more than 5 people who are not capable of self-preservation. Therefore I-1 is typically what applies to assisted living (unless fewer than 16 residents which might then qualify for R-4) and I-2 to SNFs. Each occupancy has different requirements in terms of items such as fire separation, places of refuge, construction type, and the like, resulting in construction costs approximately 2/3's more expensive for I-2 than I-1 (ICC, 2020).

### 2.2.1 COVID Issues in Skilled Nursing Facilities

In the annals of the history of the COVID-19 epidemic, we should never forget that, as noted earlier, the first major site of COVID-19 infections in the United States was at a skilled nursing facility in Washington State (Morris et al., 2020). Since that time, infections in SNFs have led to greater mortality and hospitalizations than those occurring in other locations. By January 2021, long-term care (LTC) accounted for 6% of the infections, and 38% of the deaths attributed to COVID-19 in the United States (Kaiser Family Foundation, 2021). Nursing home residents are characterized by older age, more prevalent chronic disease and comorbidities, and highly impaired physical and cognitive function that put them at the greatest risk of severe COVID-19 infections (Li et al., 2020). The growing literature on health disparities due to race makes it unsurprising that there has been a 3.3-fold higher prevalence of death in facilities serving higher percentages of non-white residents as compared to those SNFs serving predominantly white populations (Gorges & Konetzka, 2021).

Autonomy and Skilled Care: Compensation, Control, Challenge

The population in skilled care skews to those with greater needs, or in other words, those experiencing a greater decline in personal independence. Institutions are associated with a loss of personal control in exchange for greater security by having reliable supportive resources available such as care staff and a prosthetic environment. Yet it was precisely the model of care, with its reliance on staff, group programming, typically shared rooms, and lack of outdoor engagement, that led to infections spreading so efficiently once a staff member or family visitor became infected. Once present, residents had little control over responses and few compensatory resources. SNF residents experienced a precipitous drop from their already lowered sense of autonomy due to COVID-19 and the operational responses to it.

Challenges presented by the pandemic in the physical environment of SNFs included the scale and model of congregate living skilled care; poor ventilation; and lack of outdoor programming. Skilled care remains predicated on its ties to hospital design catalyzed by the Hill-Burton Act of 1954. Common characteristics of SNF designs include double-loaded corridors of up to 150 feet in length, semi-private rooms, and a centralized nursing station (Schwarz, 1997). This results in residents and care staff sharing the same spaces at relatively high densities, thereby creating a network in which airborne infectious diseases are easily spread. Vulnerabilities in the layout are exacerbated by poor ventilation systems potentially acting as distributors of infection. With the emergence of masking and social distancing as primary defenses to the spread of COVID-19, social life in SNF's was compromised due to the presence of personal protective equipment (PPE) such as masks and the inability to maintain social distancing in shared resident rooms. While private rooms have long been promoted within environmental gerontology largely due to its benefits to privacy, COVID-19 has demonstrated its utility to limit infection spread and the potential to adjust ventilation settings to create slightly negative pressure in rooms where residents are contagious (Lynch & Goring, 2020). Lastly, while we have known the importance of fresh air and its relation to good health since the Asklepion in Ancient Greece, SNFs often lack programming of their exterior spaces which may have proven salutogenic as outdoor spread of COVID-19 was very rare.

Decisions as to how to respond to the pandemic were almost all made at the organizational level, exacerbating the lack of control residents of LTC typically feel. As infections, serious illnesses, and eventual deaths mounted, the lack of security and the concomitant increase in fear made skilled care environments feel very unsafe indeed.

## Identity and Skilled Care: Connection, Continuity, Contribution

Wahl and Lang (2004) hypothesize that issues associated with personal agency, or autonomy, would become less of a focus as people age and greater energy would be spent on issues of personal identity, such as a sense of belonging. However, the interventions made due to the COVID-19 pandemic, such as restricting visitors, volunteers, and nonessential healthcare personnel and the cancelling of all group/ social activities, struck at the core of the interventions typically utilized to promote continuity, connection, and contribution. To address the recognized negative social impact of such recommendations, the CDC recommended facilitating virtual communication and identifying a staff member as a primary contact for families (CDC, 2020). While those steps help to maintain some semblance of connection, they do little in terms of continuity and contribution.

Both of these suggested changes typify the shift COVID-19 had on lessening personal control for residents and increasing the demand on staff in LTC settings. Thus, it should not be surprising that LTC staff are experiencing significant anxiety and burnout, exacerbated by a fear of infection themselves (Sarabia-Cobo et al., 2021). Chronic understaffing makes provision of basic care difficult under normal circumstances yet alone with the heightened demands on staff during this pandemic. Protocols are too often violated due to both understaffing and under training, and there is little reason to believe this is also not happening during the pandemic. Low pay, part time work, and a coercive sense of obligation to work when sick is part of a global staffing crisis in LTC (McGilton et al., 2020).

In short, we believe that the devastating outcomes related to COVID-19 in SNFs provide a tipping point for reconsidering the nature of this place type, particularly from the standpoint of care provision as families are reluctant to let older adults go into LTC (Dolan & Hamilton, 2020). There is preliminary evidence that smaller SNFs (those serving less than 50 residents) have fewer incidents and lower mortality due to COVID-19 than larger long-term care facilities (LTCFs) (Zimmerman et al., 2021). Additionally, those with a higher ratio of registered nurses and higher levels of staffing generally experienced half the infection rate among residents (Gorges & Konetzka, 2020; Harrington et al., 2020). Consistent with better COVID-19 health outcomes linked to better staffing and a better socio-environmental setting, "5-star" skilled nursing facilities on the Centers for Medicare & Medicaid Services (CMS) 5-star Quality Rating System (CMS, 2021) experienced less prevalence and subsequently less death among residents due to COVID-19 infection.

### 2.2.2  Design Opportunities in Skilled Nursing Facilities: Digital Technology

The previous discussion is suggestive of opportunities to reconsider the nature of SNFs, with a hopeful acceleration of efforts blending smaller, less dense approaches. From the resident perspective, a sense of social connectivity might be further strengthened by "low-assistive" technologies that facilitate, for instance, live streaming local public events such as parades, performances, or sporting events, as they bring the life of the community into the life of SNFs (MacDonald et al., 2021). A modicum of autonomy might be enhanced with automated pill dispensers that provide reminders and documentation of medication adherence (Testa & Pollard, 2007). There is increasing research into the potential of using robots in care settings, ranging from providing care to social support (Porkodi & Kesavaraja, 2021). Currently, logistic robots are used in some healthcare settings to assist in distribution functions, such as medications. However, personalized logistic robots make possible the eventuality that residents could ask robots to secure Chinese food from a restaurant down the block or pick up a package from an Amazon Hub Locker and thereby serve as a source of compensation (Pirhonen et al., 2020). However, while connection may be supported through digital technology, both continuity and contribution possess a stronger temporal component, demanding sustained engagement with relevant people, places, and activities.

A discussion of technological design opportunities in SNFs would not be complete without considering the levels of control and safety that caregiving staff encounter. The pandemic has seen rates of infection, absenteeism, and burnout to rise significantly among staff and has exposed the extent to which workforce stress impacts the physical and mental health of SNF residents. Edelman et al. (2020) note the significant role that technology has to play in improving the capacity that staff have to deliver care while maintaining their own safety. They note that SNF staff, comprised of teams of nurses, physical and occupational therapists, social workers, and direct care workers, often work at several different facilities, increasing risks of infection and transmission, and underscoring the need to implement ways that staff leverage technology to deliver care to SNF residents. The interface of tablets, smart devices, and remote monitoring allows for greater coordination among teams of caregivers, and telehealth platforms can significantly support staff as they work to meet the physical and mental health needs of SNF residents (Ackerman, 2020; Eghtesadi, 2020; Olsho et al., 2014).

### 2.2.3 Design Opportunities in Skilled Nursing Facilities: Physical Environment

Much has been written on infection control measures needed in SNFs in order to prevent virus transmission, such as higher ventilation rates, single occupancy rooms, private bathrooms, and regular disinfection. To begin with, single occupancy rooms with private bathrooms should be the operative norm. The flexibility this provides from contagion containment to resident placement will prove invaluable to care organizations (Lynch & Goring, 2020). Designing the supply of PPE and enhancing the accessibility of handwashing stations to suit the range of needs that residents have is also imperative (Spaetgens et al., 2020). Given the range of physical and cognitive conditions of residents, environmental factors that promote control and security should be considered on a spectrum—according to needs—rather than as a homogenous category.

In addition to design interventions that prevent disease transmission, those that impact the quality of life for both residents and staff are equally critical (Anderson et al., 2010). Chaudhury and Oswald's (2019) Integrative Framework of P-E Exchange allows us to consider design factors that support residents' sense of connection to place and continuity of self, both of which are central to promoting a sense of belonging and identity. Aspects of the environment that enable SNF residents to contribute and engage in social interaction should be considered as a way to strengthen continuity of self. It is critical for there to be a diversity of types of social spaces where residents can gather to form friendships, exercise, and maintain personal interests. A range of person-centered care activities facilitated by such spaces are of increasing importance during this time of COVID-19 (Ferdous, 2021). Lounge spaces have the potential to be retrofitted to expand the variety of types of settings, from more active work at tables around games and computing to more passive enjoyment of books, conversation, and views of nature (Diaz Moore et.al, 2006). Corridors and common spaces might be retrofitted to support indoor walking paths. Where possible, simple equipment or stations for stretching and exercise might be set up in exterior spaces. Underused indoor or outdoor areas might be retrofitted and designated as meditation or prayer spaces (Lee et.al, 2021). Installation of artwork created by residents—or displays of art created by children at local schools—can lend to the sense of generativity and help de-institutionalize the feel of interior environments.

The above suggestions are enhanced by a more intimate approach to scale. The small house or Green House provides an innovative model of small-scale nursing homes providing care in residential settings (c.f. Reinhardt et.al., 2019). These models, which are intentional in strategies to interior design, staffing and size, deinstitutionalize the feel of traditional LTCFs, and promote a sense of belonging and connection between older adults and care givers. Smaller scale skilled care facilities may also have a greater opportunity to find acceptance in surrounding communities (Forsyth et.al., 2019). Finding ways to then connect SNF environments with neighborhoods—for instance through exterior open spaces, walking paths and public transportation—increases the potential for residents, staff and visitors to connect.

## 3  Conclusion

We believe that the vulnerabilities revealed by the COVID-19 pandemic provide an inflection point to reconsider the manner in which we serve residential needs of older adults. The recent theoretical reconsideration of aging-in-place by Golant (2015) and Scharlach and Diaz Moore (2016) were prescient in raising questions that became magnified in the COVID-19 pandemic. Building upon both Chaudhury and Oswald (2019) and Scharlach and Diaz Moore (2016), we believe the concept of time needs to be moved front and center and drive innovation in the continuum of care.

The driving question of innovation in the independent housing industry should be "how supportive, and therefore inclusive, can we design dwellings to support the lifespan and diverse ability levels?" The continuous extension of inclusive design in residential environments ought to enable a more diverse population to stay independent longer in their "own homes."

Similarly, SNFs need to be designed differently depending upon the length of stay or, again, based upon time. Short-term environments may be closely designed to acute care settings and the emphasis may be on care delivery. Medium term might parallel extended stay residences or corporate housing wherein the environment facilitates autonomy through the affordance of items such as kitchen and furnishings. Long term would then focus on environmental issues of identity such as the 4 H's of history, habit, heart, and hearth.

If skilled care were to provide a smaller scale, more supportive environment and independent housing could extend the level of need it might support through inclusive design and ambient assisted living, it may well be that assisted living is no longer be considered a place type in its own right, but something enabled by evolution in both independent housing and skilled care. To do so, we believe there are four essential considerations for design innovation in the housing continuum:

1. Inclusive housing models: a diversity of residential setting types inclusively designed to enable the widest range of abilities as possible.
2. Age-friendly integration of technology: ambient-assisted living facilitated from the macro (infrastructure), the meso (building design), and the micro (proximate/product) scales of P-E transaction.
3. Environmental flexibility: movement away from tight-fit thinking to loose-fit design and significant consideration of how the physical environment and digital technologies are resilient to future, unknown threats.
4. Greater emphasis on the needs of caregivers: much of environmental gerontology has focused upon user needs (and quite rightly so), but Lawton's (1989) three functions of the environment—stimulation, maintenance, and support—are equally as relevant to caregivers, whether professional or informal.

In conclusion, the ravages of the COVID-19 pandemic call us to engage in a complete reconsideration of how society designs neighborhoods, independent housing, and skilled care moving forward. We believe a focus on place types ought to further the developmentally salient attributes of autonomy and identity. Our hope is there a radical reconsideration of the continuum of care for older adults over the coming decades, one that focuses on enhancing personal autonomy for as long as possible while promoting identity as one ages.

# References

Ackerman E. IEE Spectrum. (2020 April 15). *Telepresence Robots Are Helping Take Pressure Off Hospital Staff.* Retrieved November 6, 2021, from https://spectrum.ieee.org/automaton/robotics/medical-robots/telepresence-robots-are-helping-take-pressure-off-hospital-staff

Anderson, D. C., Grey, T., Kennedy, S., & O'Neill, D. (2010). Nursing home design and COVID-19: Balancing infection control, quality of life, and resiliency. *JAMDA, 21*(11), 1519–1524.

Antonucci, T. C., Ajrouch, K. J., & Birditt, K. S. (2014). The convoy model: Explaining social relations from a multidisciplinary perspective. *The Gerontologist, 54*(1), 82–92.

Armitage, R., & Nellmus, L. B. (2020). Emerging from COVID-19: Prioritizing the burden of loneliness in older people. *British Journal of General Practice, 70*(697), 382.

Baltes, P. B. (1997). On the incomplete architecture of human ontogeny: Selection, optimization, and compensation as foundation of developmental theory. *American Psychologist, 52*(4), 366.

Beaunoyer, E., Dupéré, S., & Guitton, M. J. (2020). COVID-19 and digital inequalities: Reciprocal impacts and mitigation strategies. *Computers in Human Behavior, 111*, 106424.

Black, K., & Oh, P. (2021). Assessing age-friendly community progress: What have we learned? *The Gerontologist, 62*(1), 6–17. https://doi.org/10.1093/geront/gnab051

Canham, S. L., Humphries, J., Moore, P., Burns, V., & Mahmood, A. (2021). Shelter/housing options, supports and interventions for older people experiencing homelessness. *Ageing & Society*, 42(11), 2615–2641.

CDC. (2020). https://www.cms.gov/newsroom/press-releases/cms-announces-new-measures-protect-nursing-home-residents-covid-19. Retrieved June 14, 2021.

Chaudhury, H., & Oswald, F. (2019). Advancing understanding of person-environment interaction in later life: One step further. *Journal of Aging Studies, 51*, 100821.

Chen, K. (2020). Use of gerontechnology to assist older adults to cope with the COVID-19 pandemic. *Journal of the American Medical Directors Association, 21*(7), 983–984.

Cicirelli, G., Marani, R., Petitti, A., Milella, A., & D'Orazio, T. (2021). Ambient assisted living: A review of technologies, methodologies and future perspectives for healthy aging of population. *Sensors, 21*(10), 3549.

CMS. (2021). https://www.cms.gov/Medicare/Provider-Enrollment-and-Certification/CertificationandComplianc/FSQRS. Retrieved June 13, 2021.

Davidson, P. M., & Szanton, S. L. (2020). Nursing homes and COVID-19: We can and should do better. *Journal of Clinical Nursing, 29*(15–16), 2758–2759.

Diaz Moore, K., Geboy, L. D., & Weisman, G. D. (2006). *Designing a better day: Guidelines for adult and dementia day services centers*. Johns Hopkins University Press.

Diaz Moore, K., Greenfield, E., & Scharlach, A. (2018). Healthy aging and its implications for public health: Healthy communities. In W. Satariano & M. Maus (Eds.), *Aging, place and health: A global perspective*. Jones & Bartlett.

Diaz Moore, K., Garcia, I., & Kim, J. Y. (2019). Healthy places and the social life of older adults. In L. Kane & C. Singer (Eds.), *Social isolation of older adults: Strategies to bolster health and Well-being* (pp. 103–118). Springer.

Dolan, J., & Hamilton, M. (2020, April 7). *Consider pulling residents from nursing homes over coronavirus, says county health director*. Los Angeles Times Communications, LLC (Nant Capital): Los Angeles Times. https://www.latimes.com/california/story/2020-04-07/coronavirus-nursing-homes-residents-remove-la-county

Edelman, L. S., McConnell, E. S., Kennerly, S. M., Alderden, J., Horn, S. D., & Yap, T. L. (2020). Mitigating the effects of a pandemic: Facilitating improved nursing home care delivery through technology. *JMIR Aging, 3*(1), e20110.

Eghtesadi, M. (2020). Breaking social isolation amidst COVID-19: A viewpoint on improving access to technology in long-term care facilities. *Journal of the American Geriatrics Society (JAGS), 68*(5), 949–950.

Ferdous, F. (2021). Social distancing vs social interaction for older adults at long-term care facilities in the midst of the COVID-19 pandemic: A rapid review and synthesis of action plans. *INQUIRY: The Journal of Health Care Organization, Provision, and Financing, 58*, 00469580211044287.

Florida, R., & Ozimek, A. (2021, 5 March). *How remote work is Reshaping America's Urban Geography*. The Wall Street Journal. Retrieved 1 December 2021, from https://www.wsj.com/articles/how-remote-work-is-reshaping-americas-urban-geography-11614960100

Forsyth, A., Molinsky, J., & Kan, H. Y. (2019). Improving housing and neighborhoods for the vulnerable: Older people, small households, urban design, and planning. *Urban Design International, 24*(3), 171–186.

Ganzer, C., & Jacobs, A. (2021). A rapid shift: Adopting gerontechnology during a pandemic. *Academia Letters, Article, 2748*. https://doi.org/10.20935/AL2748

Garcia, I., & DeLaTorre, A. (2019). *Life-space mobility: How transportation and policy can support aging in place for older adults. Project brief 1109*. Transportation Research and Education Center (TREC).

Gerst-Emmerson, K., & Jayawardhana, J. (2015). Loneliness as a public health issue: The impact of loneliness on health care utilization among older adults. *American Journal of Public Health, 105*(5), 1013–1019.

Goffman, E. (1961). *Asylums*. Anchor Books.

Golant, S. (2011). The quest for residential normalcy by older adults: Relocation but one pathway. *Journal of Aging Studies, 25*(3), 193–205. https://doi.org/10.1016/j.jaging.2011.03.003

Golant, S. M. (2015). *Aging in the right place*. Health Professions Press.

Gorges, R. J., & Konetzka, R. T. (2020). Staffing levels and COVID-19 cases and outbreaks in US nursing homes. *Journal of the American Geriatrics Society, 68*(11), 2462–2466.

Gorges, R. J., & Konetzka, R. T. (2021). Factors associated with racial differences in deaths among nursing home residents with COVID-19 infection in the US. *JAMA Network Open, 4*(2), e2037431–e2037431.

Greenfield, E. A. (2012). Using ecological frameworks to advance a field of research, practice, and policy on aging-in-place initiatives. *The Gerontologist, 52*(1), 1–12.

Harrington, C., Ross, L., Chapman, S., Halifax, E., Spurlock, B., & Bakerjian, D. (2020). Nurse staffing and coronavirus infections in California nursing homes. *Policy, Politics, & Nursing Practice, 21*(3), 174–186.

Humphries, J., & Canham, S. L. (2021). Conceptualizing the shelter and housing needs and solutions of homeless older adults. *Housing Studies, 36*(2), 157–179.

Institute of Medicine. Committee on Nursing Home Regulation. (1986). *Improving the quality of care in nursing homes* (Vol. 85, No. 10). National Academies Press.

International Code Council. (2020). *Building valuation data – August 2020*. Retrieved June 13, 2021, from https://www.iccsafe.org/wp-content/uploads/BVD-BSJ-AUG20-pdf.pdf

Inzitari, M., Risco, E., Cesari, M., Buurman, B. M., Kuluski, K., Davey, V., Bennett, L., Varela, J., & Prvu Bettger, J. (2020). Nursing homes and long term care after COVID-19: A new ERA? *The Journal of Nutrition, Health & Aging, 24*(10), 1024–1046.

Kaiser Family Foundation. (2021). COVID-19: Long-term care facilities. Retrieved January 8, 2021, from https://www.kff.org/health-costs/issue-brief/state-data-and-policy-actions-to-address-coronavirus/

Katz, S., Down, T. D., Cash, H. R., & Grotz, R. C. (1970). Progress in the development of the index of ADL. *The Gerontologist, 10*(1), 20–30.

Lawton, M. P. (1989). Three functions of the residential environment. *Journal of Housing for the Elderly, 5*(1), 35–50.

Lawton, M. P., & Brody, E. M. (1969). Assessment of older people: Self-maintaining and instrumental activities of daily living. *The Gerontologist, 9*(3), 179–186.

Lawton, M. P., & Nahemow, L. (1973). Ecology and the aging process. In C. Eisdorfer & M. P. Lawton (Eds.), *The psychology of adult development and aging* (pp. 619–674). American Psychological Association.

Lee, H., & Miller, V. J. (2020). The disproportionate impact of COVID-19 on minority groups: A social justice concern. *Journal of Gerontological Social Work, 63*(6–7), 580–584. https://doi.org/10.1080/01634372.2020.1777241

Lee, S. Y., Hung, L., Chaudhury, H., & Morelli, A. (2021). Staff perspectives on the role of physical environment in long-term care facilities on dementia care in Canada and Sweden. *Dementia, 20*(7), 2558–2572. https://doi.org/10.1177/14713012211003994

Li, Y., Temkin-Greener, H., Shan, G., & Cai, X. (2020). COVID-19 infections and deaths among connecticut nursing home residents: Facility correlates. *Journal of the American Geriatrics Society, 68*(9), 1899–1906.

Lynch, R. M., & Goring, R. (2020). Practical steps to improve air flow in long-term care resident rooms to reduce COVID-19 infection risk. *Journal of the American Medical Directors Association, 21*(7), 893–894.

Macdonald, M., Yu, Z., Weeks, L., Moody, E., Wilson, B., Almukhaini, S., Martin-Misener, R., Sim, M., Jefferies, K., Iduye, D., Neeb, D., & McKibbon, S. (2021). Assistive technologies that support social interaction in long-term care homes: A scoping review. *JBI Evidence Synthesis, 19*(10), 2695–2738. https://doi.org/10.11124/JBIES-20-00264

Maisel, J. L., Steinfeld, E., Basnak, M., Smith, K., & Tauke, M. B. (2017). *Inclusive design: Implementation and evaluation*. London: Routledge.

Mannheim, I., Schwartz, E., Xi, W., Buttigieg, S. C., McDonnell-Naughton, M., Wouters, E. J., & Van Zaalen, Y. (2019). Inclusion of older adults in the research and design of digital technology. *International Journal of Environmental Research and Public Health, 16*(19), 3718.

McGilton, K. S., Escrig-Pinol, A., Gordon, A., Chu, C. H., Zúñiga, F., Sanchez, M. G., & Bowers, B. (2020). Uncovering the devaluation of nursing home staff during COVID-19: Are we fuelling the next health care crisis? *Journal of the American Medical Directors Association, 21*(7), 962–965.

Midlarsky, E., Kahana, E., & Belser, A. (2015). Prosocial behavior in late life. In D. A. Schroeder & W. G. Graziano (Eds.), *The Oxford handbook of prosocial behavior* (pp. 415–432). Oxford University Press. https://doi.org/10.1093/oxfordhb/9780195399813.013.030

Miller, E. A. (2020). Protecting and improving the lives of older adults in the COVID-19 era. *Journal of Aging & Social Policy, 32*(4–5), 297–309. https://doi.org/10.1080/0895942 0.2020.1780104

Morris, S. C., Resnick, A. T., England, S. A., Stern, S. A., & Mitchell, S. H. (2020). Lessons learned from COVID-19 outbreak in a skilled nursing facility, Washington state. *Journal of the American College of Emergency Physicians Open, 1*(4), 563–568.

Morrison, B. A., Coventry, L., & Briggs, P. (2020). Technological change in the retirement transition and the implications for cybersecurity vulnerability in older adults. *Frontiers in Psychology, 11*, 623.

Oswald, F., & Rowles, G. (2006). Beyond the relocation trauma in old age: New trends in today's elders' residential decisions. In H.-W. Wahl, C. Tesch-Römer, & A. Hoff (Eds.), *New dynamics in old age: Environmental and societal perspectives* (pp. 127–152). Baywood Publishing.

Parmelee, P. A., & Lawton, M. P. (1990). The design of special environments for the aged. In J. E. Birren & K. W. Schaie (Eds.), *Handbook of the psychology of aging* (pp. 464–488). Academic Press. https://doi.org/10.1016/B978-0-12-101280-9.50033-4

Pirhonen, J., Melkas, H., Laitinen, A., & Pekkarinen, S. (2020). Could robots strengthen the sense of autonomy of older people residing in assisted living facilities?—A future-oriented study. *Ethics and Information Technology, 22*(2), 151–162.

Porkodi, S., & Kesavaraja, D. (2021). Healthcare robots enabled with IoT and artificial intelligence for elderly patients. *AI and IoT-Based Intelligent Automation in Robotics*, 87–108.

Poscia, A., Stojanovic, J., La Milia, D. I., et al. (2018). Interventions targeting loneliness and social isolation among the older people: An update systematic review. *Experimental Gerontology, 102*, 133–144.

Ramkissoon, H. (2020). COVID-19 place confinement, pro-social, pro-environmental behaviors, and residents' wellbeing: A new conceptual framework. *Frontiers in Psychology, 11*, 2248.

Rashidi, P., & Mihalidis, A. (2013). A survey on ambient-assisted living tools for older adults. *IEEE Journal of Biomedical and Health Informatics, 17*(3), 579–590.

Regnier, V. (2018). *Housing design for an increasingly older population: Redefining assisted living for the mentally and physically frail*. Wiley.

Reinhardt, J. P., Cimarolli, V. R., Burack, O. R., Minahan, J., Marshall, T. L., & Weiner, A. S. (2019). The small house model of long-term care: Association with older adult functioning. *Journal of the American Medical Directors Association, 20*(2), 222–223.

Robinson, J.W. (2004). Architecture of institution & home: Architecture as cultural medium. Unpublished doctoral thesis, Delft University of Technology.

Rowles, G. D. (1983). Geographical dimensions of social support in rural Appalachia. In G. Rowles & R. Ohta (Eds.), *Aging and milieu: Environmental perspectives on growing old* (pp. 111–130). Academic Press.

Rowles, G. D., & Watkins, J. F. (2003). History, habit, heart and hearth: On making spaces into places. In *Aging independently: Living arrangements and mobility* (pp. 77–96). Springer.

Rubinstein, R., & de Medeiros, K. (2004). Ecology and the aging self. *Annual Review of Gerontology and Geriatrics, 23*, 59–84. ISBN-13: 9780826117342.

Sachs-Ericsson, N., Joiner, T., Plant, E. A., & Blazer, D. G. (2005). The influence of depression on cognitive decline in community-dwelling elderly persons. *The American Journal of Geriatric Psychiatry., 13*(5), 402–408.

Salari, S. M., & Rich, M. (2001). Social and environmental infantilization of aged persons: Observations in two adult day care centers. *The International Journal of Aging and Human Development, 52*(2), 115–134.

Sarabia-Cobo, C., Perez, V., de Lorena, P., Hermosilla-Grijalbo, C., Saenz-Jalon, M., Fernandez-Rodriguez, A., & Alconero-Camarero, A. R. (2021). Experiences of geriatric nurses in nursing homes across four counries in the face of the COVID-19 pandemic. *Journal of Advanced Nursing, 77*(2), 869–878.

Scharlach, A., & Diaz Moore, K. (2016). Aging in place: Chapter 21. In V. Bengston & R. Settersten (Eds.), *Handbook of theories of aging* (pp. 407–425). Springer.

Scharlach, A., & Lehning, A. (2015). *Creating aging-friendly communities*. Oxford University Press.

Scheidt, R., & Norris-Baker, C. (2003). Many meanings of community. *Journal of Housing for the Elderly, 17*(1–2), 55–66. https://doi.org/10.1300/J081v17n01_05

Schwarz, B. (1997). Nursing home design: A misguided architectural model. *Journal of Architectural and Planning Research, 14*(4), 343–359.

Seifert, A., & Hassler, B. (2020). Impact of the COVID-19 pandemic on loneliness among older adults. *Frontiers in Sociology, 5*, 590935. https://doi.org/10.3389/fsoc.2020.590935

Smith, G. V., & Ekerdt, D. J. (2011). Confronting the material convoy in later life. *Sociological Inquiry, 81*(3), 377–391.

Spaetgens, B., Brouns, S. H., & Schols, J. M. (2020). The post-acute and long-term care crisis in the aftermath of COVID-19: A Dutch perspective. *Journal of the American Medical Directors Association, 21*(8), 1171–1172.

Stark, S., Landsbaum, A., Palmer, J. L., et al. (2009). Client-centered home modifications improve daily activity performance of older adults. *Canadian Journal of Occupational Therapy, 76*(1_suppl), 235–245. https://doi.org/10.1177/000841740907600s09

Testa, M., & Pollard, J. (2007). Safe pill-dispensing. *Studies in Health Technology and Informatics, 127*, 139.

Van Jaarsveld, G. M. (2020). The effects of COVID-19 among the elderly population: A case for closing the digital divide. *Frontiers in Psychiatry, 11*, 57742. https://doi.org/10.3389/fpsyt.2020.577427

Wahl, H.-W., & Lang, F. (2004). Aging in context across the adult life course: Integrating physical and social environmental research perspectives. *Annual Review of Gerontology and Geriatrics, 23*, 1–33. ISBN-13: 9780826117342.

Weisman, G. D., Chaudhury, H., & Moore Diaz, K. (2000). Theory and practice of place: Toward and integrative model. In R. L. Rubinstein, M. Moss, & M. H. Kleban (Eds.), *The many dimensions of aging* (pp. 3–21). Springer.

Wilder, J. (2021). The disproportionate impact of COVID-19 on racial and ethnic minorities in the United States. *Clinical Infectious Diseases, 72*(4), 707–709. https://doi.org/10.1093/cid/ciaa959

Wong, J. S., & Waite, L. J. (2016). Theories of social connectedness and aging. In V. Bengston & R. Setterson (Eds.), *Handbook of theories of aging* (3rd ed., pp. 349–363). Springer.

Yoders, J. (2021). AGC survey: Chaotic supply chain, worker shortages still plague contractors a year into pandemic. Retrieved June 19, 2021 at https://www.enr.com/articles/51400-agc-survey-chaotic-supply-chain-worker-shortages-still-plague-contractors-a-year-into-pandemic

Zimmerman, S., Dumond-Stryker, C., Tandan, M., Preisser, J. S., Wretman, C. J., Howell, A., & Ryan, S. (2021). Nontraditional small house nursing homes have fewer COVID-19 cases and deaths. *Journal of the American Medical Directors Association, 22*(3), 489–493.

# Creating a Tailored Approach: The Transformation of Jewish Senior Life

Emily Chmielewski and Melissa DeStout

## 1 Introduction

Today's senior living market is different from the past, even the recent past. Consumer preferences, advances in technology, and financial realities are resulting in new building typologies and models of care while also driving more people to age in place (Winters et al., 2019). The majority of older adults in the United States will never move into a senior living facility, primarily due to a lack of desire. In fact, 87% of people age 65 and older report they want to continue living in their community as they age (Harrell et al., 2014, p. 8). But what about those who *do* decide to move into senior living communities?

People seeking independent living housing can easily find residential-style options; there is also a growing movement to create home-like assisted living settings (Long, 2021). Yet long-term care (LTC) environments are typically more institutional in nature, both as a result of historical building practices and the more medically-focused care that is delivered in these settings. However, LTC residents desire—and deserve—residential settings, too (Shield et al., 2014). The market has been demanding it, and senior living care providers are finally responding to this call to action. Michelle Cottle (2021), a writer for *The New York Times*, noted that "among the more interesting reform possibilities being discussed is a shift toward smaller, more self-contained, unconventional facilities that reflect the evolving attitude toward aging."

These "unconventional" facilities are disruptors in a landscape of older, outdated long-term care facilities, which typically feature multiple-occupancy bedrooms with minimal privacy and communal bathing rooms that offer little dignity to residents. These outdated facilities' living/activity/dining spaces don't encourage or

E. Chmielewski (✉) · M. DeStout
Perkins Eastman, Pittsburgh, PA, USA
e-mail: e.chmielewski@perkinseastman.com; m.destout@perkinseastman.com

© The Author(s), under exclusive license to Springer Nature
Switzerland AG 2023
F. Ferdous, E. Roberts (eds.), *(Re)designing the Continuum of Care for Older Adults*, https://doi.org/10.1007/978-3-031-20970-3_15

support resident engagement (from poor acoustics to deficient furnishings); and there is often a lack of outdoor access. The dated interiors don't appeal to residents or their families, either; and the floor plan layouts are hospital-like, with long corridors of resident rooms that extend from centralized nurse stations (Perkins & Hoglund, 2013b).

More and more, new construction and renovations to existing senior living facilities are addressing these concerns. Many senior living designers are now creating facilities that not only appeal to today's market consumers but also "accommodate the physical and psychological changes that come with aging [while permitting] residents to exercise their remaining abilities as much as possible" (Perkins & Hoglund, 2013c). This chapter details one such story: the evolution of Jewish Senior Life, a senior living community located near Rochester, New York, that was redesigned in the late 2010s. When Jewish Senior Life decided to revamp their model of care to a more person-centered approach, they knew this pivot would require modernization of the physical environment to better support the new operational model and progressive delivery of care. This chapter shares that journey toward a future-oriented direction for this community.

## 2  Project Premise

Jewish Senior Life is a life plan community on a 75-acre campus near Rochester, New York. Open to residents of all faiths and ethnicities, it offers (at this writing) independent living, assisted living, memory care, LTC, short-term rehabilitation, outpatient rehabilitation, and an adult day program. Rooted in more than a century of caring for older adults, the organization's mission is "to enhance the quality of life, health, and well-being of Jewish older adults, their families, and others in [the] community, consistent with the values and traditions of our Jewish heritage" (Jewish Senior Life, 2020).

This focus on quality of life, health, and the well-being of residents was at the heart of Jewish Senior Life's decision to move to a person-centered care approach, which represents "a shift from a culture where the provider and staff dictate when people will sleep, eat, and shower, what they will eat, and what they will do for activities to honoring the individual rhythms and preferences of the [resident]" (Galiana, 2019). In other words, a person-centered care model enables residents to have a much greater role in the decision-making that affects their lives. This approach can also positively impact the direct care staff (Barbosa et al., 2014), offering them greater empowerment, more collaboration when caring and planning for residents, and the formation of deeper, more consistent relationships with residents.

As Jewish Senior Life set their sights on how a person-centered care model would apply to the physical environment, they began to renovate their facilities with features such as decentralized dining and upgraded finishes in the residential wings. However, they quickly realized their push for person-centered care needed to go further. Accordingly, Jewish Senior Life enlisted help from the designers at Perkins Eastman and consultants with The Green House Project. The three organizations worked together to address the project's four key goals: (1) create living and care environments that support a person-centered, collaborative approach; (2) right-size the skilled nursing program to be financially sustainable and provide adequate care support for the full campus community; (3) minimize disruption to existing residents during construction and the transition to new living environments; and (4) maintain and support campus community involvement in programs and activities despite a new, distributed program.

## 3 Design Process

To address these four design project goals, Jewish Senior Life hired Perkins Eastman, a global architecture firm dedicated to the idea that design can have "a direct and positive impact on people's lives and the environment," according to its mission statement (Perkins Eastman, 2021). Perkins Eastman initiated the design with a strategic visioning process called IDEAS, an acronym for integrating design, economics, assessment, and strategy. This highly collaborative process provided Jewish Senior Life with business, market position, and concept development results that were actionable and supported the organization's mission. During the IDEAS process, the design team engaged the project's stakeholders—from the executive team to direct care staff to residents—to develop a well-tested plan that was supported by group consensus as well as evidence-based decision-making. Using the qualitative and quantitative data gathered during the IDEAS process to inform their decisions, the design team developed a long-range vision with four major elements that would frame the scope of design.

First, the design called for new small house buildings to be built. A small house typically consists of 10 to 12 private residential bedrooms organized around a shared living, kitchen, and dining area. These small houses would be designed using the Green House model and would also be formally certified as Green House homes. (Refer to the *Adopting the Green House Model* section of this chapter for more information about Green Houses.) In this case, the small houses—known as cottages on this campus—would be vertically stacked, with one household per floor for 12 residents each, across three floors and three buildings to accommodate the desired 108 residential units. The design team called for three cottages to be constructed, but also included a fourth building in the new site plan to allow for future community growth.

The second part of the project's scope focused on Jewish Senior Life's existing skilled nursing building, the Farash Tower, which would undergo a major renovation that would transform its six stories into Green House-inspired neighborhoods with both short-term rehabilitation and LTC settings. A neighborhood is when two or three small houses are clustered together and organized around a singular living, kitchen, and dining area as well as shared staff support spaces. The Farash Tower's floors were converted from one large unit to two Green House-inspired neighborhoods per floor, with a total of 22 residents per neighborhood. This plan reduced the number of residences in the building from 362 to 220 private rooms. By reducing the bed count, the design team not only adapted the space to be similar to Green House spatial standards but also helped right-size Jewish Senior Life's program, which was a major goal of the overall design project (Fig. 1).

The third design approach focused on updating the entry sequence at the Farash Tower. That meant modernizing the interior aesthetics, from porte cochere to lobby, and creating a more welcoming experience to support the whole campus community's involvement in programs and activities despite the new, decentralized housing program. The design team also looked at the Jewish Senior Life campus as a whole, such that the fourth component of the design was about developing a site plan that considered the new building elements being added to the campus as well as the future of the community.

Another important part of the overall process was to minimize disruptions during the public-space upgrades and when moving residents into the new cottages and renovated wings of the Farash Tower. The new cottages were built first as a result, allowing half the Farash Tower residents to move into them. That move then opened

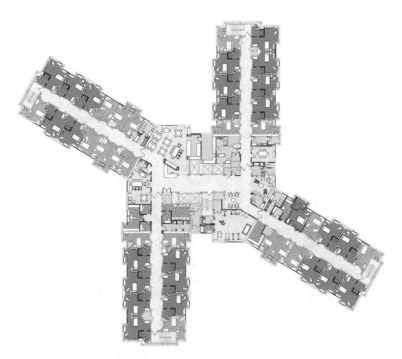

**Fig. 1** Farash Tower renovation typical floor plan (2015). © Perkins Eastman. The renovations to the Farash Tower reconfigured the layout such that there are now two Green House-inspired neighborhoods per floor, where each resident has a private room and shower, among many other person-centered design improvements

up space for renovations in the tower. Construction in the tower took place in phases, as well, to further minimize disruptions.

The design project took nearly a decade to complete. The initial strategic planning began in 2011; site work and construction of the cottages started in 2016; and the tower renovations were completed in early 2020. Perkins Eastman collaborated with Jewish Senior Life administrators, staff, and residents and their families throughout the process to tailor the project to their needs. The design team also sought to make evidence-based design decisions as the project progressed, exploring the existing knowledge base of senior living research and also referencing their own pre- and post-occupancy evaluations from past projects to make data-informed decisions.

Further, during the design documentation phase of the project, Perkins Eastman built and tested two full-scale mock-ups to further hone their plans. One was a resident room in the Farash Tower, which was constructed using the actual specified materials, was fully furnished, and had working fixtures. A resident moved into the mock-up room, and staff provided care there to test its utility. The other mock-up was a small house kitchen, built with sturdy foam boards, to demonstrate the spatial configuration and location of key design features. Both mock-ups were built on the Jewish Senior Life campus and remained in place for several weeks (Fig. 2).

Multiple direct care staff members had daily interactions with the mocked-up resident room, and all were encouraged to tour the kitchen mock-up to act out their day-to-day routines. The design team collected feedback throughout the testing period and used this information to make evidence-based decisions to tweak the

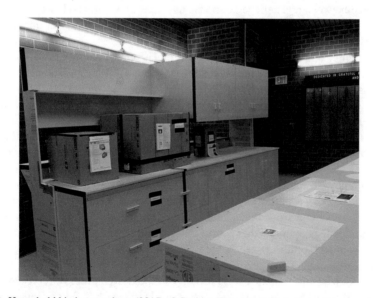

**Fig. 2** Household kitchen mock-up (2015). © Perkins Eastman. Full-scale mock-ups, such as the household kitchen mock-up pictured here, were built so the design team could collect feedback from users to fine-tune the design

design. For instance, staff suggested several changes to the resident bathroom, including adjusting the angle of the mirror to better accommodate someone in a wheelchair, selecting a different faucet for a more residential feel, and recessing the paper towel dispenser, among a few other modifications. They also recommended adjustments to the medicine server cabinet to better suit their needs, such as modifying shelving heights to accommodate the size of pill packs and adding a pull-out shelf under the counter to offer additional workspace. The resident room mock-up also allowed for changes to the design, such as the coordination of electrical outlets to furnishings and testing an overhead lift system to determine where this costly feature would best be used. In these respects, Perkins Eastman used this process as another opportunity to help tailor the design specifically to the needs of Jewish Senior Life.

## 4  Adopting the Green House Model

The Green House Project was another active collaborator in the design for Jewish Senior Life, acting as a consultant on this ambitious project. The non-profit organization, which helps care providers build and operate Green Houses for older adults, focuses on "destigmatizing aging and humanizing care for all people through the creation of radically non-institutional eldercare environments that empower the lives of people who live and work in them" (The Green House Project, n.d.-a). A Green House is a specific version of the small house building typology. The main difference between a generic small house and a certified Green House home is the prescriptive design and operational practices that come along with adopting the Green House model.

Although "facilities don't have to be part of The Green House Project to adopt a culture that puts the needs of the resident first" (Singer, 2017), embracing the Green House model gives senior care providers guidelines and support as they strive to achieve person-centered care. Jewish Senior Life felt that by working with The Green House Project, they would not only get authoritative advice on the person-centered care model but they would also be held accountable to adopting this new model of care to the fullest extent possible. They also wanted to take advantage of The Green House Project's long history of continual improvement, where a significant amount of research has gone into its operational guidelines, standard floor plans, and the impacts that built Green Houses have had on operations and the people who live and work there. In fact, The Green House Project states, it's the only "culture change model that is backed by ongoing research that evaluates quality of care, quality of life, and financial viability" (The Green House Project, n.d.-c).

There were many other benefits to adopting this model, including Perkins Eastman's own fruitful history with it. Early in the design process, representatives from Jewish Senior Life and Perkins Eastman toured several Green House homes across the country and interviewed associated stakeholders to understand where the model could be tailored to Jewish Senior Life's unique community and resident needs. The Perkins Eastman design team additionally tapped into the work they had previously completed with The Green House Project, which included design projects for other clients and a 2010 partnership with The Green House Project and NCB Capital Impact to develop The Green House Prototype Design Package (The Green House Project, n.d.-d). Together, Jewish Senior Life, Perkins Eastman, and The Green House Project were able to implement a tailored design to support person-centered care practices.

## 5   The Cottages: Breaking the Mold

The Green House Project and Perkins Eastman collaborated with Jewish Senior Life to develop its three new Green House-certified cottage buildings, which embody the principles of person-centered care. But from the early stages of design, Perkins Eastman recognized there would have to be certain aspects of the cottages' plans that pushed the boundaries of the usual Green House architecture. For instance, Green House homes are usually single-story, stand-alone buildings similar in scale to a large, market-rate residential house. Each Jewish Senior Life cottage, however, was going to be three vertically stacked small houses within one building. As described by an Administrator at Jewish Senior Life in an interview with the authors, the decision to make the Green Houses multi-story went beyond site restrictions. It also "revolved around the staffing and the outdoor elements" (Anonymous Jewish Senior Life staff member, A, personal communication, October 14, 2021).

The vertical nature of the cottages required some design modifications because they are larger in scale than a typical Green House, so the floor plan had to be adapted for these multi-story buildings. The design team had to rethink how the

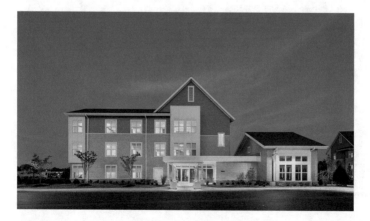

**Fig. 3**  Cottage exterior (2017). © Sarah Mechling/Perkins Eastman. The cottage building designed for Jewish Senior Life, with its three vertically stacked small houses and ground floor Community Room, is a departure from the typical one-story Green House model

small houses would connect to each other and how the cottages would connect to the rest of the campus. A ground floor main entrance vestibule was one of the solutions; it creates a transitional space between the building and the broader campus, providing an interior space protected from the elements but still separate from the small houses (Fig. 3).

The vestibule also connects the small houses to a shared Community Room, which is another unique element to the Green Houses at Jewish Senior Life. Before the cottage construction and Farash Tower renovations began, residents were accustomed to gathering in common areas for events like performances, guest speakers, and celebrations, and they wanted to preserve this kind of experience. The ground floor Community Room in each cottage affords opportunities for smaller versions of these events, which are also open to residents in adjacent buildings (Fig. 4).

The entry sequence is also different in the Jewish Senior Life cottages because how people enter a multi-story building is inherently different than approaching the

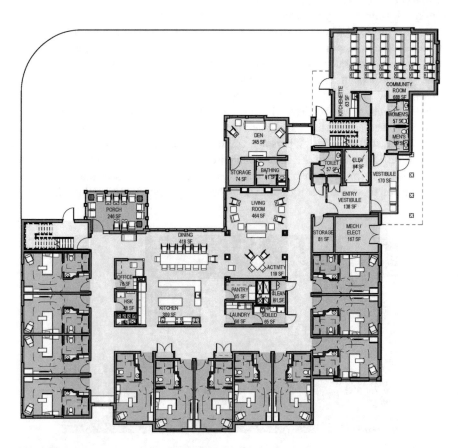

**Fig. 4** Cottage ground floor plan (2015). © Perkins Eastman. The ground floor of a Jewish Senior Life cottage includes a Community Room, access to a shared outdoor garden, and a vestibule/elevator lobby that provides access to the households on the upper floors

front door to a single-family home. At a typical Green House home, a person would knock or ring a door bell at a front door to be let into the small house, where the first space entered would be an entry hall (just like someone would experience entering a single-family market-rate house). At Jewish Senior Life, however, the entry experience begins at the sidewalk, which leads to a covered entrance that provides protection from the elements upon leaving a vehicle. The covered entrance opens into the building at an interior vestibule that connects the residents in all three small houses to the ground floor shared Community Room. This vestibule also connects to the elevator lobby that, at each floor, opens onto the front door to each of the small houses, thereby functioning as the typical Green House home's front door with doorbell.

Most single-story Green House homes also have a back door that is accessed through a garage. In the three-story cottages at Jewish Senior Life, however, the single front entrance to each household has to serve multiple purposes: It offers an attractive entrance for residents, staff, and visitors but also must function as a holding area for back-of-house functions, such as delivery storage and trash removal. The original design of the cottages included a closet just inside each household entry for back-of-house purposes, but it was found to be disruptive to the home environment. The design team pivoted as a result, repurposing a closet in the elevator lobby just outside the household's entrance.

Outdoor access also required careful consideration given the multi-story nature of the cottages. To address this important need, the design team created a shared courtyard that can be reached from both the ground floor small house and via the shared Community Room. The residents of the three vertically stacked small houses all have access to this courtyard and adapt its use based on their personal interests (e.g., vegetable and flower gardening, picnics, group events). In addition, each small house has a four-season porch off its living room, providing further connection to the outdoors.

# 6   The Tower: Further Adaptations

The existing Farash Tower offered another opportunity to introduce person-centered care environments to the Jewish Senior Life campus. But instead of vertically stacked small houses, the design team opted for a neighborhood plan, where small house-style wings are connected through shared common areas. The plan adopts certain Green House features though it doesn't achieve full Green House certification. This approach was intentional, given that the existing building lent itself to a certain kind of renovation and also because it created more choices among living environments for Jewish Senior Life to offer its community. Because Farash Tower includes so many levels of care (LTC, short-term rehabilitation, memory care, and a neurobehavioral unit), some areas have a more residential interior style, whereas others offer a hospitality approach more suited to short-term stays.

In the short-term rehabilitation neighborhoods (where people typically have just a few weeks stay), the state-of-the-art rehabilitation gym is located close to the elevator lobby, with large glass doors to emphasize and celebrate the journey to wellness. Further, the living rooms and dining areas in these neighborhoods were designed to feel more like a café and a space where visitors and rehab guests could spend time comfortably. Additional staff areas and spaces for family meetings were also designed into these neighborhoods to facilitate conversations around care and next steps. In contrast, for the LTC neighborhoods (where residents may spend years), the designers employed a more residential interior style to create a sense of home. "It really isn't 'home-like'… it's establishing a real home so that you or I would feel comfortable being here," said Susan Ryan, Senior Director of The Green House Project (Spicer, 2017).

The ambiance inside the tower was just one factor in establishing an overall feel for the building. The design team paid a lot of attention to the exterior façade as well, and how Farash Tower was situated on the grounds. Originally, the six-story brick building loomed over the main approach from the campus entrance. Although it was surrounded by large expanses of grass, residents, staff, and visitors often commented on how its presence felt overwhelming. The approach to the building was not human-scaled and didn't provide residents with any natural connection to a relaxing outdoor space. To remedy this, thoughtful site work, new landscaping, and some minor façade modifications combined to create a low-cost yet impactful solution. A new gazebo also provides a pleasing community connection on the path between the cottages and the tower, establishing a visual focus along the campus entrance drive as it winds through the newly planted landscaping around the buildings.

The design team also aimed to enhance wayfinding and orientation throughout the campus and within the tower. To mitigate the confusing layout within the existing Farash Tower building, Perkins Eastman implemented various design elements on each floor to indicate the transition into each neighborhood, such as opening up walls to create views into adjacent spaces, strategically varying the ceiling heights, changing the flooring and wall finishes, and installing distinct furnishings. Newly open lounge spaces with windows, furthermore, replaced closed-off rooms that once surrounded the elevator lobbies, exposing residents and staff to ample daylight and broad campus views toward orienting landmarks for wayfinding reference points. These design decisions were evidence-based, as research indicates that brighter light and outside views can help older adults' wayfinding ability (Jiang & Verderber, 2017; Tuaycharoen, 2020). The design team also improved the daylighting in the tower's living room areas since research indicates that greater daylight exposure can help regulate circadian rhythms, prevent sleep disorders, reduce sundowning among people with Alzheimer's disease or other dementias, and counteract seasonal depression (Khachiyants et al., 2011; Leibrock, 2000).

## 7 Project Impact

When Jewish Senior Life adopted a progressive, person-centered care model and worked with Perkins Eastman and The Green House Project to update their facilities, they saw a number of positive effects. The new cottages, the renovation of the Farash Tower, and site work around the campus have all combined to help Jewish Senior Life align the physical environment to their goals for a person-centered approach.

### 7.1 Interior Aesthetics

"We're really working on deinstitutionalizing the nursing home," Jewish Senior Life President and CEO Michael King has explained (Spicer, 2017). This is embodied by the new cottages and their residential aesthetic as well as the Farash Tower's mix of residential and hospitality environments, where the open and welcoming spaces, with their contemporary and airy aesthetic and enhanced fenestration, are a pleasant departure from the building before the renovation. Now, each cottage and several neighborhoods in the tower are designed like a single-family home, with customized finishes, accessories, and artwork that work together to afford personalization and enhance wayfinding.

   "The residents love it, and I love it too, because it's like you're going to work in somebody's home. The residents feel more comfortable and secure and safe with us," said a direct care staff member who works in one of the Jewish Senior Life cottages (Anonymous Jewish Senior Life staff member, B, personal communication, October 14, 2021). A Social Worker at Jewish Senior Life agreed. "If we can do institutional work but in a home setting, it's the best of both worlds" (Anonymous Jewish Senior Life staff member, C, personal communication, October 14, 2021).

### 7.2 Independence

Another benefit of a person-centered care model coupled with supportive environments that are designed as a home is that residents feel like they truly are at home. They have the confidence and security to go about their day as they see fit. At Jewish Senior Life, residents are encouraged to be as independent as possible. A resident in one of the Jewish Senior Life cottages confided to the authors about how she loves ice cream, for example. "In the middle of the afternoon I go to the kitchen and help myself to a bowl of ice cream. I just feel like this is my home and I can do what I want to do," she explained (Anonymous Jewish Senior Life resident, personal communication, October 14, 2021). A Social Worker at Jewish Senior Life added, "In the cottages, we can encourage independence and the staff fill in where the dependence needs are. I think the residents age better in the cottages because [it's their] home" (Anonymous Jewish Senior Life staff member, C, personal communication, October 14, 2021).

Resident independence also means a continuation of meaningful roles. As a resident of a Jewish Senior Life cottage described it, "I help [the staff] cook and I help with laundry. I'm independent; I walk and so I get up early, I make my bed, take out the garbage. It's just like living at home… Whenever I need help, I ask for it and they come in and help me; otherwise, I try to do as much as I can" (Anonymous Jewish Senior Life resident, personal communication, October 14, 2021). This level of resident empowerment and independence is beneficial to residents' long-term well-being (Phinney et al., 2007).

## 7.3 Privacy

Privacy was another important consideration for the design of the residential spaces at Jewish Senior Life. The cottage bedrooms are designed so that none open onto the household's common living/dining/kitchen areas—a departure from the typical Green House model, but an important move in this case so residents could enjoy more privacy and retreat from the noise and activity of the household. As a resident of a Jewish Senior Life cottage described it to the authors, "I have my privacy; I can just shut the door when I'm having a bad day and no one's going to bother me" (Anonymous Jewish Senior Life resident, personal communication, October 14, 2021). Privacy was also key in the Farash Tower. Before the renovation, there had been a mix of semi-private and private resident rooms, but nearly all of them lacked private showers. Now, every bedroom is private and enjoys an en suite bathroom.

The new design also benefits the staff, who told the authors they no longer have to wait for one roommate to finish using the bathroom before helping the other. They also noted how the private showers support residents' dignity because residents no longer have to share a bathing area that would often be far from their bedrooms, said a Jewish Senior Life direct care staff member (Anonymous Jewish Senior Life staff member, B, personal communication, October 14, 2021). A Social Worker at Jewish Senior Life added that they no longer have to be referees in arguments between roommates or help residents hunt down personal items. Now they can focus their attention and energy into caring for the residents, she said (Anonymous Jewish Senior Life staff member, C, personal communication, October 14, 2021).

## 7.4  Sense of Community

Since the new construction and renovations to the Jewish Senior Life campus, LTC residents are now in smaller groupings. The staffing under the person-centered care model is also now more consistent, with direct care staff typically designated to just one household or neighborhood. This allows for deeper and more meaningful connections to develop, both between residents as well as among residents and staff. As a Jewish Senior Life Administrator described it, there was some initial hesitation by the staff when moving into the new spaces and working under a new model of care, but people quickly adapted. Staff now understand that "because of the work they do and the [small] number of residents they care for, they build better relationships" (Anonymous Jewish Senior Life staff member, A, personal communication, October 14, 2021).

The staff value their relationships with residents—not just so they can monitor their well-being, but also because these close interactions give meaning and fulfillment to their work. The family-style dining table and the kitchen counter seating in the cottages and neighborhoods are design features that foster these relationships, where conversations happen during normal daily activities. The COVID-19 pandemic, in fact, underscored how important these interactions had become. A Jewish Senior Life direct care staff member observed that, before the pandemic, the direct care staff would join the residents for meals—a time when residents would typically open up about how they were feeling. Pandemic restrictions no longer allowed the staff to share meals with residents, however, because they couldn't unmask around them. "We miss that," a Jewish Senior Life direct care staff member stated

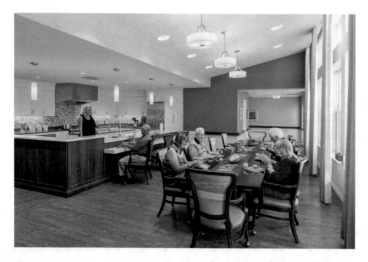

**Fig. 5**  Cottage interior (2017). © Sarah Mechling/Perkins Eastman. The family-style dining table and kitchen counter seating in the Jewish Senior Life households foster relationships among residents and staff

(Anonymous Jewish Senior Life staff member, B, personal communication, October 14, 2021) (Fig. 5).

When a Social Worker at Jewish Senior Life described her day-to-day interactions to the authors, she stated that it felt like she "lived in the cottages… [which] allowed me to be more involved in the minutiae of day-to-day activities; allowed me to share more with families who aren't here. It just makes those engagements that much more meaningful." Since the pandemic, however, things have understandably changed. She described how many conversations were happening over the telephone with families who couldn't be there and that she spent a lot of time arranging window-visits and video calls. "It is a family among families. Our most happy residents have happy families and have staff around them who truly care about them" (Anonymous Jewish Senior Life staff member, C, personal communication, October 14, 2021).

The Community Rooms on the ground floor of each cottage have been particularly successful in facilitating resident and family gatherings, both before and during the pandemic. Jewish Senior Life has been able to host small group events and family visitations in a safe and controlled setting, a Jewish Senior Life Administrator explained (Anonymous Jewish Senior Life staff member, A, personal communication, October 14, 2021). Further, the Community Rooms have also provided a safe space for staff training sessions and visits from outside guests—without anyone ever having to enter the households.

The exterior site work at Jewish Senior Life also promotes community with more walkable grounds, pleasing landscapes, and outdoor gathering areas. "We use a lot more of our grounds than we ever did before," a Social Worker at Jewish Senior Life explained. "Those outdoor spaces—the gazebo, the walkways, the pond, the overlooks—they're used year-round" (Anonymous Jewish Senior Life staff member, C, personal communication, October 14, 2021).

## 7.5   Well-being

Beyond dramatic improvements to residents' independence, privacy, and socialization, staff also have reported that the new small houses have led to better sleep among the residents. "Within a couple of days, one of the first things we noticed was people were sleeping in longer," said King. "Instead of waking up at seven o'clock because that's when we [served] breakfast over at the tower, we're now able to provide breakfast and meals whenever they want it. It's been a great change" (Singer, 2017).

Even better, small house facilities, such as the new and renovated homes at Jewish Senior Life, fared better during the pandemic than their more institutional peers (Cottle, 2021). Research into this phenomenon found that "nontraditional Green House/small NHs [nursing homes] have better outcomes than traditional NHs in numerous areas; evidence now demonstrates they have lower rates of COVID-19 and COVID-19 mortality than other NHs as well. As such, they are an especially promising model as NHs are reinvented post-COVID" (Zimmerman et al., 2021).

At Jewish Senior Life, the Green House cottages and the switch to all private rooms in the tower helped the campus manage and avoid COVID-19 spread, while the dedicated staff assignments to each residential unit further limited the potential for spreading disease across households (Cottle, 2021). At this writing, the Jewish Senior Life cottages had been COVID-free, a Social Worker at Jewish Senior Life explained, because everyone has their own room and can stay spread apart in the spacious common areas, maximizing all the different spaces in the households and neighborhoods (Anonymous Jewish Senior Life staff member, C, personal communication, October 14, 2021). "I feel very fortunate we did the design we did, especially because of the pandemic. I do believe that helped," a Jewish Senior Life Administrator said (Anonymous Jewish Senior Life staff member, A, personal communication, October 14, 2021).

## 7.6 Staffing

Beyond limiting the spread of disease, research has shown that assigning a dedicated staff to groups of residents in LTC has broad value, encouraging bonds with these groups and allowing staff to become closely attuned to their routines, so they are more likely to notice subtle signs when something is amiss (Advancing Excellence, n.d.). In addition, direct care staff who work within the new small houses and neighborhoods at Jewish Senior Life have expressed that they feel more supported and confident in their work. "It makes you feel good to be in the Green House and to take control of your own home," a Jewish Senior Life direct care staff member told the authors. "It's my home; I'm in charge. It gives you the confidence. All the aids have the confidence to be in charge of their home and do what needs to be done" (Anonymous Jewish Senior Life staff member, B, personal communication, October 14, 2021).

Direct care staff have also developed a sense of pride in their work and the environments they work in. This was evidenced when a Jewish Senior Life direct care staff member explained how everything looks similar to the day they moved in: "We keep everything clean. [We] want to keep it as fresh as possible" (Anonymous Jewish Senior Life staff member, B, personal communication, October 14, 2021). This passion for the upkeep of the environment is an extension of their pride in working there and the ownership they feel over the space. Anne Marie Cook, CEO of Lifespan of Greater Rochester, explained, "'Once you change the environment and put a design in that fosters the kind of culture change that makes it more of a home, more of a person-centered environment, it pushes some of the other culture change activities'" (Singer, 2017).

# 8 Conclusion

Using a combination of certified Green House cottages and Green House-inspired neighborhoods, a person-centered care environment was created for Jewish Senior Life. Designed using a collaborative and tailored approach, the cottages' small houses and the neighborhoods within the Farash Tower are both adaptations to the typical Green House model. However, both provide the physical environments needed to support the person-centered care that Jewish Senior Life aimed to provide. Residents are now afforded more autonomy, greater privacy, and a homier, more personalized environment, while staff and the new person-centered model of care are also better supported.

Jewish Senior Life is now better positioned for the future with these person-centered changes, both in operations and to the physical environment. It took a lot of hard work, a Jewish Senior Life Administrator told the authors, from careful planning and thoughtful designing to educating staff, residents, and families about the changes. There were speed bumps along the way, she added, but people quickly adapted and learned to love their new environment (Anonymous Jewish Senior Life staff member, A, personal communication, October 14, 2021). "It's a different way of doing it. I think it's a better way of doing it," a Social Worker at Jewish Senior Life explained. "It is the right way of taking care of our elders" (Anonymous Jewish Senior Life staff member, C, personal communication, October 14, 2021).

If a design can be measured by how well the environment meets an organization's mission-driven project goals and the positive impact it has on occupants' lives, then Jewish Senior Life can be deemed a success. "What greater compliment could I give than to express the *humanity* of your design?" a resident wrote in a thank you letter to the design team (B. Smith, personal communication, September 17, 2017). Ted Donsky, another resident, was equally impressed. "'I can't begin to tell you how wonderful it is. I wake up to a fantasy. My favorite part? The whole thing'" (Spicer, 2017).

The design project for Jewish Senior Life achieved the goals of creating a person-centered care environment, right-sizing the program, minimizing disruption to the residents during construction and relocation, and maintaining and supporting community involvement across multiple buildings. Further, this project shows how a community with a tailored design approach, rooted in the principles of person-centered care and supported by evidence-based decision-making, can transform a community for the better.

# References

AARP. (n.d.). *The Green House Project COVID study report*. Retrieved October 20, 2021, from AARP: https://www.aarp.org/content/dam/aarp/caregiving/2020/09/green-house-homes-report-summary-09-21.pdf

Advancing Excellence. (n.d.). *Fast facts: Consistent assignment*. Retrieved October 26, 2021, from PHI National: https://phinational.org/wp-content/uploads/2017/07/Consumer-Fact-Sheet-Consistent-Assignment.pdf

Barbosa, A., Sousa, L., Nolan, M., & Figueiredo, D. (2014). Effects of person-centered care approaches to dementia care on staff: A systematic review. *American Journal of Alzheimer's Disease & Other Dementias, 30*(8), 713–722.

Building Design and Construction. (2011, March 17). *Perkins Eastman launches the Green House prototype design package*. Building Design and Construction. Retrieved October 19, 2021, from https://www.bdcnetwork.com/perkins-eastman-launches-green-house-prototype-design-package

Chmielewski, E. (2018). DFAR14 insights and innovations. In *Dsesign for aging review 14: AIA design for aging knowledge community*, (pp. 174–203). Images Publishing.

Cottle, M. (2021, August 1). Nobody wants to live in a nursing home. Something's got to give. *The New York Times*. Retrieved October 21, 2021, from https://www.nytimes.com/2021/08/01/opinion/aging-nursing-homes.html

Galiana, J. (2019). Person-centered long-term care. In *Aging well* (pp. 29–58). Springer. Retrieved from https://link.springer.com/content/pdf/10.1007%2F978-981-13-2164-1_4.pdf

Harrell, R., Lynott, J., Guzman, S., & Lampkin, C. (2014). *What is livable? Community preferences of older adults*. AARP Public Policy Institute.

Jewish Senior Life. (2020, March 10). *History, mission, vision & values*. Jewish Senior Life. Retrieved August 2, 2021, from https://jewishseniorlife.org/about/history

Jiang, S., & Verderber, S. (2017). On the planning and design of hospital circulation zones: A review of the evidence-based literature. *HERD: Health Environments Research & Design Journal, 10*(2), 124–146.

Khachiyants, N., Trinkle, D., Son, S. J., & Kim, K. Y. (2011). Sundown syndrome in persons with dementia: An update. *Psychiatry Investigation, 8*(4), 275–287.

Leibrock, C. (2000). *Design details for health: Making the most of interior design's healing potential*. Wiley.

Long, C. (2021, September 22). Home sweet home: Thinking differently about senior living as an asset class. *Forbes*. Retrieved from https://www.forbes.com/sites/forbesrealestatecouncil/2021/09/22/home-sweet-home-thinking-differently-about-senior-living-as-an-asset-class/?sh=1294ee464257

Perkins Eastman. (2021, July 14). *Human by design*. Perkins Eastman. Retrieved August 2, 2021, from https://www.perkinseastman.com/

Perkins, B., & Hoglund, J. D. (2013a). Senior living today. In B. Perkins & J. D. Hoglund (Eds.), *Building type basics for senior living* (2nd ed., p. 6). Wiley.

Perkins, B., & Hoglund, J. D. (2013b). *Building type basics for senior living* (2nd ed.). Wiley.

Perkins, B., & Hoglund, J. D. (2013c). Renovation, restoration, and adaptive reuse. In I. B. Perkins & J. D. Hoglund (Eds.), *Building type basics for senior living* (2nd ed., pp. 299–306). Wiley.

Phinney, A., Chaudhury, H., & O'Connor, D. L. (2007). Doing as much as I can do: The meaning of activity for people with dementia. *Aging & Mental Health, 11*(4), 384–393.

Shield, R. R., Tyler, D., Lepore, M., Looze, J., & Miller, S. C. (2014). Would you do that in your home? Making nursing homes home-like in culture change implementation. *Journal of Housing for the Elderly, 28*(4), 383–398.

Singer, P. (2017, September 27). *Take a look inside $83 million nursing home project*. Democrat and Chronicle. Retrieved August 2, 2021, from https://www.democratandchronicle.com/story/news/2017/09/26/senior-living-jewish-senior-life-cottages-brighton/704753001

Spicer, V. (2017, September 27). Jewish senior life's Green House cottages give residents 'real home'. *Rochester Business Journal*. Retrieved August 2, 2021, from https://rbj.net/2017/09/27/jewish-senior-lifes-green-house-cottages-give-residents-realhome

The Center for Health Design. (n.d.). *What is evidence-based design (EBD)?* The Center for Health Design. Retrieved October 19, 2021, from https://www.healthdesign.org/certification-outreach/edac/about-ebd

The Green House Project. (n.d.-a). *Who we are*. The Green House Project. Retrieved August 2, 2021, from https://thegreenhouseproject.org/about/visionmission

The Green House Project. (n.d.-b). *Building a Green House home*. The Green House Project. Retrieved October 19, 2021, from https://thegreenhouseproject.org/solutions/build-a-green-house/

The Green House Project. (n.d.-c). *Backed by evidence*. The Green House Project. Retrieved October 19, 2021, from https://thegreenhouseproject.org/resources/research

The Green House Project. (n.d.-d). *Announcing the Green House prototype design package*. The Green House Project. Retrieved October 19, 2021, from https://blog.thegreenhouseproject.org/announcing-the-green-house-prototype-design-package/

Tuaycharoen, N. (2020). Lighting to enhance wayfinding for Thai elderly adults in nursing homes. *Journal of Daylighting, 7*(1), 25–36.

Winters, M., Chmielewski, E., Moldow, L., Cinelli, D., Hoglund, J. D., & Skoda, J. (2019). *Clean slate project*. Perkins Eastman.

Zimmerman, S., Dumond-Stryker, C., Tandan, M., Preisser, J. S., Wretman, C. J., Howell, A., & Ryan, S. (2021, March 1). Nontraditional small house nursing homes have fewer COVID-19 cases and deaths. *Journal of Post-Acute and Long-Term Care Medicine, 22*(3), 489–493. Retrieved October 21, 2021, from https://www.jamda.com/article/S1525-8610(21)00120-1/fulltext

# Flexible and Enriched Environments for Senior Living and Aging-in-Place in Dense Urban Environments

Upali Nanda and Grant Warner

## 1 Outline

### 1.1 Countering Ageism and Promoting Brain Health

The World Health Organization (WHO) defines institutionalized ageism as the stereotyping, prejudice, and discrimination against people based on their age (WHO, n.d.). Age stereotypes can detrimentally impact older populations' performance on physical or mental tasks such as memory, handwriting skills, walking, and overall cognitive performance (Abrams et al., 2006). In fact, one common misconception we hold is that our cognitive abilities decline steadily as we age. However, studies in neuroscience have made a compelling case for how the brain can continue to grow, even as we age (Cohen, 2005). Countering the perception that cognitive decline is inevitable can help curtail ageist stereotypes and promote healthy aging. A key strategy is to change the conversation from preventing decline to promoting brain health. According to the WHO (n.d.), brain health is a state in which every individual can realize their own abilities and optimize their cognitive, emotional, psychological, and behavioral functioning to cope with life situations. Creating environments that support healthy aging and stimulate brain health needs to be a goal for the design community.

U. Nanda (✉) · G. Warner
HKS Architects, Dallas, TX, USA
e-mail: unanda@hksinc.com

## 2   Enriched Environments

Environmental enrichment (EE) is defined as a "housing condition in which animals benefit from the sensory, physical, cognitive, and social stimulation provided, on brain and cognitive functions usually impaired during aging"(Sampedro-Piqeuro & Begega, 2017; p.1). The concept of EE, which was born out of animal studies, has now been extensively studied in adult populations. Leon and Woo (2018) argue that the loss of hearing, vision, and mastication skills, olfactory impairment, and motoric decline all accompany cognitive loss. However, enriched environments can aid in the improved functioning of these systems, as well as the restoration of the cognitive abilities in older adults. HKS and Hume (2021) identified four key elements that define the enriched environment from a recent review of the literature:

1. Sensory stimuli (taste, olfactory, tactile, visual, auditory, and proprioceptive).
2. Motor (locomotion and physical activity).
3. Social (social interaction).
4. Cognitive and affective (cognition, learning, and emotion).

The ability to provide EE can significantly change how design can support the range of needs that define aging.

## 3   Flexible Environments

Aging is a spectrum of physical, sensory, and cognitive abilities. Environments must respond to this spectrum, which is the fundamental premise of flexibility. In the design of environments, flexibility is often used as a catch-all phrase, but there is extensive research on this subject that divides flexibility into four levels (Nanda et al., 2019):

1. Versatility: environments where many functions can take place without requiring any physical modification.
2. Modifiability: environments that can be modified *by the user* in a simple way to allow a wider range of use.
3. Convertibility: environments that can be converted to a new function by small renovations.
4. Scalability: environments that can grow or shrink based on evolving needs.

Creating senior living communities that can address flexible aging-in-place environments are key, especially when we consider the "environmental docility hypothesis" (Lawton & Simon, 1968) that argues that the less competent the individual, the greater the impact of environmental factors on that individual. When we think of the person-environment fit, we must consider a range of environmental affordances to meet the range of personal competencies. These affordances must be both in terms of enrichment and flexibility to meet the range of competencies needed by an aging population. The case study below illustrates this.

## 4 A Case Study of an Enriched and Flexible Environment Allowing Aging-in-Place

CC Young is a senior living continuum of care community in East Dallas. In the 1990s, they commenced a transformation that resulted in some positive changes but also some unfortunate consequences. As part of a prior master plan, the community was spread out around the periphery of a central park creating a beautiful open space, but also social disconnection and operational challenges. In 2012, under a new leadership team, CC Young began to reconsider the master plan and look for ways to redirect and improve the equitable sense of connection and community. The complex included licensed healthcare services, skilled nursing long-term care, rehabilitation, memory support, assisted living, and hospice. The licensed care units were located in four separate buildings spread across the large campus. In addition, most of the healthcare services were located on a significant slope down toward the spillway to the lake. The owner realized that consolidation of these services into a single efficient complex would improve market penetration, quality of care, and efficiency, as well as reduce staff turnover. The challenge was that the campus was land-locked, surrounded by a light-rail line for the Dallas Area Rapid Transit (DART) system, a single-family home neighborhood, Mockingbird Lane, Lawther Road, and a mixed-use development. A small open area with a small parking lot on the steepest part of the 20-acre site was chosen to add a new high-rise building to consolidate all licensed healthcare services as Phase 1 of the new master plan (CC Young, 2021). They hired HKS Inc., a large global firm with a senior living focus to take on this challenge of consolidation and transformation.

CC Young was subject to a planned development ordinance (PD). While support in East Dallas is unusually strong for a senior living community, there was some opposition to the PD amendment that would allow for the implementation of their new master plan. This was partly due to proximity to a single-family neighborhood, but more vociferously from those opposed to development anywhere around White Rock Lake. Through public engagement, townhall meetings, committee meetings, and discussions with city leaders, a compromise was reached to recognize the critical services CC Young provides to the community and balance the concerns from the "Save the Lake" organization. This compromise included an absolute height limit, severe setback requirements, and density limits.

***Stakeholder Engagement*** Extensive engagement with stakeholders including owners and board members, care partners, residents/family, neighbors, peer providers, state licensing officials, and the local fire marshal was done through user group meetings as well as on-site observation (i.e., staying for 1 day and night at the Lawther Point East skilled nursing and rehabilitation building). Through this process of engagement and observation, as well as a process of renovating the existing assisted living building, insights were generated that informed the design process.

***A Flexible Infrastructure*** The building takes full advantage of the steep 30 ft. slope to create entrances on three levels for different purposes. The building is ten stories, with nine above ground and a parking garage below. Several floors are devoted to specific and/or shared uses with pairs of flexible residential small households to allow CC Young to support residents who are aging-in-place, adapt to changing senior needs, and reassign state licenses for each individual household to respond to unknown challenges in the future. Though no one could have foreseen the COVID-19 pandemic, this flexibility has already proven highly useful in responding to that horrific challenge. The flexible households were used to adapt to outbreaks, serve as rapid response isolation areas, temporarily house key care partners, and create layers of defense against the virus with some elements defined as clean transition and disinfection zones. As dining areas were forced to close, the distributed country and commercial kitchens stacked throughout the core of the building were instrumental in close support for continuing high-quality food services (Fig. 1).

# 5   Institution to Home

The building not only improves efficiency and modernizes care but also strives to transform a large, otherwise institutional program into a vertical neighborhood of flexible small households with smaller, more family-like resident groupings. It uses three key strategies to translate the scale of the institution into the experience of home:

1. **Create Households and Vertical Neighborhoods:** The project consolidated the licensed care environments of four buildings into one. To address the daunting challenge of taking a large program and making it feel residential, The Vista was broken down into two small households of 16 residents per floor. These pairings allowed the design to share hidden support services to minimize the disruptions and presence of unknown staff that might interrupt the feeling of home while increasing security. Each household is independent, with smaller residentially scaled spaces, hidden support services, private areas, and flexible apartments for resident personalization (Fig. 2).

2. **Flexibility to Adapt and Allow Aging-in-Place:** The project used a flexible chassis to prepare for the rapidly evolving needs of senior living. Every household was designed and constructed to the most stringent code and licensing requirements in Texas so that each could adapt independently. At the same time, the finishes and design allowed the overall aesthetic to remain residential. Layouts were designed to give residents the ability to personalize their surroundings and bring furniture from their homes. The flexibility of the chassis allowed one of the floors to be changed more extensively during construction.

3. **Provide Access to Amenities, Nature, and Vibrant Common Areas.** A shared amenity and support floor encouraged socialization, excursions, dining choices, activities, events, and the freedom – especially for the frailest people – to "get out of their household" for a little while. The large open rehabilitation gym space

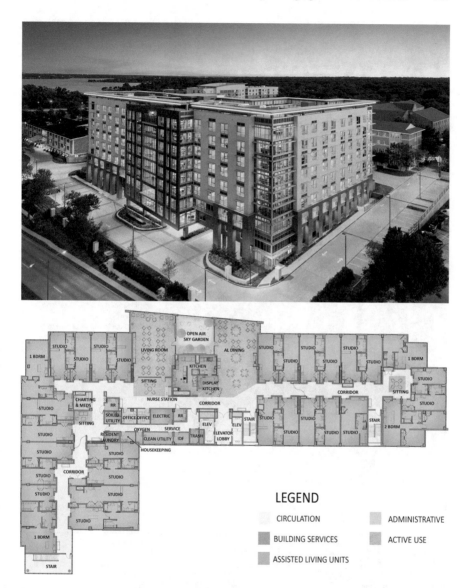

**Fig. 1** External view and typical unit plan showing a flexible chassis. © HKS Inc

divides into smaller, more residentially scaled spaces, all arrayed around an indoor walking loop that centers on a residential training kitchen that residents can relate to because of the home-like decor. The large parking garage remains hidden below the tower to maximize outdoor garden space for residents, care partners, and visitors. A lazy river for grandchildren in the aquatics gym promotes inter-generational social interaction (Figs. 3 and 4).

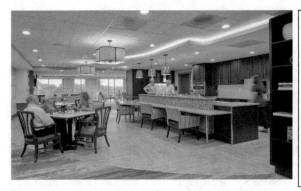

**Enrichment**

**Physical:** Mobility supported by open, barrier free, wheel-chair accessible spaces;
**Social:** Spaces to congregate in daily activity and feel connected;
**Sensory:** natural light, views, fresh food;
**Cognitive:** Range of choices to engage with- cook, view nature, meet others.
*Flexibility:* Versatile for multiple uses and modifiable for rapid reconfiguration

**Fig. 2** Unit level neighborhood. © HKS Inc.

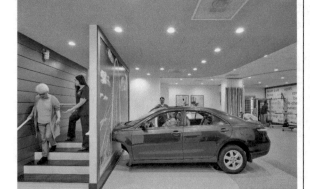

**Enrichment**

**Physical:** Mobility supported by engaging walking paths & exercise equipment;
**Social:** Open layout to be able to see others engaging in exercise;
**Sensory:** Colors, lighting, art accents;
**Cognitive:** Range of choices to engage with. Wall art with inspirational messages.

*Flexibility*

Versatile for multiple uses

**Fig. 3** A flexible and enriched rehab space

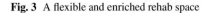

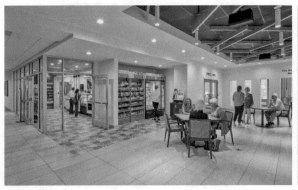

**Enrichment**

**Physical:** Mobility supported by minimum level changes and easy access
**Social:** Spaces to congregate
**Sensory:** View to nature; smell of fresh baked goods
**Cognitive:** Optimal complexity to engage

*Flexibility*
Versatile for multiple uses and modifiable to rapidly reconfigure for different densities

**Fig. 4** Amenity-rich social areas with environmental enrichment and flexibility

# 6 Summary and Key Takeaways

Environments for aging and environments for all of us. As the aging population rises the shift to creating environments where we can age-in-place is also becoming vital. As real estate and health costs continue to grow, such solutions often have to be considered in dense, amenity-rich environments. In this chapter, we shared a case study of a senior living environment that provides enriched and flexible environments that can meet the diverse demands that define our aging process in a positive and meaningful way:

1. Design enriched environments where physical, social, cognitive, and sensory stimuli are provided to create a range of affordances for a range of personal needs and competencies, via amenities, access to nature, and vibrant common areas.
2. Design environments for flexibility at room, unit, and building scale, so that the owner/operator, as well as the user/inhabitant, can change and transform as needed via a flexible plan chassis, flexible interiors, and user-friendly furniture.
3. Ensure that environmental enrichment and flexibility work side by side to support the evolving range of personal competencies that defines the aging process.

# 7 Conclusion

The need for health and well-being has never been greater for our aging communities. Enriched environments that provide physical, social, sensory, and cognitive stimuli are essential to live enriched lives. In many senior living facilities, environmental enrichment can become challenging due to an overwhelming focus on functional needs. However, when environments are designed in a flexible way, allowing users as well as operators to change the environment when needed, environmental enrichment becomes an attainable goal. The coming together of a clear framework for environmental enrichment and one for flexibility creates a new opportunity for designers to design for physical, social, and cognitive health, across the aging spectrum.

# References

Abrams, D., et al. (2006). An age apart: The effects of intergenerational contact and stereotype threat on performance and intergroup bias. *Psychology and Aging, 4,* 691–702.

Cohen, G. D. (2005). *The mature mind: The positive power of the aging brain.* Basic Books.

HKS Inc and HUME. (2021, June 24). *Enriched environments for brain health that foster creativity, promote positivity, and reduce stress: A neurogenesis hypothesis.* https://www.HKSinc.com/how-we-think/research/enriched-environments-for-brain-health-that-foster-creativity-promote-positivity-and-reduce-stress-a-neurogenesis-hypothesis/

CC Young. (2021, March 15). *Our senior community story: CC young*. CC Young Senior Living. Retrieved February 24, 2022, from https://www.ccyoung.org/our-story/

Leon, M., & Woo, C. (2018). Environmental enrichment and successful aging. *Frontiers in Behavioral Neuroscience, 12*, 155.

Sampedro-Piquero, P., & Begega, A. (2017). Environmental enrichment as a positive behavioral intervention across the lifespan. *Current Neuropharmacology, 15*, 459.

Lawton, M. P., & Simon, B. (1968). The ecology of social relationships in housing for the elderly. *Gerontologist, 8*, 108–115.

Nanda, U., Essary, J., Hoelting, M., & Park, G. (2019). *FleXX: A study of flexibility in outpatient settings*. Center for Advanced Design Research and Evaluation.

World Health Organization. (n.d.). *Ageing and health unit*. World Health Organization. Retrieved January 8, 2022, from https://www.who.int/ageing/ageism/en/

# Envisioning Innovative Post-COVID Approaches Toward LTCF Design in Dense Urban Areas: Exploring an Evidence-Based Design Prototype

Hui Cai, Caroline Coleman, and Dani Kolker

## 1 Introduction

Long-term care facilities (LTCFs), including nursing homes (NHs) and skilled nursing facilities (SNFs), have been disproportionally affected by the COVID-19 pandemic. As of June 2021, nearly one-third of US coronavirus deaths included LTCF residents (New York Times, 2021). While all LTCFs suffer from the difficulties that arise from increased COVID-19 infections rates, LTCFs within dense urban settings pose additional unique challenges which undermine LTCF residents'well-being.

### 1.1 Unique Challenges of LTCFs in Dense Urban Environments

As cities are rapidly growing, the aging population and urbanization are two global trends shaping the twenty-first century. Senior living communities in urban locations are an increasingly popular choice for older Americans (World Health Organization, 2007). A survey of 3000 adults residing among 10 large North American cities revealed a majority of respondents wanted to remain

H. Cai (✉)
Department of Architecture, University of Kansas, Lawrence, KS, USA
e-mail: huicai@ku.edu

C. Coleman
The Beck Group, Dallas, TX, USA
e-mail: carolinecoleman@beckgroup.com

D. Kolker
EYP, Dallas, TX, USA
e-mail: dkolker@eypae.com

309

F. Ferdous, E. Roberts (eds.), *(Re)designing the Continuum of Care for Older Adults*, https://doi.org/10.1007/978-3-031-20970-3_17

where they currently live (Welltower, 2017). As such, roughly 70% of city dwellers and 80% of Baby Boomers wish to live in their current city beyond 80 years old. It is likely that respondents value the advantages that cities have to offer including increased healthcare resources, transportation, and making new friends (Welltower, 2017).

There are also challenges unique to LTCFs in dense urban settings which were exacerbated by the pandemic. In Canada, mortality rates were significantly higher in high-rise apartments in dense urban areas than in other dwelling types (e.g., single-detached houses and semi-detached houses) (Yang & Aitken, 2021). A study of nearly 10,000 NHs in the USA revealed the urban location and larger facility size were associated with a higher probability of a COVID-19 case, relative to smaller facilities in non-urban areas (Abrams et al., 2020). These findings may be attributed to limited indoor spaces to move around and a lack of access to nature and outdoor spaces. Widespread lockdown measures prolonged resident isolation which challenged healthy living conditions. It is imperative that urban LTCFs are designed in a manner that aligns with rapidly growing trends while addressing the pandemic-like conditions for a more resilient future. Forthcoming design prototypes should balance these needs to improve older adults' quality of life and safety and support staff and visitors' needs and safety. Even though the design for rural LTCFs is equally important and has its own challenges, this chapter will focus on the LTCF design in the urban context to address its unique challenges to balance residents' quality of life (QoL) and pandemic resiliency.

## 2 Research Objectives

This chapter proposes innovative approaches in a more pandemic-resilient care environment for older adults and their caregivers in the post-COVID-19 era. Proposed approaches aim to support healthy aging, effective provision of healthcare delivery, and a resilient environment for potential future pandemics. This chapter is composed of three parts: (1) a comprehensive literature review on LTCFs' recent experiences responding to the COVID-19 pandemic, capturing lessons learned to develop evidence-based design guiding principles for future senior care environments; (2) an evaluation of past and current design trends that benefit older adults, staff, and visitors in senior care settings during pandemics; and (3) a prototype design for an LTCF as part of an intergenerational continuing care community located in a dense urban setting in the post-COVID era. The prototype design was a result of a research-based, graduate student capstone studio project which incorporated secondary research findings and LTCF design principles into a design example.

## 3   Literature Review

An extensive explorative literature review was conducted in the Web of Science database to gather lessons learned in the past 2 years regarding LTCFs' responses to the COVID-19 pandemic with respect to design. The search covers studies from January 2020 to December 2021, including search terms as listed in Table 1. Only peer-reviewed journal articles written in English were included in the review. The initial search resulted in 214 articles. After screening the titles, a total of 86 articles were selected for abstract and full-text review. Among them, 15 articles specifically addressed space and design issues in LTCFs during the COVID-19 pandemic. Literature review results were categorized based on the impacts of COVID-19 on LTCF in six areas: LTCF residents' physical health and safety, psychological well-being, family and visitors of LTCF residents, healthcare personnel, infection control, and the physical LTCF environment.

### 3.1   The Impacts of COVID-19 on LTC Residents' Physical Health and Safety

The COVID-19 pandemic severely affected LTC residents' physical health and safety. Nearly one-third of US coronavirus deaths are linked to LTCFs (New York Times, 2021). Infectious diseases are not new to the LTC environments. Infectious diseases, like those caused by influenza, pneumonia, respiratory syncytial virus, norovirus, and methicillin-resistant *Staphylococcus aureus*, are problematic in LTCFs (Lai et al., 2020). The current COVID-19 pandemic further revealed LTC residents were at a greater risk of infection and mortality than the general population. Due to the greater number and severity of chronic diseases, disabilities, and immunocompromised conditions, LTC residents are among the most vulnerable populations with poor health outcomes due to COVID-19 (D'Adamo et al., 2020).

LTC residents at an increased risk of morbidity during infectious disease outbreaks due to several underlying factors: (1) LTC residents tend to have multiple chronic diseases and are frail, which make them more susceptible to infection; (2) the residents in the congregated senior living environment share the same sources of air, food, and water, which may facilitate the transmission of infectious agents

**Table 1**  Search terms that were used for the literature search

| Domain | Keywords |
| --- | --- |
| Pandemic-related | "COVID-19" OR "Pandemic" |
| Settings | "Long-term care" OR "Nursing home" OR "Skilled nursing" OR "Assisted living" OR "Independent living" OR "CCRC" OR "Continuous care retirement community" OR "Senior housing" OR "Senior living" |
| Design | "Design" OR "Facilities" OR "Physical environment" OR "Architecture" |

among vulnerable residents; (3) crowding of the environment; (4) sharing of bathroom facilities; (5) gathering in common areas such as large dining rooms; (6) caregivers move from room to room to assist residents and/or provide medical care, which further provides challenges in limiting the spread of infection; (7) the frequent movement of outside visitors, practitioners, and residents can potentially introduce pathogens from around the facility and the community; and (8) low preparedness for infection control (Barnett & Grabowski, 2020; Davidson & Szanton, 2020).

Several studies explored LTCF characteristics associated with COVID-19 outbreaks and mortality among residents (Abrams et al., 2020; Costa et al., 2021). Noteworthy characteristics include facility size, LTCF location, and resident living quarters. Larger LTCFs were associated with the increased probability of viral outbreaks (Abrams et al., 2020; Costa et al., 2021; Ibrahim et al., 2021; Wang et al., 2021; White et al., 2020). Other reports observed lower density or lower occupancy rate could mitigate the incidence and severity of COVID-19 cases (Brown et al., 2021; Simoni-Wastila et al., 2021). The urban location of LTCFs was significantly associated with an increased probability of having a COVID-19 case (Abrams et al., 2020; Ibrahim et al., 2021). Facilities with shared bedrooms and bathrooms were associated with larger outbreaks (Brown et al., 2021; Ibrahim et al., 2021). Increased share of private rooms and larger living area per licensed bed (in sq. ft) were significantly associated with reductions in COVID-19 cases, deaths, and transmissibility among residents (Zhu et al., 2021).

There are mixed results with respect to LTCF quality ratings as a predictor of COVID-19 cases, mortality, and persistence (He et al., 2020; Li et al., 2020; Williams et al., 2021; Abrams et al., 2020; Wang et al., 2021). Studies also showed the importance of integrating healthcare services in residential senior living models and access to telemedicine to provide more effective safety and medical service coordination during the pandemic (Ferdous, 2021a; Kolakowski et al., 2021; Verdoorn et al., 2021; Wang, 2021).

## 3.2 The Impacts of COVID-19 on LTC Residents' Psychological Well-being

Pandemics impose a significant psychosocial impact on LTC residents. Isolating residents within LTCFs is an effective precaution during the pandemic in order to protect the residents' physical health while reducing viral transmission. However, such safety precautions come at the expense of resident autonomy and psychological well-being. Social isolation, fewer social relationships, and loneliness are considered serious health risks for older Americans (Paulin, 2020). Social isolation and loneliness are associated with higher rates of clinical depression, anxiety, and suicidal ideation (Chen & Feeley, 2014). Moreover, these factors have a greater influence on mortality than smoking, obesity, and high blood pressure (National Academies of Sciences & Medicine, 2020).

With the increased isolation during the pandemic, a heightened sense of loneliness, depression, and mental illness warrants greater concern among senior residents. Social distancing, though a major strategy to fight COVID-19, is also a major contributor of loneliness in LTCF settings (Banerjee, 2020). A cross-sectional study in Turkey compared anxiety, life satisfaction, and depression observed that LTCF residents when compared to community-dwelling older adults experienced higher psychological distress and decreased life satisfaction because of social isolation due to prolonged confinements (Arpacioglu et al., 2021). LTC residents were confined to their rooms, subjected to limited social interactions with decrease congregate dining, group physical activities, and in-person family visits. Studies have shown LTCF residents' decline in cognitive and functional scores and increased depression following the social distancing precautions enacted (Greco et al., 2021; Noguchi et al., 2021; Pereiro et al., 2021). Among residents living with dementia, increased social isolation during the COVID-19 pandemic reduced QoL, increased neuropsychiatric symptoms, more psychotropic drug use, and accelerated dementia progression (Curelaru et al., 2021).

The pandemic also restricted access to essential medical, mental health, and other therapeutic services (Agronin, 2020). Restricting movement presents a significant loss of independence, with psychological and physical harms associated with social isolation and immobility (Courtin & Knapp, 2017). Residents in LTCFs would lack exercise, access to direct sunlight and fresh air, and the social benefits of a group living facility (Anderson et al., 2020). The loss of freedom, social life, and loss of mobility can lead to a decreased sense of belonging and boredom (Kaelen et al., 2021). LTC residents rely upon staff personnel to facilitate video calls with family and loved ones (Agronin, 2020). In the absence of visits (in-person or virtual), residents'perception of loneliness is perpetuated throughout their time in the LTCFs. Masks, robes, and face shields also undermine communication efforts for residents with hearing and vision loss.

Several studies identified strategies to mitigate social isolation amid the pandemic. Maintain contact with families and friends via telecommunication or safe face-to-face visit approaches, and participate in safe shared social activities (Arpacioglu et al., 2021; Bethell et al., 2021), physical activities (Bethell et al., 2021; Curelaru et al., 2021), indoor or outdoor gardening (Bethell et al., 2021), virtual immersive garden experiences (Hsieh et al., 2021), tele-technology to access various modes of behavioral and mental health therapies (Curelaru et al., 2021), and application of robotic companion pets in LTCFs (Fogelson et al., 2021) that are found to be effective in mitigating the impacts of the lockdown on social isolation and depression. Similarly, based on a rapid systematic literature review, Ferdous (2021b) highlighted interventions and strategies to improve residents' social interaction during and after the COVID-19 pandemic: technological advancement, remote communication, therapeutic care/stress management, and preventive measures.

### 3.3 The Impact of COVID-19 on Families and Visitors of LTCF Residents

Restricted in-person visit policies during COVID-19 affected the emotional well-being of the families and relatives of LTCF residents (Monin et al., 2020; O'Caoimh et al., 2020; Prins et al., 2021; Wammes et al., 2020; Yeh et al., 2020). Synchronous methods of communication like the phone and email between families and LTC residents are effective in maintaining emotional well-being when in-person visits are restricted (Monin et al., 2020). Families and visitors have a higher level of satisfaction when communicating with LTCF residents by telephone, behind glass dividers, outside, and multiple modalities to remain connected with residents (Wammes et al., 2020).

LTCFs should consider the positive effects of family visits as a means for exploring strategies that restore in-person visits (Verbeek et al., 2020) or alternative methods for families to connect with residents. Wang (2021) shared some strategies such as providing registration spaces for visitor screening and designated areas for visitors' stay to protect both residents' and visitors' safety during the visits. Shepley et al. (2021) also proposed a strategy to provide a visitors' room with interior windows or glass partitions to allow safe in-person visits during pandemics.

### 3.4 The Impact of COVID-19 on LTC Healthcare Workers

LTC healthcare workers are impacted greatly as they are subject to rapidly evolving work circumstances while caring for a vulnerable population. LTCFs inherently struggle with staff recruitment and retention, in part, because of unfavorable compensation and a demanding work environment. During the pandemic, LTC healthcare worker illness and quarantine precautions created staffing shortages and worsened an already demanding work environment for the remaining staff (Barnett & Grabowski, 2020).

A recent study that evaluated healthcare workers (HCWs)' mental health and quality of life during the COVID-19 pandemic through a national survey revealed that more than half of the 1685 participating HCWs reported at least mild psychiatric symptoms and approximately 40% reported symptoms suggesting a clinically significant emotional disorder (Young et al., 2021). A study in Ireland also reported moderate-severe post-traumatic stress disorder symptoms among 45.1% of LTC staff (Brady et al., 2021). Nurses in LTCFs are reported to experience overwhelming workload, high infection risk, job burnout, psychological distress, and depression (Fisher et al., 2021; Havaei et al., 2021; Navarro Prados et al., 2022; Sarabia-Cobo et al., 2021; White et al., 2021).

Facility characteristics influence occupational safety and physical health. Facilities with lower resident density (Ryskina et al., 2021) and higher staff-to-resident ratios (Li et al., 2020; Ryskina et al., 2021) are associated with decreased

COVID-19 infection risk among staff. Dedicated staff spaces can mitigate the spread of COVID-19 through the facility (Vandoorn et al., 2021). Examples include separate break rooms, conference rooms, and laundry facilities separate from residential common areas. Dedicated areas for staff's on-site accommodation can help reduce the risk of virus transmission between the staff and the outside community (Wang, 2021). Reducing density in nurse stations (Olson & Albensi, 2021), using mobile workstations (Verdoorn et al., 2021), or decentralized nurse stations (Anderson et al., 2020), or adjusting staffing schedule (Ferdous, 2021a) to avoid crowding in nurse station was important to control the transmission of the virus among staff and between staff and residents. Regarding LTC workers' psychological distress, current approaches used to address mental health challenges focused on intuitional support and coping strategies. More efforts should be placed on exploring the role of the physical environment of LTCFs in mitigating staff stress and burnout and improving protection for staff safety.

## 3.5  Infection Control

SARS-CoV-2, the virus that causes COVID-19, is primarily transmitted by air droplets by means of the respiratory tract (CDC, 2021). It is imperative to establish infection controls in LTCFs and SH facilities to protect residents, staff, and visitors. Providing comprehensive infection control in senior living facilities requires multi-tier design strategies at the site, the building, and the room levels to keep COVID-19 from entering the facility, prevent COVID-19 from spreading in the facility, and manage infection and illness (Wang, 2021). Infection prevention and control strategies are summarized into five categories: hand hygiene, disinfection, social distancing, PPE (personnel protective equipment), and symptom screening (Telford et al., 2021). Empirical data suggests lower COVID-19 infection rates are associated with screening (Krone et al., 2021), social distancing (Telford et al., 2021), cohort isolation (Collison et al., 2020; Krone et al., 2021; Wang, 2021), and PPE (Simoni-Wastila et al., 2021; Telford et al., 2021). Contact limitation, daily monitoring of the staff's health conditions, and the usage of information and communication technology were effective in reducing the number of residents' visits to medical facilities without increasing the risk of emergencies (Ohta et al., 2021).

Another important aspect of infection control is indoor air quality. Dedicated air-conditioning systems by zones (contaminated, semi-clean, and clean zones) (Wang, 2021), decoupling thermal space conditioning from ventilation provision, and the application of packaged terminal air-conditioners (PACT) for resident rooms (Dietz et al., 2020) have been proposed as strategies to control the transmission of COVID-19 in the indoor environment. Low-dose far-UVC lighting was also proven effective to reduce SARS-CoV-2 aerosol transmissions (Buchan et al., 2020). Suggestions have been made to adapt strategies from negative-pressure isolation rooms in acute care facilities to convert existing LTC rooms to be negative-pressure by installing supplemental exhaust ventilation through dedicated exhaust portals, in order to reduce the potential for the spread of infectious airborne droplets into surrounding areas (Lynch & Goring, 2020).

Developing an LTC COVID-19 unit with dedicated physical space, personnel, and equipment can facilitate the conservation of PPE and reduce the risk of transmission (Verdoorn et al., 2021). Specific strategies to adapt the LTC space to be a COVID-19 unit include installing a negative-pressure air exchanger, physically separating the unit with a dedicated entrance/exit and anteroom for PPE donning/doffing (areas to safely put on/take off PPE), dedicated facilities (break room, conference room, laundry facility), and private rooms (Verdoorn et al., 2021).

## 3.6  The Physical Environment of LTC and Residents' Quality of Life (QoL) and Safety During and After the COVID-19 Pandemic

According to the World Health Organization (2007), special design considerations to improve QoL, access, and safety include pleasant and clean environments, green space, rest areas, age−/mobile-friendly pavements, safe pedestrian crossings, and walkways and cycle paths (World Health Organization, 2007). It has been argued that the current LTCFs do not support QoL of aging adults as facility design measures do not properly uphold infection control measures to protect a vulnerable population (Olson & Albensi, 2021).

Some studies proposed design strategies for LTCs to balance the resident QoL and safety. During the pandemic, Anderson and others (2020) proposed a framework for LTCFs at all scales: macro-scale to integrate with community resources (overall urban setting); meso-scale to provide an accessible, walkable, and activity-friendly neighborhood and public realm (neighborhoods and districts); and micro-scale to support both resident and staff safety and wellness needs (site/building design). Shepley and others (2021) offered a range of recommendations that include technology (touchless device and telemedicine), spatial territoriality at the site level, access to outdoor spaces, unit and room design and furnishing (e.g., small neighborhoods of resident clusters, private rooms, visit rooms, smart and flexible furniture arrangement, cleanable surfaces), air quality, and private food delivery. However, these two studies were mainly based on gray literature, best-practice publications, and expert opinions, as limited peer-reviewed publications and research evidence on senior living during COVID-19 were available at the time of publications.

Based on previous "dementia-friendly" design models and best-practice examples in the non-nursing community model and LTC nursing model, Olson and Albensi (2021) summarized several design features to support QoL, improve safety, and reduce stress for residents with dementia and staff. The design features include small cluster design, exposure to natural light, selective use of color and tonal contrast, access to outdoor spaces, using racetrack layout and centralized kitchen/dining/living area to support wayfinding, person-centered home-like design, spaces for recreational activities, indoor air quality and temperature control, and the use of technology. Ferdous (2021a) built upon existing evidence and proposed an interdisciplinary approach for redesigning memory care facilities in preparation for future pandemics, which included encouraging outdoor space and activities, dedensification of staff workspace and community space for residents' social activities, personalized interior and furniture layouts, and leveraging technology for video chats, social media, virtual reality technology, and telehealth.

## 4 Design Principles for LTCFS During and After the COVID-19 Pandemic

The literature review revealed the pandemic has fundamentally challenged the existing building typology, form, and environment of senior living and LTCFs. Issues regarding physical and mental health, wellness and healthy living, infection control, and pandemic resiliency are increasingly prominent. A safer and more resilient environment for older adults is warranted that takes into account these issues.

The literature review points to critical areas for prospective LTC design efforts that balance the needs for QoL and pandemic resilience while supporting the physical, social, and psychological well-being of older adults, families, and LTC staff. The evidence-based design strategies are summarized based on design goals to support key stakeholders' (residents, families and visitors, and staff) needs (Table 2).

## 5 Lessons Learned From Recent LTCF Design Trends

Recent trends of LTCF design provide alternative solutions for future LTC design. These design principles have characteristics that fulfill the aforementioned design goals. The following section details the design trends and conceptualization within urban contexts.

### 5.1 Intergenerational Community

There has been an increasing trend of shifting from age-restricted retirement communities to intergenerational communities in the past decade. The shift is a result of the demographic change and a growing understanding of the importance of intergenerational interactions on healthy aging. A growing body of evidence suggests each age group benefits when different generations come together. Older adults, children, and families share common needs and interests.

**Table 2** Evidence-based design features that support LTCF residents, families, visitors, and staff during and post-COVID-19

| Stakeholders | Design goals | Evidence-based design strategies |
| --- | --- | --- |
| Residents | Improve quality of life and support independence | Walkability and bike-ability of surrounding neighborhood Anderson et al. (2020) |
| | | Access to outdoor space Anderson et al. (2020), Ferdous (2021a), Olson and Albensi (2021) and Shepley et al. (2021) |
| | | Smaller unit with lower resident density and higher staffing ratio Olson and Albensi (2021) and Shepley et al. (2021) |
| | | Natural light Anderson et al. (2020), Olson and Albensi (2021) and Shepley et al. (2021) |
| | | Indoor air quality Anderson et al. (2020), Olson and Albensi (2021) and Shepley et al. (2021) |
| | | Private rooms with bathrooms Anderson et al. (2020), Ferdous (2021a), Olson and Albensi (2021) and Shepley et al. (2021) |
| | | Personalized and flexible interior and furniture layout Ferdous (2021a), Olson and Albensi (2021) and Shepley et al. (2021) |
| | | Spaces for recreational activities Ferdous (2021a) and Olson and Albensi (2021) |
| | | Leveraging on technology Ferdous (2021a), Olson and Albensi (2021) and Shepley et al. (2021) |
| | Mitigate social isolation and psychological distress | Telecommunication and virtual visits Arpacioglu et al. (2021), Bethell et al. (2021) and robotic companion pets Fogelson et al. (2021) |
| | | Safe in-person visits Arpacioglu et al. (2021) and Bethell et al. (2021) |
| | | Physical activities Bethell et al. (2021) and Curelaru et al. (2021) |
| | | Gardening either indoor or outdoor Bethell et al. (2021) and Farhana (2021b) or virtual reality immersive garden experience Hsieh et al. (2021) |
| | | Telehealth for behavioral and mental health therapies Curelaru et al. (2021) |
| | Infection control and prevention | Separate entry/exit Verdoorn et al. (2021), Wang (2021) and separate circulation Anderson et al. (2020) |
| | | Screening Telford et al. (2021) and Krone et al. (2021) |
| | | Smaller unit size Abrams et al. (2020), Costa et al. (2021), Ibrahim et al. (2021), Wang et al. (2021), White et al. (2020) and less density Brown et al. (2021), and Simoni-Wastila et al. (2021) |
| | | Single bedroom with dedicated bathroom Brown et al. (2021) and Ibrahim et al. (2021) |
| | | Cohort isolation Collison et al. (2020), Krone et al. (2021), Wang (2021) |
| | | Decentralized dining and social activity spaces Barnett and Grabowski (2020), Davidson and Szanton (2020) and Farhana (2021b)) |
| | | Social distancing in dining and social activity spaces Farhana (2021a) and Telford et al. (2021) |
| | | PPE storage and utilization Simoni-Wastila et al. (2021), Telford et al. (2021) and ante room for dedicated PPE donning/doffing area Verdoorn et al. (2021) |
| | | Hand hygiene Telford et al. (2021) |
| | | Indoor air quality control: Negative pressure rooms Lynch and Goring (2020), Verdoorn et al. (2021); dedicated air-conditioning system by zones Wang (2021) and separate air-conditioner for resident rooms Dietz et al. (2020) |
| | | Low dose far-UVC lighting to disinfect (Buchan et al., 2020) |

| | | |
|---|---|---|
| Families and visitors | Mitigate psychological distress | Telecommunication and virtual visits Monin et al. (2020) and Wammes et al. (2020) |
| | | Safe in-person visits Wammes et al. (2020) |
| | Infection control and prevention | Separate visitor area Wang (2021) |
| | | Safe indoor visits behind glass Wammes et al. (2020) |
| | | Outdoor contact while maintaining social distancing Wammes et al. (2020) |
| Staff | Mitigate psychological distress | Dedicated staff facilities such as break room, conference room, laundry facility Vandoorn et al. (2021) and onsite lodging and accommodation Wang (2021) |
| | Infection control and prevention | Smaller unit with lower resident density and higher staffing ratio |
| | | Reduce density in nurse station and staff work areas |
| | | Dedicated staff facilities such as break room, conference room, laundry facility Vandoorn et al. (2021), and on-site lodging and accommodation Wang (2021) |
| | | PPE storage and utilization Simoni-Wastila et al. (2021), Telford et al. 2021) and ante room for dedicated PPE donning/doffing area Verdoorn et al. (2021) |
| | | Hand hygiene Telford et al. (2021) |
| | | Indoor air quality control: Negative pressure rooms Lynch and Goring (2020), Verdoorn et al. (2021), dedicated air-conditioning system by zones Wang (2021) and separate air-conditioner for resident rooms Dietz et al. (2020) |

The key components of a community that the older adults strive for are the same components younger generations want: safe and walkable neighborhoods, acceptable transportation options, affordable housing options, and nearby services including childcare, senior centers, parks, grocery stores, and healthcare facilities (Ghazaleh et al., 2011). Intergenerational communities are inclusive and build on the positive resources that both young and old can offer (Hatton-Yeo and Ohsako, 2000). A systemic review of available literature found that intergenerational communities promote the physical and social health of older adults and extend throughout society (Zhong et al., 2020). There are multiple ways to achieve intergenerational community, such as creating shared sites (Jarrott & Bruni, 2007; Kuehen & Kaplan, 2001; Ruggiano, 2012), and/or intergenerational programs (Newman, 2014).

One example of integrating intergenerational activities in dense urban settings is the Clare Tower at Water Tower Place located in Chicago, Illinois, USA. The Clare is a 53-story building designed by Perkins and Will. It is one of the tallest buildings designed specifically for senior citizens in the USA. As a vertical CCRC, it stacked 326 units of skilled care, assisted living, independent living units, amenities, and their respective support functions within a uniform 12,600-square-foot floorplate. The strategic stacking of the building programs placed the higher acuity senior living units closer to the ground level while placing the independent living units on the highest levels. In addition to senior living, the Clare also includes 50,000 square feet of classroom space belonging to Loyola University Chicago. This connection with Loyola University provides residents an environment for continued development of the intellect, spirit, and skills essential to spiritual growth (Gosalia, n.d.). It also provides natural opportunities for intergenerational interactions with the local community.

The current pandemic presented some barriers to intergenerational connections. However, collocating different generations of residents in a vertical intergenerational community create opportunities to maintain visual connections between different age groups while physically separating older adults from others (e.g., through separate entry/exits, separate circulation paths, and separate floors). It also has the potential to provide safe outdoor areas for intergenerational interactions.

## 5.2 Small Household Model for the Home-Like Environment and Person-Centered Care

Creating a home-like environment in long-term care facilities is part of the major culture change movement that is transforming formerly institutional healthcare facilities into more person-centered homes offering long-term care (LTC) services. A study completed to understand how the quality of the built environment can impact QoL, and the sense of home of senior care residents identified four key themes that influence the sense of home – (1) physical view; (2) mobility and accessibility; (3) space, place, and personal belonging; and (4) the social environment and activities (Van Hoof et al., 2015). These characteristics help serve as a baseline to determine how residents individually perceive their surroundings. Additionally, through the study, residents reported appreciation for the ability to move around independently and that loss of mobility created a significant lack of freedom (Van Hoof et al., 2015). The study also revealed that having the ability to customize a space with personal belongings allows for residents to feel nostalgic and have a greater sense of home, as they have personalized their rooms with fond memories (Van Hoof et al., 2015). Lastly, having dedicated activity spaces for social activities engage residents with other residents, the care team, and visitors. The dining room is a space that residents find most crucial to creating a social environment (Van Hoof et al., 2015). These themes provide opportunities in improved LTC models that continue the shift toward less institutional and more home-like environments.

One emerging model that aims to create a comfortable and welcoming home-like environment for LTC residents is the Green House (GH) model (Ragsdale & McDougnall, 2008; Xu et al., 2013). The National Green House Project was established in 2002 to aid organizations in moving away from a medical model toward a social model of care in LTC settings (Ragsdale & McDougnall, 2008). The organizational structure of the GH Model is fundamentally different from traditional LTC models because these homes are small, self-contained, and self-sufficient with the residents at the center surrounded by a self-managed care team. Key attributes of the Green House model include designing spaces that remove the feeling of being institutionalized and instead focus on creating an environment that feels more like a home for residents. Each neighborhood has its own activity room and large common space facing toward the exterior of the building with outdoor views that bring natural sunlight. Through a person-centered care approach, the GH model emphasizes autonomy and intimacy through private rooms/bathrooms and the ability to move throughout shared, social areas freely (Li, 2021). Additionally, the introduction of green life and warmth in the GH model encourages social engagement and nurtures a sense of comfort. Traditional medical components such as medical signs and visible nurse care team stations are also concealed (Li, 2021).

One of the first examples of the application of the GH model in an urban context is the Leonard Florence Center for Living at the Chelsea Jewish Lifecare in Chelsea, MA. The facility featured five floors with two homes on every level, each including ten resident rooms with private bathrooms. Residents share a common living and dining space within the home and have access to a dedicated outdoor space. The living and dining spaces were positioned to allow natural daylighting through windows that created a connection between the private homes and the outdoors (Hodges, 2019). Integrating the GH model for Chelsea Jewish Lifecare residents was intended to allow residents to create a family-like bond within their homes as the units provide space for more communal activities. Hidden between each home, there is an area for staff care team functions, support spaces, and laundry. This provides staff the ability to aid residents without taking away their independence. Examples such as the Leonard Florence Center for Living demonstrate the success in implementing the GH model to improve resident and staff experience. It has been reported that design outcomes are linked to increased resident satisfaction, better staff rapport with residents, and less resident psychological distress (Hodges, 2019; Semuels,

2015). Studies in other similar GH projects also showed that GH helps improve residents' QoL (Cutler & Kane, 2009; Kane et al., 2007).

The GH model can not only provide higher resident satisfaction due to the positive correlation between resident experience and the home-like environment; it also may create increased opportunity for protection against COVID-19 or other infectious disease outbreaks. A recent study on 219 facilities across 43 organizations revealed that COVID-19 cases and mortality rates are less in GH model organizations than those in traditional senior care facilities (Zimmerman, et al., 2021). The differences might be due to the smaller unit size, better privacy, and more attention from staff in the small household model LTCFs than those in large facilities (Zimmerman, et al., 2021).

## 5.3   Biophilic Design

Biophilic design was formed to promote the integration of natural systems into the design (Gillis & Gatersleben, 2015). Biophilic design principles can be applied to create direct connections to natural systems through the use of natural light, air, water, plants, and natural landscapes. It can also be applied to create indirect connections that mimic natural systems, such as images of nature, natural materials and colors, simulating natural light and air, or evoking nature (Ryan et al., 2014).

The biophilia theory suggests that humans are genetically predisposed to be attracted to nature, and consequently this connection can lead people to be healthier and happier. Although the design philosophy primarily aims to create connections to nature, it also places emphasis on the experience of space and place, such as transitional spaces, organized complexity, and mobility and wayfinding. Evidence shows that biophilic environments, both natural and artificial, exert a healing effect on the human body and can improve QoL, human health, and well-being (Gillis & Gatersleben, 2015).

There is a growing interest in applying biophilic design in LTC and SH environments (Miller & Burton, 2020). An increased amount of natural light in the built environment has been shown to positively influence residents in LTC. Due to the extensive amount of time that people spend indoors, it is important to consider how light, both natural and artificial, is being used in the built environment to ensure that it supports the health and well-being of building occupants (White et al., 2013). Studies show that natural light can help to alleviate symptoms of depression and reduce stress, due to the link between light and the human circadian rhythm (White et al., 2013). Furthermore, residents may experience depression, difficulty sleeping, frequent daytime napping, and loss of cognitive abilities as a result of circadian disruption. An in-depth literature review has revealed the benefits of visual connection, non-visual connection, and non-rhythmic connection to nature for LTC residents (Peters & Verderber, 2021). Residents in LTCFs can benefit from bringing nature indoors, as physical impairments may limit their exposure and access to the outdoors.

Incorporating more opportunities for connections to nature can provide significant benefits to not only LTC residents' but also staff's physical and psychological well-being. One study used a quantitative approach and demonstrated the positive impacts of biophilic design features, such as daylight and greenery on workplace performance and staff well-being (Sanchez et al., 2018).

An example of incorporating biophilic design in dense urban settings is De Bouwmeester designed by LEVS Architecten located at the edge of the new Springer Park, in one of the renewal districts in Utrecht, the Netherlands. Completed in 2013, this building is a mixed-use, multigenerational building designed to meet the needs of its various residents as well as encourage interaction between resident groups. Starting at the ground level as a brick base, the form rises from two to seven stories around a spacious courtyard. Each level offers a space for a communal terrace with panoramic views of the surrounding city and nature. These outdoor spaces are key features of the design used for daylighting and improved health of residents. Residents in the facilities claim that the amount of green space is what attracted them to this facility and that the balconies make them feel as if they are sitting in the trees (Singhal, 2013). The programs are organized with more private spaces moving from the base of the building to the upper levels. The ground floor contains spaces such as the child daycare and communal courtyard, while the upper levels contain private residences. The ground floor provides access to the central courtyard via large glass doors. Here, meeting areas and spatial sight relations create a place where both, young and old, come together; protected. Together, the organic building form and the access and views of nature throughout the building help to create a facility that promotes community engagement and resident mental and physical well-being.

Biophilic design can be applied in LTCFs during and after the COVID-19 pandemic to mitigate psychological distress caused by social isolation and improve QoL. It can also enable opportunities for safe visitation and social interactions in outdoor spaces with physical distancing. Design strategies include designing spaces that provide multisensory connections to nature and landscape, natural ventilation, natural lighting, and more direct interior-exterior connections (Peters & Verderber, 2021).

These recent design trends/principles in LTCFs shed light on some innovative ideas to redesign these facilities to balance the needs for QoL and independence, mitigate social isolation and psychological distress, and manage infection control during the current and future pandemics (Fig. 1).

## 6 Translating Research to Design: An Urban Vertical Continuous Care Intergenerational Community Prototype Design

These design principles and strategies were further translated into a vertical continuous care intergenerational community (CCIC) prototype (Fig. 2). The project was a research-based graduate capstone studio project that intended to design a

**DESIGN GOALS**          **DESIGN TRENDS/PRINCIPLES**

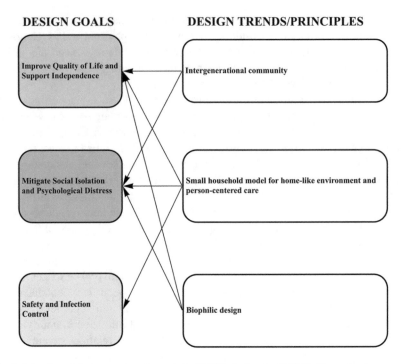

**Fig. 1** Mapping of design goals and trends for LTCFs during the COVID-19 pandemic

hypothetical prototype to provide a safer and more resilient environment for residents and staff post-COVID. The prototype was designed over a semester, by the second and third authors of the chapter, and guided by the first author, who was the instructor of the studio.

The proposed prototype is a visual illustration comprising evidence-based design solutions applied within a dense urban setting. The prototype design considered macro-, meso-, and micro-levels following the multi-tier framework (Anderson et al., 2020). The designers based their design decisions on findings from the secondary research on the best available evidence and best practices. The design received the 2021 Healthcare Environment Award Honorable Mention under the student work category.

## 6.1 Macro-level (Overall Urban Setting)

At the macro-level, the setting for this prototype is a dense urban location at the Hyde Park neighborhood in Chicago, directly across from the Chicago Museum of Science and Industry. It is along the Lake Michigan shoreline just a short distance from downtown Chicago and the University of Chicago. It is embedded in a mature

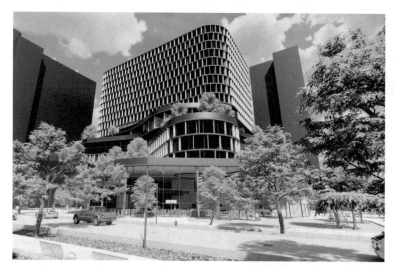

**Fig. 2** Exterior rendering of the vertical CCRC prototype design

neighborhood with natural potential for intergenerational activities. It has easy access to local resources such as healthcare and emergency services from the University of Chicago medical system.

## 6.2 Meso-level (Neighborhoods and Districts)

At the meso-level, the site provides access to a walkable and activity-friendly neighborhood. It offers easy access to the shoreline and green open spaces with pedestrian- and bike-friendly paths. In addition, its close proximity to public transportation supports the mobility of older adults. Moreover, the lower floors of the vertical CCIC are designed with shared programs that are open to the community in surrounding neighborhoods. The mixed-use retail and social programs integrate the CCIC with existing neighborhoods and create natural opportunities for intergenerational activities and interactions.

## 6.3 Micro-level (Site/Building)

The design principles and strategies we identified previously were applied throughout the site and building design.

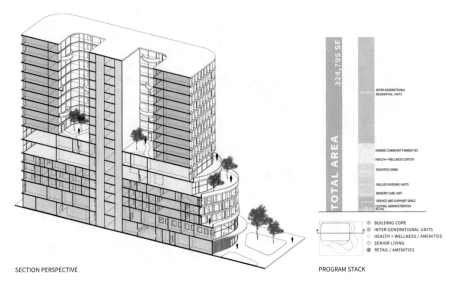

SECTION PERSPECTIVE                                    PROGRAM STACK

**Fig. 3** Sectional perspective and stack diagram of space programs of the vertical CCRC prototype

### 6.3.1 Intergenerational Programs and Amenities

This program includes one memory care unit with 24 rooms, 1 LTC unit with 24 rooms, 30 assisted living units, 170 intergenerational residential units, a health and wellness center, and other amenities such as a library, café, and daycare center into one building to serve both senior residents and the surrounding community. The facilities programs were strategically grouped together, which were stacked based on use and acuity levels (Fig. 3). Levels One and Two include retail space, community amenities, and administration. Levels Three, Four, and Five house LTC, memory care, and assisted living. Levels Six and Seven are the health and wellness center and more community amenities. The health and wellness center provides residents access to many different health amenities including a health clinic, a rehabilitation clinic, a telehealth space, a pool, and a 24-hour fitness studio. These two floors with shared amenities act as both the separator and connector between the senior care floors and intergenerational living units (Levels Eight through Eighteen). The integration of recreational activities, intergenerational programs, and healthcare prevention and management services aim to encourage spontaneity, community, and capability to address the three plagues of senior care environments: boredom, loneliness, and helplessness (Thomas, 2003).

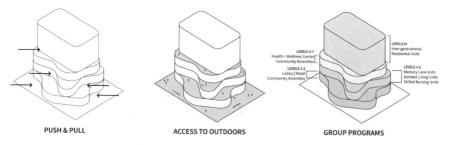

PUSH & PULL            ACCESS TO OUTDOORS            GROUP PROGRAMS

**Fig. 4** Parti diagrams of the vertical CCRC prototype to achieve a harmonious relationship between humans and nature

### 6.3.2 Biophilic Design

The key design concepts incorporated biophilic design throughout the building. The overall form of the building was designed to reflect a harmonious relationship between humans and nature. The building took its shape intending to maximize residents' view and access to nature, light, and the view of the Lake of Michigan (Fig. 4). The ground level of the building was shaped to become organic in form and maximize green space on the site. The building form was molded to create various outdoor terraces and encourage outdoor activities for different age groups and ability levels, beyond just residents. The two terraces on Level Three are dedicated to LTC and dementia unit residents. The terraces on Levels Six and Seven can be used for the public, family visitors, and residents. Level Six terraces provide opportunities for outdoor dining and family visits. There are two terraces on Level Seven: one is connected with the fitness center and can offer outdoor exercise space; the other one connected to a health café is a gardening area with planters.

Access to natural light is another important biophilic design feature incorporated in the design. Natural daylight floods through the two atriums located in the intergenerational residential towers, illuminating throughout the interior corridors. The connection between nature and natural light is emphasized in order to promote residents' and staff's physical and psychological well-being while decreasing buildings' total energy consumption. The atriums also contain small balconies on each level to provide residents fresh air and views of nature without having to travel far from their units. It was intended that these atriums would make impactful contributions to the social engagement of residents and to the overall natural aesthetic of the building.

### 6.3.3 Small Household Model

Each senior care floor was designed based on the evidence behind the GH model/ small household model (Fig. 5). Each floor comprises three neighborhoods, with each housing eight patient rooms, a staff and service space, a community den, and a shared central space for the living room, dining room, and care team stations. To

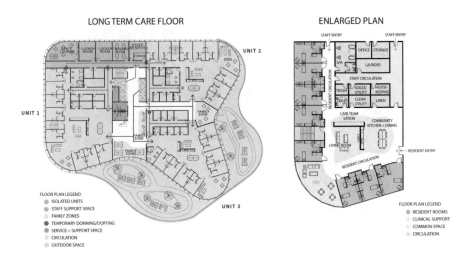

**Fig. 5** Typical LTC floor plan and enlarged plan for each household of the LTC unit

align with the design goal of building a sense of community, spontaneity, and capability, the center of the unit was designed with three sides. First, the kitchenette promotes community by allowing residents to eat and cook together. Next, the living room allows for spontaneity as residents may walk by and see what's on TV and decide if that is where they'd like to spend time. Lastly, the hidden care team station promotes capability by allowing residents to feel independent, while the care team remains co-located. The teamwork area is spacious to avoid crowding. The variety of different spaces will allow residents to choose how they want to spend their time outside of their private patient rooms. Moreover, two outdoor terraces are dedicated to LTC residents and staff on this floor to provide easy access to nature in a dense urban setting.

### 6.3.4 Multi-tier Infection Control and Pandemic-Resilient Design

To better prepare for future pandemics, special consideration was given to infection control and prevention. With consideration to different users, separate public and private entrances were created for privacy and safety. The staff has a separate entrance from both visitors and residents. The staff entry leads directly to the area of lockers for disinfection and hygiene and an area that can turn into a screening area during pandemics. Each small neighborhood within the senior care units could be isolated, if needed, to create cohort isolation and limit the spread of possible infection. Each neighborhood is equipped with a separate air-conditioning system that can turn it into a negative pressure zone. Within each neighborhood, there is a PPE storage space that can be converted into a donning and doffing zone to put on and remove PPE safely to reduce the risk of cross-contamination among different neighborhoods.

The layout also allows for separate circulation for residents and staff to prevent cross-contamination. All rooms are single occupancy with a dedicated bathroom to reduce the risk of infection among residents. Decentralized group activity areas with flexible furniture allow residents to continue small group activities with social distancing. Dedicated outdoor terraces for LTC residents offer not only opportunities for view and access to nature but also provide alternative settings for group dining, physical and social activities, as well as family visitation areas during pandemics to counter the effect of social isolation. Outside of each isolated unit, there are family zones to provide safe visitation without a guest having to enter the unit. Telecommunication and telemedicine technology are also applied to support social interaction and access to healthcare and behavioral health services. A private staff respite area is also included to promote staff health and well-being, both physically and mentally.

By maximizing access to nature, creating smaller neighborhood clusters, and including spaces that encourage social interactions, independence, and choice, the design aligns with proven evidence-based design principles and best practices that can lead to positive residents, family, and staff experiences.

## 7 Conclusions

As this chapter has demonstrated, the COVID-19 pandemic highlighted many challenges to older adults, especially those living in congregated senior living and LTC environments in dense urban settings. As the aging population continues to grow exponentially and the world recovers from the COVID-19 pandemic, the building typology and environment of senior living and LTCFs need to be rethought to better respond to the needs of a vulnerable population.

This chapter illustrates evidence-based innovative approaches for a pandemic-resilient environment within in a dense urban setting. An extensive review was conducted in the literature, evaluating experience of congregated senior living and care in the context of the COVID-19 pandemic using recent LTCF design trends. The trends intend to promote physical and mental wellness, community engagement, safe and efficient delivery of healthcare services, resiliency for future pandemics, and an intergenerational community that will lead to a positive resident, family, and staff experience. The recommendations can also be adapted to non-urban environments.

This chapter adds to the body of knowledge by summarizing the latest research evidence regarding LTCFs design to respond to the pandemic with a focus on the design of the built environment. This study can help provide the designers and decision-makers with both secondary research findings and visual examples to inform future designs to address the balance between QoL and pandemic-resilient LTCF design. More robust post-occupancy evaluations should be performed to evaluate the effectiveness of the design features described.

# References

Abrams, H. R., Loomer, L., Gandhi, A., & Grabowski, D. C. (2020). Characteristics of US nursing homes with COVID-19 cases. *Journal of the American Geriatrics Society, 68*(8), 1653–1656. https://doi.org/10.1111/jgs.16661

Agronin, M. E. (2020, November 10). *The impact of covid-19 on mental health in long-term care settings.* Psychiatric Times. Retrieved August 20, 2021, from https://www.psychiatrictimes. com/view/the-impact-of-covid-19-on-mental-health-in-long-term-care-settings

Anderson, D. C., Grey, T., Kennelly, S., & O'Neill, D. (2020). Nursing home design and COVID-19: Balancing infection control, quality of life, and resilience. *Journal of the American Medical Directors Association, 21*(11), 1519–1524. https://doi.org/10.1016/j.jamda.2020.09.005

Arpacioglu, S., Yalcin, M., Turkmenoglu, F., Unubol, B., & Celebi Cakiroglu, O. (2021). Mental health and factors related to life satisfaction in nursing home and community-dwelling older adults during COVID-19 pandemic in Turkey. *Psychogeriatrics, 21*(6), 881–891. https://doi. org/10.1111/psyg.12762

Banerjee, D. (2020). 'Age and ageism in COVID-19': Elderly mental health-care vulnerabilities and needs. *Asian Journal of Psychiatry, 51*, 102154.

Barnett, M. L., & Grabowski, D. C. (2020). NHs are ground zero for COVID-19 pandemic. *JAMA Health Forum, 1*(3), e200369–e200369. https://doi.org/10.1001/jamahealthforum.2020.0369

Bethell, J., Aelick, K., Babineau, J., Bretzlaff, M., Edwards, C., Gibson, J.-L., Colborne, D. H., Iaboni, A., Lender, D., Schon, D., & McGilton, K. S. (2021). Social connection in long-term care homes: A scoping review of published research on the mental health impacts and potential strategies during COVID-19. *Journal of the American Medical Directors Association, 22*(2), 228-+. https://doi.org/10.1016/j.jamda.2020.11.025

Brady, C., Fenton, C., Loughran, O., Hayes, B., Hennessy, M., Higgins, A., Leroi, I., Shanagher, D., & McLoughlin, D. M. (2021). Nursing home staff mental health during the Covid-19 pandemic in the Republic of Ireland. *International Journal of Geriatric Psychiatry.* https://doi. org/10.1002/gps.5648

Brown, K. A., Jones, A., Daneman, N., Chan, A. K., Schwartz, K. L., Garber, G. E., Costa, A. P., & Stall, N. M. (2021). Association between nursing home crowding and COVID-19 infection and mortality in Ontario, Canada. *Jama Internal Medicine, 181*(2), 229–236. https://doi. org/10.1001/jamainternmed.2020.6466

Buchan, A. G., Yang, L., & Atkinson, K. D. (2020). Predicting airborne coronavirus inactivation by far-UVC in populated rooms using a high-fidelity coupled radiation-CFD model. *Scientific Reports, 10*(1), 19659. https://doi.org/10.1038/s41598-020-76597-y

CDC. (2021). *Centers for disease control and prevention scientific brief: SARS-CoV-2 transmission.* Centers for Disease Control and Prevention Retrieved Janurary 2 from https:// www.cdc.gov/coronavirus/2019-ncov/science/science-briefs/sars-cov-2-transmission. html?CDC_AA_refVal=https%3A%2F%2Fwww.cdc.gov%2Fcoronavirus%2F2019- ncov%2Fscience%2Fscience-briefs%2Fscientific-brief-sars-cov-2.html

Chen, Y., & Feeley, T. H. (2014). Social support, social strain, loneliness, and well-being among older adults: An analysis of the health and retirement study. *Journal of Social and Personal Relationships, 31*(2), 141–161.

Collison, M., Beiting, K. J., Walker, J., Huisingh-Scheetz, M., Pisano, J., Chia, S., Marrs, R., Landon, E., Levine, S., & Gleason, L. J. (2020). Three-tiered COVID-19 cohorting strategy and implications for memory-care. *Journal of the American Medical Directors Association, 21*(11), 1560–1562. https://doi.org/10.1016/j.jamda.2020.09.001

Costa, A. P., Manis, D. R., Jones, A., Stall, N. M., Brown, K. A., Boscart, V., Castellino, A., Heckman, G. A., Hillmer, M. P., Ma, C., Pham, P., Rais, S., Sinha, S. K., & Poss, J. W. (2021). Risk factors for outbreaks of SARS-CoV-2 at retirement homes in Ontario, Canada: A population-level cohort study. *Canadian Medical Association Journal, 193*(25), E969–E977. https:// doi.org/10.1503/cmaj.202756-f

Courtin, E., & Knapp, M. (2017). Social isolation, loneliness and health in old age: A scoping review. *Health & Social Care in the Community, 25*(3), 799–812. https://doi.org/10.1111/hsc.12311

Curelaru, A., Marzolf, S. J., Provost, J.-C. K. G., & Zeon, H. H. H. (2021). Social isolation in dementia: The effects of COVID-19. *Journal for Nurse Practitioners, 17*(8), 950–953. https://doi.org/10.1016/j.nurpra.2021.05.002

Cutler, L. J., & Kane, R. A. (2009). Post-occupancy evaluation of a transformed nursing home: The first four green house® settings. *Journal of Housing for the Elderly, 23*(4), 304–334.

D'Adamo, H., Yoshikawa, T., & Ouslander, J. G. (2020). Coronavirus disease 2019 in geriatrics and long-term care: The ABCDs of COVID-19. *Journal of the American Geriatrics Society, 68*(5), 912–917.

Davidson, P. M., & Szanton, S. L. (2020). NHs and COVID-19: We can and should do better. *Journal of Clinical Nursing, 29*(15–16), 2758–2759. https://doi.org/10.1111/jocn.15297

Dietz, L., Horve, P. F., Coil, D. A., Fretz, M., Eisen, J. A., & Van Den Wymelenberg, K. (2020). 2019 novel coronavirus (COVID-19) pandemic: Built environment considerations to reduce transmission. *Msystems, 5*(2), e00245–e00220. https://escholarship.org/content/qt6136m08m/qt6136m08m.pdf?t=qak2tt

Ferdous, F. (2021a). Redesigning memory care in the COVID-19 era: Interdisciplinary spatial design interventions to minimize social isolation in older adults. *Journal of Aging & Social Policy, 33*(4–5), 555–569. https://doi.org/10.1080/08959420.2021.1924345

Ferdous, F. (2021b). Social distancing vs social interaction for older adults at long-term care facilities in the midst of the COVID-19 pandemic: A rapid review and synthesis of action plans. *Inquiry-the Journal of Health Care Organization Provision and Financing, 58*, 00469580211044287. https://doi.org/10.1177/00469580211044287

Fisher, E., Cardenas, L., Kieffer, E., & Larson, E. (2021). Reflections from the "forgotten front line": A qualitative study of factors affecting wellbeing among long-term care workers in New York City during the COVID-19 pandemic. *Geriatric Nursing, 42*(6), 1408–1414. https://doi.org/10.1016/j.gerinurse.2021.09.002

Fogelson, D. M., Rutledge, C., & Zimbro, K. S. (2021). The impact of robotic companion pets on depression and loneliness for older adults with dementia during the COVID-19 pandemic. *Journal of Holistic Nursing, 40*, 08980101211064605. https://doi.org/10.1177/08980101211064605

Ghazaleh, R. A., Greenhouse, E., Homsy, G. C., & Warner, M. (2011). *Using smart growth and universal design to link the needs of children and the aging population.*

Gillis, K., & Gatersleben, B. (2015). A review of psychological literature on the health and well-being benefits of biophilic design. *Buildings, 5*(3). https://doi.org/10.3390/buildings5030948

Gosalia, S. (n.d.). *Loyola University Chicago.* Introducing The Clare Corner: Community Relations: Loyola University Chicago. Retrieved August 20, 2021, from https://www.luc.edu/communityrelations/stories/archive/llnwtc/introducingtheclarecorner/

Greco, G. I., Noale, M., Trevisan, C., Zatti, G., Dalla Pozza, M., Lazzarin, M., Haxhiaj, L., Ramon, R., Imoscopi, A., Bellon, S., Maggi, S., & Sergi, G. (2021). Increase in frailty in nursing home survivors of coronavirus disease 2019: Comparison with noninfected residents. *Journal of the American Medical Directors Association, 22*(5), 943-+. https://doi.org/10.1016/j.jamda.2021.02.019

Hatton-Yeo, A., & Ohsako, T. (2000). *Intergenerational programmes: Public policy and research implications—An international perspective.*

Havaei, F., Smith, P., Oudyk, J., & Potter, G. G. (2021). The impact of the COVID-19 pandemic on mental health of nurses in British Columbia, Canada using trends analysis across three time points. *Annals of Epidemiology, 62*, 7–12. https://doi.org/10.1016/j.annepidem.2021.05.004

He, M., Li, Y., & Fang, F. (2020). Is there a link between nursing home reported quality and COVID-19 cases? Evidence from California skilled nursing facilities. *Journal of the American Medical Directors Association, 21*(7), 905–908. https://doi.org/10.1016/j.jamda.2020.06.016

Hodges, E. (2019, November 5). *Architecture with care*. DiMella Shaffer. Retrieved September 21, 2021, from https://www.dimellashaffer.com/blog/architecture-with-care/

Hsieh, C.-H., Chen, C.-M., Yang, J.-Y., Lin, Y.-J., Liao, M.-L., & Chueh, K.-H. (2021). The effects of immersive garden experience on the health care to elderly residents with mild-to-moderate cognitive impairment living in nursing homes after the COVID-19 pandemic. *Landscape and Ecological Engineering*. https://doi.org/10.1007/s11355-021-00480-9

Ibrahim, J. E., Li, Y., McKee, G., Eren, H., Brown, C., Aitken, G., & Pham, T. (2021). Characteristics of nursing homes associated with COVID-19 outbreaks and mortality among residents in Victoria, Australia. *Australasian Journal on Ageing, 40*(3), 283–292. https://doi.org/10.1111/ajag.12982

Jarrott, S. E., & Bruno, K. (2007). Shared site intergenerational programs: A case study. *Journal of Applied Gerontology, 26*(3), 239–257.

Kaelen, S., van den Boogaard, W., Pellecchia, U., Spiers, S., De Cramer, C., Demaegd, G., Fouqueray, E., Van den Bergh, R., Goublomme, S., Decroo, T., Quinet, M., Van Hoof, E., & Draguez, B. (2021). How to bring residents' psychosocial well-being to the heart of the fight against Covid-19 in Belgian NHs-A qualitative study. *PLoS One, 16*(3), e0249098–e0249098. https://doi.org/10.1371/journal.pone.0249098

Kane, R. A., Lum, T. Y., Cutler, L. J., Degenholtz, H. B., & Yu, T. C. (2007). Resident outcomes in small-house nursing homes: A longitudinal evaluation of the initial green house program. *Journal of the American Geriatrics Society, 55*(6), 832–839.

Kolakowski, H., Shepley, M. M., Valenzuela-Mendoza, E., & Ziebarth, N. R. (2021). How the COVID-19 pandemic will change workplaces, healthcare markets and healthy living: An overview and assessment. *Sustainability, 13*(18), 10096. https://doi.org/10.3390/su131810096

Krone, M., Noffz, A., Richter, E., Vogel, U., & Schwab, M. (2021). Control of a COVID-19 outbreak in a nursing home by general screening and cohort isolation in Germany, March to May 2020. *Eurosurveillance, 26*(1), 22–29, Article 2001365. https://doi.org/10.2807/1560-7917.Es.2021.26.1.2001365

Kuehne, V., & Kaplan, M. (2001). Evaluation and research on intergenerational shared site facilities and programs: What we know and what we need to learn. In *Generations United background paper. Project SHARE*. Generations United.

Lai, C.-C., Wang, J.-H., Ko, W.-C., Yen, M.-Y., Lu, M.-C., Lee, C.-M., & Hsueh, P.-R. (2020). COVID-19 in long-term care facilities: An upcoming threat that cannot be ignored. *Journal of Microbiology, Immunology, and Infection, 53*(3), 444.

Li, X. (2021). *Sustaining long-term care model: Green house experiences in COVID-19*. Retrieved October 15, 2021, from http://scrjournal.org/SCR Spring 2021/4_Green House Xiaoli Li.pdf

Li, Y., Temkin-Greener, H., Shan, G., & Cai, X. (2020). COVID-19 infections and deaths among connecticut nursing home residents: Facility correlates. *Journal of the American Geriatrics Society, 68*(9), 1899–1906. https://doi.org/10.1111/jgs.16689

Lynch, R. M., & Goring, R. (2020). Practical steps to improve air flow in long-term care resident rooms to reduce COVID-19 infection risk. *Journal of the American Medical Directors Association, 21*(7), 893–894. https://doi.org/10.1016/j.jamda.2020.04.001

Miller, E., & Burton, L. O. (2020). Redesigning aged care with a biophilic lens: A call to action. *Cities & Health*, 1–13. https://doi.org/10.1080/23748834.2020.1772557

Monin, J. K., Ali, T., Syed, S., Piechota, A., Lepore, M., Mourgues, C., Gaugler, J. E., Marottoli, R., & David, D. (2020). Family communication in long-term care during a pandemic: Lessons for enhancing emotional experiences. *American Journal of Geriatric Psychiatry, 28*(12), 1299–1307. https://doi.org/10.1016/j.jagp.2020.09.008

National Academies of Sciences, Engineering & Medicine. (2020). *Social isolation and loneliness in older adults: Opportunities for the health care system*. The National Academies Press. https://doi.org/10.17226/25663

Navarro Prados, A. B., Jimenez Garcia-Tizon, S., & Carlos Melendez, J. (2022). Sense of coherence and burnout in nursing home workers during the COVID-19 pandemic in Spain. *Health & Social Care in the Community, 30*(1), 244–252. https://doi.org/10.1111/hsc.13397

Newman, S. (2014). *Intergenerational programs: Past, present and future.* Taylor & Francis.

Noguchi, T., Kubo, Y., Hayashi, T., Tomiyama, N., Ochi, A., & Hayashi, H. (2021). Social isolation and self-reported cognitive decline among older adults in Japan: A longitudinal study in the COVID-19 pandemic. *Journal of the American Medical Directors Association, 22*(7), 1352. https://doi.org/10.1016/j.jamda.2021.05.015

O'Caoimh, R., O'Donovan, M. R., Monahan, M. P., Dalton O'Connor, C., Buckley, C., Kilty, C., Fitzgerald, S., Hartigan, I., & Cornally, N. (2020). Psychosocial impact of COVID-19 nursing home restrictions on visitors of residents with cognitive impairment: A cross-sectional study as part of the engaging remotely in care (ERiC) Project. *Frontiers in Psychiatry, 11*, 585373. https://doi.org/10.3389/fpsyt.2020.585373

Ohta, R., Ryu, Y., & Sano, C. (2021). Effects of implementation of infection control measures against COVID-19 on the condition of Japanese rural nursing homes. *International Journal of Environmental Research and Public Health, 18*(11), 5805. https://doi.org/10.3390/ijerph18115805

Olson, N. L., & Albensi, B. C. (2021). Dementia-friendly "design": Impact on COVID-19 death rates in long-term care facilities around the world. *Journal of Alzheimers Disease, 81*(2), 427–450. https://doi.org/10.3233/jad-210017

Paulin, E. (2020, September 3). *Is isolation killing america's NH residents?* AARP. Retrieved August 20, 2021, from https://www.aarp.org/caregiving/health/info-2020/covid-isolation-killing-nursing-home-residents.html

Pereiro, A. X., Dosil-Diaz, C., Mouriz-Corbelle, R., Pereira-Rodriguez, S., Nieto-Vieites, A., Pinazo-Hernandis, S., Pinazo-Clapes, C., & Facal, D. (2021). Impact of the COVID-19 lockdown on a long-term care facility: The role of social contact. *Brain Sciences, 11*(8), 986. https://doi.org/10.3390/brainsci11080986

Peters, T., & Verderber, S. (2021). Biophilic design strategies in long-term residential care environments for persons with dementia. *Journal of Aging and Environment*, 1–29. https://doi.org/10.1080/26892618.2021.1918815

Prins, M., Willemse, B., van der Velden, C., Pot, A. M., & van der Roest, H. (2021). Involvement, worries and loneliness of family caregivers of people with dementia during the COVID-19 visitor ban in long-term care facilities. *Geriatric Nursing, 42*(6), 1474–1480. https://doi.org/10.1016/j.gerinurse.2021.10.002

Ragsdale, V., & McDougall, G. J., Jr. (2008). The changing face of long-term care: Looking at the past decade. *Issues in Mental Health Nursing, 29*(9), 992–1001.

Ruggiano, N. (2012). Intergenerational shared sites: An examination of socio-physical environments and older adults' behavior. *Research on Aging, 34*(1), 34–55.

Ryan, C. O., Browning, W. D., Clancy, J. O., Andrews, S. L., & Kallianpurkar, N. B. (2014). Biophilic design patterns: Emerging nature-based parameters for health and well-being in the built environment. *ArchNet-IJAR: International Journal of Architectural Research, 8*(2), 62.

Ryskina, K. L., Yun, H., Wang, H., Chen, A. T., & Jung, H.-Y. (2021). Characteristics of nursing homes by COVID-19 cases among staff: March to august 2020. *Journal of the American Medical Directors Association, 22*(5), 960–965. https://doi.org/10.1016/j.jamda.2021.02.004

Sanchez, J. A., Ikaga, T., & Sanchez, S. V. (2018). Quantitative improvement in workplace performance through biophilic design: A pilot experiment case study. *Energy and Buildings, 177*, 316–328. https://doi.org/10.1016/j.enbuild.2018.07.065

Sarabia-Cobo, C., Perez, V., de Lorena, P., Hermosilla-Grijalbo, C., Saenz-Jalon, M., Fernandez-Rodriguez, A., & Alconero-Camarero, A. R. (2021). Experiences of geriatric nurses in nursing home settings across four countries in the face of the COVID-19 pandemic. *Journal of Advanced Nursing, 77*(2), 869–878. https://doi.org/10.1111/jan.14626

Semuels, A. (2015, April 21). *Building better nursing homes.* The Atlantic, Retrieved on Feburary 11, 2021, https://www.theatlantic.com/business/archive/2015/04/a-better-nursing-home-exists/390936/

Shepley, M. M., Kolakowski, H., Ziebarth, N., & Valenzuela-Mendoza, E. (2021). How COVID-19 will change health, hospitality and senior facility design. *Frontiers in Built Environment, 7*, 740903. https://doi.org/10.3389/fbuil.2021.740903

Simoni-Wastila, L., Wallem, A., Fleming, S. P., Le, T. T., Kepczynska, P., Yang, J., & Qato, D. M. (2021). Staffing and protective equipment access mitigated COVID-19 penetration and spread in US nursing homes during the third surge. *Journal of the American Medical Directors Association, 22*(12), 2504–2510. https://doi.org/10.1016/j.jamda.2021.09.0301525-8610

Singhal, S. (2013, November 20). *De Bouwmeester gives golden touch in Utrecht, the Netherlands by Levs Architecten.* ArchShowcase. Retrieved August 20, 2021, from https://www10.aeccafe.com/blogs/arch-showcase/2013/11/20/de-bouwmeester-gives-golden-touch-in-utrecht-the-netherlands-by-levs-architecten/

Telford, C. T., Bystrom, C., Fox, T., Holland, D. P., Wiggins-Benn, S., Mandani, A., McCloud, M., & Shah, S. (2021). COVID-19 infection prevention and control adherence in long-term care facilities, Atlanta, Georgia. *Journal of the American Geriatrics Society, 69*(3), 581–586. https://doi.org/10.1111/jgs.17001

The New York Times. (2021, June 1). https://www.nytimes.com/interactive/2020/us/coronavirus-nursing-homes.html

Thomas, W. H. (2003). Evolution of Eden. *Journal of Social Work in Long-Term Care, 2*(1–2), 141–157. https://doi.org/10.1300/J181v02n01_10

Van Hoof, J., Verhagen, M. M., Wouters, E. J. M., Marston, H. R., Rijnaard, M. D., & Janssen, B. M. (2015). Picture your NH: Exploring the sense of home of older residents through photography. *Journal of Aging Research, 2015*, 312931. https://doi.org/10.1155/2015/312931

Verbeek, H., Gerritsen, D. L., Backhaus, R., de Boer, B. S., Koopmans, R. T. C. M., & Hamers, J. P. H. (2020). Allowing visitors Back in the nursing home during the COVID-19 crisis: A Dutch national study into first experiences and impact on well-being. *Journal of the American Medical Directors Association, 21*(7), 900–904. https://doi.org/10.1016/j.jamda.2020.06.020

Verdoorn, B. P., Bartley, M. M., Baumbach, L. J., Chandra, A., McKenzie, K. M., De la Garza, M. M., Pellecer, D. E. S., Small, T. C., & Hanson, G. J. (2021). Design and implementation of a skilled nursing facility COVID-19 unit. *Journal of the American Medical Directors Association, 22*(5), 971–973. https://doi.org/10.1016/j.jamda.2021.02.001

Wammes, J. D., Kolk, D., van den Besselaar, J. H., MacNeil-Vroomen, J. L., Buurman-van Es, B. M., & van Rijn, M. (2020). Evaluating perspectives of relatives of nursing home residents on the nursing home visiting restrictions during the COVID-19 crisis: A Dutch cross-sectional survey study. *Journal of the American Medical Directors Association, 21*(12), 1746–1750. https://doi.org/10.1016/j.jamda.2020.09.031

Wang, Z. (2021). Use the environment to prevent and control COVID-19 in senior-living facilities: An analysis of the guidelines used in China. *Herd-Health Environments Research & Design Journal, 14*(1), 130–140, Article 1937586720953519. https://doi.org/10.1177/1937586720953519

Wang, X., Wilson, C., & Holmes, K. (2021). Role of nursing home quality on COVID-19 cases and deaths: Evidence from Florida nursing homes. *Journal of Gerontological Social Work, 64*(8), 885–901. https://doi.org/10.1080/01634372.2021.1950255

Welltower. (2017). *2017 aging in cities survey.* Aging In Cities Survey. Retrieved August 20, 2021, from http://agingincities.com/

White, M. D., Ancoli-Israel, S., & Wilson, R. R. (2013). Senior living environments: Evidence-based lighting design strategies. *HERD: Health Environments Research & Design Journal, 7*(1), 60–78. https://doi.org/10.1177/193758671300700106

White, E. M., Kosar, C. M., Feifer, R. A., Blackman, C., Gravenstein, S., Ouslander, J., & Mor, V. (2020). Variation in SARS-CoV-2 prevalence in US skilled nursing facilities. *Journal of the American Geriatrics Society, 68*(10), 2167–2173. https://doi.org/10.1111/jgs.16752

White, E. M., Wetle, T. F., Reddy, A., & Baier, R. R. (2021). Front-line nursing home staff experiences during the COVID-19 pandemic. *Journal of the American Medical Directors Association, 22*(1), 199–203. https://doi.org/10.1016/j.jamda.2020.11.022

Williams, C. S., Zheng, Q., White, A. J., Bengtsson, A. I., Shulman, E. T., Herzer, K. R., & Fleisher, L. A. (2021). The association of nursing home quality ratings and spread of COVID-19. *Journal of the American Geriatrics Society, 69*(8), 2070–2078. https://doi.org/10.1111/jgs.17309

World Health Organization. (2007). *Global age-friendly cities: A guide.* World Health Organization.

Xu, D., Kane, R. L., & Shamliyan, T. A. (2013). Effect of nursing home characteristics on residents' quality of life: A systematic review. *Archives of Gerontology and Geriatrics, 57*(2), 127–142.

Yang, FJ., & Aitken, N. (2021). People living in apartments and larger households were at higher risk of dying from COVID-19 during the first wave of the pandemic, government report catalogue. In *StanCan COVID-19: Data to insights for a better Canada, issued by Statistics Canada*, Retrieved on Sep. 25, 2021, https://publications.gc.ca/pub?id=9.898602&sl=0

Yeh, T.-C., Huang, H.-C., Yeh, T.-Y., Huang, W.-T., Huang, H.-C., Chang, Y.-M., & Chen, W. (2020). Family members' concerns about relatives in long-term care facilities: Acceptance of visiting restriction policy amid the COVID-19 pandemic. *Geriatrics & Gerontology International, 20*(10), 938–942. https://doi.org/10.1111/ggi.14022

Young, K. P., Kolcz, D. L., O'Sullivan, D. M., Ferrand, J., Fried, J., & Robinson, K. (2021). Health care workers' mental health and quality of life during COVID-19: Results from a mid-pandemic, National Survey. *Psychiatric Services (Washington, D.C.), 72*(2), 122–128. https://doi.org/10.1176/appi.ps.202000424

Zhong, S., Lee, C., Foster, M. J., & Bian, J. (2020). Intergenerational communities: A systematic literature review of intergenerational interactions and older adults' health-related outcomes. *Social Science & Medicine (1982), 264*, 113374. https://doi.org/10.1016/j.socscimed.2020.113374

Zhu, X., Lee, H., Sang, H., Muller, J., Yang, H., Lee, C., & Ory, M. (2021). Nursing home design and COVID-19: Implications of guidelines and regulation. *Journal of the American Medical Directors Association.* https://doi.org/10.1016/j.jamda.2021.12.026

Zimmerman, S., Dumond-Stryker, C., Tandan, M., Preisser, J. S., Wretman, C. J., Howell, A., & Ryan, S. (2021). Nontraditional small house NHs have fewer COVID-19 cases and deaths. *Journal of the American Medical Directors Association, 22*(3), 489–493. https://doi.org/10.1016/j.jamda.2021.01.069

# Realizing the Future of Intergenerational Environments for Aging Through Design Research

**Tama Duffy Day, Stella Donovan, Laura Latham, Tim Pittman, Sofia Song, and Nicholas Watkins**

## 1 Introduction

We are living in an age of increased longevity and vitality. It is projected that by 2050, 16% of the world's population will be 65 years old or over. This increase will represent more than a doubling of the individuals 65 or older—from 727 million in 2020 to 1.5 billion in 2050 (United Nations, 2020). Additionally, the number of adults 100 years of age or older will increase to 3.7 million by 2050 (Stepler, 2016). As countries around the world shift toward demographically older populations, rethinking how and where people will live and age presents an unprecedented opportunity to reimagine the later decades of the life course.

The Organisation for Economic Co-operation and Development finds that in its 38 member nations, 43.2% of adults aged 65 years or older live in cities. This older and urban population is at increased risk of mortality, depression, loss of autonomy, boredom, loneliness, and reduced quality-of-life and well-being because of current and popular living situations, such as long-term care institutions or living alone (Feng et al., 2016; Haugan et al., 2020). Given these findings and projections, it is essential to have a deeper understanding of older adults' experiences in urban environments. This imperative is the guiding principle behind Gensler's championing of intergenerational communities or communities that "provide opportunities for interaction, engagement, and support across more than two generations" (Cushing & van Vliet, 2018).

Gensler is a global architecture, design, and planning firm with 50 locations across Asia, Europ, Australia, the Middle East, and the Americas. Founded in 1965, the firm serves more than 3500 active clients in virtually every industry.

T. D. Day (✉) · S. Donovan · L. Latham · T. Pittman · S. Song · N. Watkins
Gensler, Washington, DC, USA
e-mail: Tama_DuffyDay@gensler.com; stella_donovan@gensler.com; laura_latham@gensler.com; Tim_pittman@gensler.com; sofia_song@gensler.com; nick_watkins@gensler.com

F. Ferdous, E. Roberts (eds.), *(Re)designing the Continuum of Care for Older Adults*, https://doi.org/10.1007/978-3-031-20970-3_18

337

Guided by determined optimism, we believe the power of design can spark positive change and create a future that promotes equity, resilience, and well-being for everyone. Within Gensler, the Gensler Research Institute consists of a global, collaborative network of researchers focused on a common goal: to generate new knowledge. The current chapter is an example of the Gensler Research Institute's design research process as illustrated with the development, validation, and application of a framework that addresses the needs of intergenerational communities for aging or the Boomtown framework. First, a systematic review of available literature found that intergenerational communities promote the physical and social health of older adults and extend further benefits throughout society (Zhong et al., 2020). With additional support through funding and programs, intergenerational communities can reduce housing costs and caregiver burnout while contributing to increases in social trust and connectivity (Suleman & Bhatia, 2021).

From the systematic review, the Boomtown framework was developed. The Boomtown framework is an intergenerational community model that outlines recommendations and targeted interventions for physical architecture; social architecture; and economics, and policy to promote longevity and connection among its residents (Duffy Day et al., 2019). Then, the Boomtown framework was further supported by Gensler's ongoing City Pulse Surveys, which have been used to test and validate the Boomtown framework with survey data from actual cities across the globe. A City Pulse Survey asks urban residents questions on how they interact with their environments. The results provide insights into the preferences and behaviors of a global dataset of adults aged 55 and over (Gensler Research Institute, 2020a, b). To conclude the chapter, three case studies are presented that demonstrate how age-friendly designs and interventions inspired by the Boomtown framework can apply to existing communities around the world.

## 2 The Boomtown Framework

Boomtown is a progressive community framework that integrates people and property types to sustain opportunities for individuals of all ages. Specifically, Boomtown is a place where neighbors leverage and expand intergenerational engagement within a mixed-use urban landscape—inclusive of age, gender, ability, cultural background, and economic status.

Boomtown's name is inspired by two sources. The research team first referenced the towns that had sprung up to support the new frontiers explored during the 1849 gold rush (Romich et al., 2016). The name also honors the generation of adults currently 57–75 years of age, colloquially known as Baby Boomers. Boomtown signals the new frontier or "fourth epidemiological shift" presented by the increased health and vitality of these older adults and a cultural revolution in attitudes toward aging (Olshansky & Ault, 1986; Aronson, 2019).

## 2.1 The Creation of the Boomtown Framework

Gensler's Boomtown framework culminated from 3 years of secondary and qualitative research, supported by Gensler's system of internal research grants. In the first year, we examined secondary resources on aging in communities and relevant project work for older adults. The team quickly identified that strong intergenerational connections promote the well-being, contributions, and mutual support of all age groups in a community (Suleman & Bhatia, 2021). In addition, the team conducted 11 expert interviews across industries ranging from real estate developers to healthcare practitioners. Finally, the team explored trends and policies in community development, health and wellness, and living and working environments for older adults. This was accomplished through partnerships with the Milken Institute's Center for the Future of Aging, a nonprofit think tank that "promotes healthy, productive, and purposeful aging" (Milken Institute, 2021).

In the second phase of the project, the team engaged thought leaders external to Gensler in a roundtable event in Washington, D.C. The experts included operators of communities for individuals aged 55 and over, venture capitalists, and representatives from Generations United and the American Association of Retired Persons (AARP). They considered obstacles to solutions that grow intergenerational communities. The three lenses through which the obstacles were viewed were physical place, social programming, and economics. Documentation collected from the event was synthesized into the Boomtown community framework.

In the final phase of the secondary and qualitative research, the research team expanded to include Gensler design teams in Los Angeles and Washington, D.C. The designers and design researchers incorporated the Boomtown framework into visualizations and conceptual designs based on actionable interventions for the communities of MacArthur Park (Los Angeles) and Ivy City (Washington, D.C.). Both communities were selected by the Milken Institute and Gensler as case studies because of their diversity, substantial building development, desire to improve community health conditions through urban design, and interest in growing intergenerational communities. The visioning harnessed compelling trends at the intersection of aging, urbanization, and inclusive economic development. The resulting renderings offer practical and intuitive guidelines for policymakers, municipal leaders, and urban innovators to apply an age-forward, comprehensive strategy within existing communities. Both conceptual designs demonstrate that by integrating existing infrastructure and human capital resources to an age cohort of adults aged 55 and over, cities may effectively navigate a world that is becoming more diverse and more economically stratified (Duffy Day et al., 2019).

## 2.2   The Elements of the Boomtown Framework

The Boomtown framework leverages solutions across three elements of community: physical architecture; social architecture and infrastructure; and community economics and policy. Integrated within these components of community are 6 subareas of focus. Please see Fig. 1 for an illustration of the Boomtown framework's three elements of community and additional details.

Within the Boomtown framework, physical architecture is defined as the design of the built environment, including urban planning, buildings of all scales, and

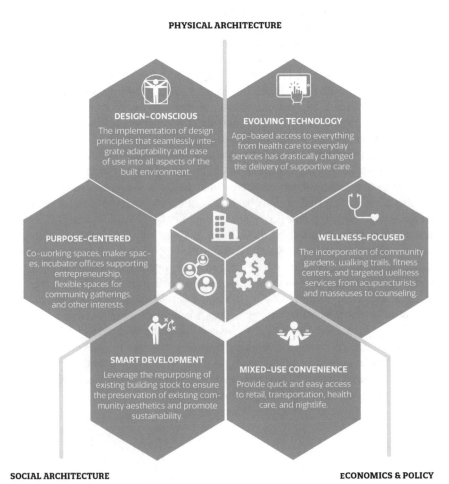

**Fig. 1** The Boomtown framework

interiors. Intentional approaches to the physical architecture of communities address issues that pose high risk to older adults' well-being and wellness, such as gentrification, displacement, homelessness, and climate change (Crewe, 2017; Gamble et al., 2013). Such design interventions allow adults over the age of 55 to live longer, and better, in their chosen environments.

Social architecture and infrastructure encompass the design of services and programs to support interactions across generations, cultures, and socioeconomic groups. Such considerations are vital as a recent survey revealed that 19% of older adults feel isolated some of the time. In addition, 22% report they lack companionship some of the time (Waite et al., 2019). Older adults who are socially isolated or lonely have increased risks of depression, Alzheimer's disease, and stroke (Donovan & Blazer, 2020).

Economics and policy address the regulations and financial structures affecting communities and housing, workforce development, and income inequality. Half of Americans over the age of 65 that live alone are unable to afford basic needs (Mutchler et al., 2019). For intergenerational communities to thrive, policies are needed that drive and support housing affordability, diverse housing options, regulations on new builds, home modification programs, and accessible urban environments. Additionally, policies that combat ageism/age discrimination in the workplace, provide flexible working arrangements, and offer opportunities for skills training are essential to ensure that adults have access to employment throughout the life course (Servat & Super, 2019).

## 2.3   The Subareas of the Boomtown Framework

Within the framework, there are six subareas of focus that drive the development of effective intergenerational communities.

### Design-Conscious Principles

The framework defines design-conscious principles as "the implementation of principles that seamlessly integrate adaptability and ease of use into all aspects of the built environment" (Duffy Day et al., 2019), such as the incorporation of universal and inclusive design principles. Universal design principles enable individuals to easily interact with their environments regardless of physical, sensory, and cognitive abilities (The Center for Universal Design, 2008). The principles promote mobility, accessibility, and neurodiversity—key issues that not only benefit older adults but are inclusive of individuals across generations. Eighty-seven percent of adults over the age of 65, and 71% of individuals aged 50–65 want to stay in their current home and community as they age (AARP Public Policy Institute, 2014). Construction using universal design principles creates new or retrofits existing building stock so that older adults can age in their current homes and communities (Carr et al., 2013).

**Wellness-Focused Community Design**
Within the Boomtown framework, wellness-focused community design is defined as "the incorporation of community gardens, walking trails, fitness centers, and targeted wellness services" within intergenerational communities. According to *Global Age-friendly Cities: A Guide*, outdoor environments "have a major impact on the mobility, independence, and quality of life of older people" (World Health Organization, 2007). Access to outdoor green spaces that are clean, well-maintained, and safe is an important contributor to well-being. Additionally, installing frequent places to rest throughout the community and maintaining age-friendly pavements are a universal benefit to all urban dwellers.

**Purpose-Centered Spaces**
The Boomtown framework defines purpose-centered spaces as "co-working spaces, maker spaces, incubator offices supporting entrepreneurship, flexible spaces for community gatherings, and other interests" (Duffy Day et al., 2019). Purpose-centered spaces support aging adults through opportunities to connect with others, such as intergenerational volunteer cohorts, continuing education programs, and work. Older adults successfully engage these opportunities to connect with others when they are available. For example, Age UK, the United Kingdom's largest charity for older adults, reports that nearly 4.9 million people aged 65 and over in England participate in volunteering or civic engagement (Agile Ageing Alliance, 2019). According to the Bureau of Labor Statistics, employment of US workers aged 65 or older has grown by 117% in a span of 20 years (Toossi & Torpey, 2017).

The development of hubs for volunteering, learning, and working across generations will ensure that cities benefit from their active and experienced aging populations while decreasing harmful levels of social isolation (Klinenberg, 2018). These hubs encourage services and programs that build social capital or "a collective asset in the form of shared norms, values, beliefs, trust, networks, social relations, and institutions that facilitate cooperation and collective action for mutual benefit around common interests, passions, and intentions" (Bhandari & Yasunobu, 2009).

**Mixed-Use Convenience**
The Boomtown framework defines mixed-use convenience as "quick and easy access to retail, transportation, healthcare, and nightlife" (Duffy Day et al., 2019). Being able to easily access a variety of care, service, and leisure activities within a close proximity has profound implications for physical health and social connectivity. Studies demonstrate that "older adults living in mixed-use, better connected, and more compact [neighborhoods] are more likely to be active as the walking distances between destinations and homes are shortened" (Chau & Jamei, 2021). Additionally, providing a wide variety of mobility and transportation options is key to helping older adults maintain their social lives. Older adults who are unable to drive or have stopped driving are three times less likely to socialize with friends and family and participate in social outings (Pristavec, 2016).

**Smart Development**

Within the Boomtown framework, smart development entails leveraging the "repurposing of existing building stock to ensure the preservation of existing community aesthetics and promote sustainability" (Duffy Day et al., 2019). In the United States alone, 49% of energy consumption is associated with the built environment (Architecture 2030, 2021). Reusing existing buildings can reduce their environmental impact by 46% (National Trust for Historic Preservation, 2011). Prioritizing building reuse and disassembly over new construction and demolition creates resilient and sustainable communities. This is critical for older adults, who are one of the populations most vulnerable to the effects of climate change (Gamble et al., 2013). Additionally, such community-focused development helps combat displacement and gentrification of existing communities that can result in a variety of adverse outcomes for older adults. These include homelessness; the loss of social networks; lack of access to affordable housing; and increased rates of cancer, diabetes, and cardiovascular disease, among other health issues (Crewe, 2017).

**Evolving Technology**

The Boomtown framework defines evolving technology as any advancement that has "drastically changed the delivery of supportive care" (Duffy Day et al., 2019). From app-based access to everyday services to the rise of telemedicine accelerated by the pandemic, the arrival of new technologies is constantly changing the landscape of care. For example, if current trends stay on pace, autonomous mobile robots (AMRs) will soon perform critical caregiving, delivery, security, and cleaning functions (Fragapane et al., 2021). Modifications such as slopes and ramps, non-slip flooring, levers that require little force to operate, and filmed glass that reduces glare can improve accessibility for people of all ages and abilities while also making environments more navigable for robots (Howard et al., 2020).

## 2.4 Processes and Partnerships

Intergenerational communities can boost social connectedness, increase generational empathy, and promote the well-being of all residents (Suleman & Bhatia, 2021). However, in current community planning, creating places that easily accommodate people of all ages and abilities is not always part of the planning process. There's an urgent need to explore innovative collaborations among experts in physical design, social programs, and policy.

To advance inclusive design processes and innovative collaborations, the Boomtown framework identifies three types of community champions that create momentum for intergenerational living: catalysts, partners, and individuals. Each category of champions was identified during the expert roundtable. Catalysts such as researchers, designers, and urban innovators must first see the urgency for intergenerational communities. Then they must engage partners—including policymakers, municipal leaders, and both not-for-profit and for-profit companies—who are willing to take calculated risks, spend money, and test and implement the new community model. Finally, individual residents like community leaders, local service providers, and local business owners must work toward the common goal of realizing and maintaining a healthy intergenerational community.

## 3   Testing the Boomtown Framework

It is essential that theories and frameworks represent the reality they explain. As part of its design research process, the Gensler Research Institute routinely tests and validates its frameworks with survey responses from actual respondents in urban communities. A recently conducted survey presented an ideal opportunity to test and validate the six subareas of the Boomtown framework with survey data from residents of ten cities. Launched February 2021, this City Pulse Survey of ten cities sought to measure the human experience relative to a city's physical, social, and economic environments (Gensler Research Institute, 2020a, b). Therefore, several of the questions on the survey address the three elements and six subareas of the Boomtown framework. The anonymous, panel-based surveys were conducted online and received 500 respondents per city. The ten cities were Atlanta, Austin, Denver, London, Mexico City, New York City, Paris, San Francisco, Shanghai, and Singapore. By focusing on a subset of the data – adults 57 years of age or older – the research team saw how older adults across the globe feel about a variety of important urban metrics.

Overall, the analyses of the survey data tested and elaborated on the six subareas of the Boomtown framework by identifying their corresponding latent constructs from exploratory and confirmatory factor analyses. Twenty-nine statistically acceptable latent variables emerged and serve as the basis for scores to compare international cities' performance on Boomtown framework criteria. Table 1 shares each latent variable within the context of its corresponding Boomtown subarea of focus.

In addition to those from the qualitative and secondary research, the survey findings for the six subareas of the Boomtown framework then helped inform two conceptual designs within the existing communities of Ivy City (Washington, D.C.) and MacArthur Park (Los Angeles, California) and an ongoing project in Lancaster, Pennsylvania. For illustrative purposes, findings for the Boomtown framework subarea of mixed-use convenience will be briefly discussed to share findings that helped inform the three case studies.

### 3.1   Results for Mixed-Use Convenience

Respondents 57 years of age or older prefer neighborhoods that are mostly residential with some mixed use. Their ideal neighborhood consists of buildings that have a wide variety of sizes and scales, vary in age, and consist of multiple design and

**Table 1** Latent variables and their corresponding subareas of focus

| Boomtown subareas of focus | Cities pulse survey 3 – latent variables |
|---|---|
| Design-conscious principles | Aging in place |
| | Inclusivity of neighborhood |
| | Navigability of neighborhood |
| | Post-pandemic comfort with activities |
| | Satisfaction with city transit |
| | Urban stressors |
| Purpose-centered spaces | Civic engagement |
| | Downtown vibrancy |
| | Financial stability |
| | Intent to move |
| | Neighborhood appeal |
| | Neighborhood community |
| Smart development | Climate change response by the City |
| | Not in my backyard (NIMBY) attitudes |
| | Prestige of neighborhood |
| | Quality of physical infrastructure |
| | Post-pandemic reclamation of the public realm |
| | Streetscape enhancements |
| Evolving technology | Hybrid worship |
| | Virtual entertainment after the pandemic |
| | Virtual routines after the pandemic |
| Mixed-use convenience | Access to city services |
| | Ease of running errands |
| | Important places for access in 20 minutes |
| Wellness-focused community design | Continuance of precautionary pandemic behaviors |
| | Growth of micromobility opportunities |
| | Neighborhood explorability |
| | Perceived safety through neighborhood characteristics |
| | Symptoms of anxiety and depression |

architectural styles. Green space is also important to them, as is having a mixture of retail, civic, and institutional buildings in their neighborhoods. When asked which amenities were the most important to have within a 20-minute walk: grocery stores, parks, and transit stops ranked within the top four choices for both US and non-US older adults.

That said, adults aged 57 years or older have limited access to these mixes of services and the purpose-driven opportunities that come with them. Case in point (refer to Latent Variables table 19.1), "Neighborhood Explorability" for individuals 57 years or older was the lowest among age groups. Their neighborhoods lack those spaces and activities that support having fun, relaxation, discovery, and connecting with others. "Civic Engagement in the Neighborhood" and access to community settings such as libraries and restaurants are limited for adults 57 years and older when compared to other age groups. Also, adults aged 57 or older are the least likely of any age group to participate in community planning decisions. The data shows they are the least likely of any age group to indicate that improvements to their city are intended for them. Altogether, this means that across the globe, adults 57 years of age or older are missing out on valuable opportunities to build social capital (Klinenberg, 2018).

Access to walkable communities and adequate public transit are two likely contributors to improved access. Adults 57 years of age and older are the least likely of any age group to feel that their neighborhoods prioritize people over cars. Across all cities, older adults want better public transit to be a priority. They are also the least likely to feel comfortable using mass transit, bikeshares, or rideshare services.

# 4    Applied Case Studies of the Boomtown Framework

The qualitative, secondary, and survey research in support of the Boomtown framework inform two conceptual designs within the existing communities of Ivy City (Washington, D.C.) and MacArthur Park (Los Angeles, California) and an ongoing project in Lancaster, Pennsylvania. These case studies emerged during the timeline of the research and apply the elements and subareas of the Boomtown framework across a variety of contexts and communities.

## 4.1   Mosaic via Willow Valley

Mosaic is located in Lancaster, Pennsylvania, one of the oldest towns of the United States. Surrounded by countryside, the 7 square miles of Downtown Lancaster act as a hub of modern life, featuring a convenience of mixed uses appealing to adults of all ages including fine dining, food tours, festivals, the Central Market, and boutique shopping (Fig. 2).

The mixed-use convenience of Downtown Lancaster allows Willow Valley to diversify its offerings for older adults to include an active, urban lifestyle. The infusion of older adults into the Downtown with Mosaic is intended to further activate the downtown community with thoughtful synergies; expand and elevate the highest standard of quality and life care; and catalyze development in downtown Lancaster. Grounded in Lancaster's traditions and revitalization of historical building structures, Mosaic's design concept is guided by nine Lancaster-inspired "muses" that guide both programmatic and aesthetic decisions: freedom, craftsmanship, nature, tradition, humility, connection, community, heritage, and bounty.

Mosaic's tower embodies the design conscious principles of the Boomtown framework. In total, there are 147 units, with sizes ranging from two to three bedrooms. Consistent with City Pulse Survey findings that older adults outside the United States are more satisfied with their multifamily living conditions versus their

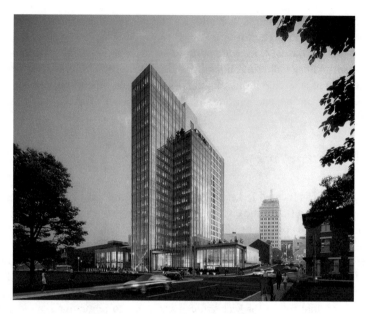

**Fig. 2** Mosaic via Willow Valley

US counterparts who are more likely to live alone and in single-family homes, units are designed with universal, adaptable, and multi-generational accommodations.

Every unit has floor-to-ceiling glass to take advantage of panoramic views and operable windows. A high volume of residences are designed as corner units to maximize daylight exposure and views of the downtown and greenery. Enhanced HVAC systems have MERV (or minimum efficiency reporting value) filtering that prevents the spread of fine particulates. Altogether, these features ensure a high standard of indoor environmental quality. Open kitchen/dining room layouts and barrier-free showers are universal design features that promote aging in place.

In addition to the wellness center on the premises, numerous outdoor amenity spaces and gardens connect the indoor experience to the outdoors, thereby promoting connectedness with others and the outdoors, physical activity, and independence. Specifically, three lobbies take advantage of existing street slopes to ensure secure and easy access for residents enjoying the city, meeting friends for lunch and a show, going for bike rides, or returning from dinner in town.

Mixed-use convenience is exemplified by accessible destinations for diverse interests and multiple age groups from the Lancaster community. The mix of communal amenities is housed in a two-floor podium scaled to the neighboring urban fabric and representative of smart development principles. A club lounge with a jazz bar, ballroom, plaza garden, fitness and wellness center, spa, and tower bar is public-facing and makes a 24/7 presence in the community. The ballroom is available for resident lectures, luncheons, reunions, and receptions and is also available to the public. Retail space will be occupied by a local French bakery and coffee shop, providing a taste of Lancaster's vibrant food scene. The mixed-use convenience is complemented by frictionless technologies and the security afforded by touch-free doorways and resident monitoring.

Of the mix of spaces, several are purpose-centered by supporting learning opportunities, community gathering, hobbies, and interests, and volunteering opportunities. These include a wine room, clinic, 50-seat theater, bike room, library, elevated dog run, chef's garden, and a professional kitchen suitable for cooking classes.

## 4.2 MacArthur Park

MacArthur Park is located in Los Angeles in one of the most populated immigrant and aging communities in the city. The area currently has 26 senior living facilities, but little affordable housing or Internet. Though the area has a diverse service-based economy, it largely relies on nonprofit organizations for age-friendly programs and services (Servat & Super, 2019). The conceptual design seeks to help residents of this community avoid displacement and homelessness as a result of gentrification, which is already being observed in nearby neighborhoods (Fig. 3).

The conceptual future for MacArthur Park seeks to reimagine how it serves its community by creating a hub that highlights the area's most valuable offerings: the people and cultures that share the space. By focusing on improving street safety, walkability, and community identity, the reimagined MacArthur Park seeks to improve its residents' health, access, and longevity.

The site currently adjoins a busy street with limited crosswalks. The conceptual design expands and widens the pedestrian walkway, using clearly marked pavement

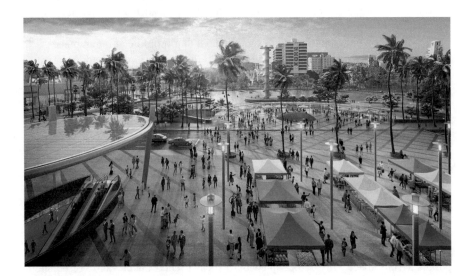

**Fig. 3** MacArthur Park

transitions for visitors. The intersections also use audible signals to alert pedestrians to the flow of the traffic.

The neighborhood is currently utilized by street vendors who sell their wares outside of the nearby transit system. The conceptual design supports these local businesses by creating a canopy system for the merchandise stalls and installing new lighting around the vendors. These well-lit structures create safe, accessible hubs for intergenerational interaction and engagement.

Aligning with the City Pulse Survey findings that many older adults feel their neighborhoods lack spaces that support fun, relaxation, and connection, the conceptual design for MacArthur Park includes ample space is provided for community-conscious programming of events and festivals to combat isolation and promote interaction across generations and cultures. Finally, the history and culture of the surrounding neighborhood are celebrated through design elements that honor the spirit of the area. A new tower in the community provides views of the surrounding city, providing an opportunity for placemaking and discovery.

## 4.3  Ivy City

Ivy City is located in Washington, D.C., situated on the New York Avenue corridor. Once home to thriving warehouse and manufacturing operations in the mid-twentieth century, the area now has a high level of poverty (Fig. 4).

The conceptual design for the future of Ivy City seeks to reimagine "spaces and programs to better meet residential, healthcare, and educational needs" (Servat & Super, 2019). This entails rethinking how existing space can be used to maximize the experience of community residents of all ages. Currently, a large amount of space in the community is allocated to industrial parking, making the creation of new city blocks for a variety of residential typologies a key priority (Duffy Day et al., 2019). By instituting vertical parking structures for industrial vehicles, the conceptual design creates space for affordable residential options that embrace the diversity of community members.

To provide purpose-centered spaces for older adults, the conceptual design consolidates industrial and municipal facilities to create hubs for healthcare, creative work environments, centralized public space, mixed-use residential, and education. Additionally, commercial space is created for co-working, maker spaces, and continued learning.

To foster wellness, a rooftop community garden creates spaces for shared affinities across generations. The design also revitalizes existing residential areas with green pocket parks; softens and buffers major adjacent highways and railyards with green space; and provides a centralized, easily accessible health and wellness center to promote healthy living. Ample public space is devoted to community programming with outdoor exercise equipment for all ages.

To foster civic and social engagement within the community, the conceptual design expands and revitalizes the historic Crummel School with a new extension

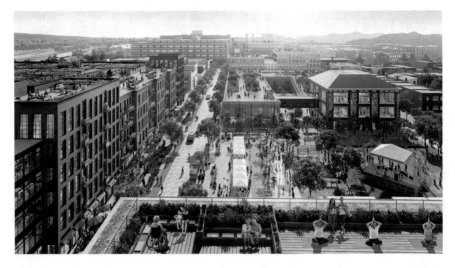

**Fig. 4** Ivy City

that connects directly to the community center. This is a crucial intervention, as findings from the City Pulse Survey reveal that many older adults feel that they lack opportunities for civic engagement in their neighborhoods and access to community settings. The survey also found that older adults value the ability to access a mixture of retail, civic, and institutional buildings within their neighborhood.

## 5    Conclusion

Aging is a universal reality. Traditional practices of relegating older adults to the periphery of communities in siloed, isolated institutions risk a variety of poor mental and physical health outcomes. As this chapter has demonstrated, communities that promote connection, health, and longevity benefit not only older adults but people of all generations and abilities (regardless of present or future care needs). By researching and designing age-inclusive communities, and prioritizing age-friendly design decisions at every phase of the planning and building process, we can help ensure an equitable future for every member of society.

## References

AARP Public Policy Institute. (2014). *What is livable? Community preferences of older adults.* Retrieved from https://www.aarp.org/content/dam/aarp/research/public_policy_institute/liv_com/2014/what-is-livable-report-AARP-ppi-liv-com.pdf

Agile Ageing Alliance. (2019). *Neighbourhoods of the future: Creating a brighter future for our older selves.* Retrieved from NeighbourhoodsoftheFuture2019_250119.pdf (agileageing.org)

Architecture 2030. (2021). *The 2030 challenge.* Retrieved from https://architecture2030.org/2030_challenges/2030-challenge/

Aronson, E. (2019). *Elderhood: Redefining aging, transforming medicine, Reimagining life.* Bloomsbury Publishing.

Bhandari, H., & Yasunobu, K. (2009). What is social capital? A comprehensive review of the concept. *Asian Journal of Social Science, 37*, 480–510. https://doi.org/10.1163/1568531

Carr, K., Weir, P. L., Azar, D., & Azar, N. R. (2013). Universal design: A step toward successful aging. *Journal of Aging Research, 2013*, 324624. https://doi.org/10.1155/2013/324624

Chau, H.-W., & Jamei, E. (2021). Age-friendly built environment. *Encyclopedia, 1*, 781–791. https://doi.org/10.3390/encyclopedia1030060

Crewe, S. E. (2017). Aging and gentrification: The urban experience. *Urban Social Work, 1*(1), 53–64.

Cushing, D. F., & van Vliet, W. (2018). Intergenerational communities as healthy places for meaningful engagement and interaction. In S. Punch, R. M. Vanderbeck, & T. Skelton (Eds.), *Families, intergenerationality, and peer group relations* (pp. 239–265). Springer.

Donovan, N. J., & Blazer, D. (2020). Social isolation and loneliness in older adults: Review and commentary of a National Academies Report. *The American Journal of Geriatric Psychiatry: Official Journal of the American Association for Geriatric Psychiatry, 28*(12), 1233–1244. https://doi.org/10.1016/j.jagp.2020.08.005

Duffy Day, T., Hampton, S., Hiatt, W., Latham, L., Lindahl, L. Sommerhalder, O., ... Zhou, D. (2019). *Designing intergenerational communities.* Retrieved from https://www.gensler.com/gri/designing-intergenerational-communities?q=designing%20intergenerational%20communities

Feng, Z., Falkingham, J., Liu, X., & Vlachantoni, A. (2016). Changes in living arrangements and mortality among older people in China. *SSM Population Health, 3*, 9–19. https://doi.org/10.1016/j.ssmph.2016.11.009

Fragapane, G., de Koster, R., Sgarbossa, F., & Strandhagen, J. O. (2021). Planning and control of autonomous mobile robots for intralogistics: Literature review and research agenda. *European Journal of Operational Research, 294*(2), 405–426. https://doi.org/10.1016/j.ejor.2021.01.019

Gamble, J. L., Hurley, B. J., Schultz, P. A., Jaglom, W. S., Krishnan, N., & Harris, M. (2013). Climate change and older Americans: State of the science. *Environmental Health Perspectives, 121*(1), 15–22.

Gensler Research Institute. (2020a). *Gensler research catalogue* (Vol. 3). ORO Editions.

Gensler Research Institute. (2020b). *Impact by design.* Gensler.

Haugan, G., Eide, W., André, B., Wu, V., Rinnan, E., Taasen, S., et al. (2020). Joy-of-life in cognitively intact nursing home patients: The impact of the nurse-patient interaction. *Scandinavian Journal of Caring Sciences, 35*, 208. https://doi.org/10.1111/scs.12836

Howard, A., Scheidt, N., Engels, N., Gonzalez, F., Shin, D., Rodriguez, M., & Brown, K. (2020). *"Excuse me, robot...": The rules of human-centric space in the 21st century.* Retrieved from https://www.gensler.com/gri/excuse-me-robot-the-rules-of-human-centric-space-in-the-21st?q=excuse%20me%20robot

Klinenberg, E. (2018). *Palaces for the people: How social infrastructure can help fight inequality, polarization, and the decline of civic life.* Crown.

Milken Institute. (2021). Retrieved from https://milkeninstitute.org/centers/center-for-the-future-of-aging

Mutchler, J., Li, Y., & Velasco Roldán, N. (2019). *Living below the line: Economic insecurity and older Americans, insecurity in the states 2019.* Center for Social and Demographic Research on Aging Publications.

National Trust for Historic Preservation. (2011). *The greenest building: Quantifying the environmental value of building reuse.* Retrieved from https://living-future.org/wp-content/uploads/2016/11/The_Greenest_Building.pdf

Olshansky, S. J., & Ault, A. B. (1986). The fourth stage of the epidemiologic transition: The age of delayed degenerative diseases. *The Milbank Quarterly, 64*(3), 355–391. https://doi.org/10.2307/3350025

Pristavec, T. (2016). Social participation in later years: The role of driving mobility. *The Journals of Gerontology Series B: Psychological Sciences and Social Sciences, 73*, gbw057. https://doi.org/10.1093/geronb/gbw057

Romich, E., Civittolo, D., & Bowen, N. (2016). *Characteristics of a Boomtown*. The Ohio State University. Retrieved from https://ohioline.osu.edu/factsheet/cdfs-sed-2

Servat, C., & Super, N. (2019). *Age-forward cities for 2030*. Retrieved from https://milkeninstitute.org/sites/default/files/reports-pdf/Age%20Forward%202030_FINAL_DIGITAL_WEB_Dec%202_0.pdf

Stepler, R. (2016). *World's centenarian population to grow eightfold by 2050*. Pew Research Center. Retrieved from https://www.pewresearch.org/fact-tank/2016/04/21/worlds-centenarian-population-projected-to-grow-eightfold-by-2050/

Suleman, R., & Bhatia, F. (2021). Intergenerational housing as a model for improving older-adult health. *BC Medical Journal, 63*(4), 171–173.

The Center for Universal Design. (2008). *Universal design history*. Retrieved from https://projects.ncsu.edu/ncsu/design/cud/about_ud/udhistory.htm

Toossi, M., & Torpey, E. (2017). *Older workers: Labor force trends and career options*. Retrieved from https://www.bls.gov/careeroutlook/2017/article/older-workers.htm

United Nations. (2020). *World population ageing 2020*. Retrieved from https://www.un.org/development/desa/pd/sites/www.un.org.development.desa.pd/files/undesa_pd-2020_world_population_ageing_highlights.pdf

Waite, L., Cagney, K., Dale, W., Hawkley, L., Huang, E., Lauderdale, D., ... Schumm, L. P. (2019). *National Social Life, health and aging project (NSHAP): Round 3, [United States], 2015–2016*.

World Health Organization. (2007). *Global Age-friendly Cities: A Guide*. Retrieved from https://www.who.int/ageing/publications/Global_age_friendly_cities_Guide_English.pdf

Zhong, S., Lee, C., Foster, M. J., & Bian, J. (2020). Intergenerational communities: A systematic literature review of intergenerational interactions and older adults' health-related outcomes. *Social Science & Medicine, 264*, 113374. https://doi.org/10.1016/j.socscimed.2020.113374

# Epilogue

**Keith Diaz Moore**

As this volume makes clear, for those living through the COVID-19 pandemic—with its economic shutdown, social isolation, racial tensions and senseless international aggression—it is hard to imagine the journey of lives being unchanged. This is particularly true for those in greatest precarity, including older adults. There is a general sense in the collection that the very designs purposely built for older adults were often unsatisfactory prior to COVID-19; but the issues of an airborne pandemic were actually exacerbated by these settings—congregate living with shared ventilation, affording low levels of privacy/isolation with low-SES staff likely to come and go from high-risk social networks—that proved to be perfect petri dishes for the spread of the virus. With this as a backdrop, reading through the preceding chapters, two themes keep recurring. First is an unmistakable proposition that place types for older adults will hybridize, fragment, and redefine themselves over the coming decades. Second is that the manner in which place-making occurs must become much more process-oriented.

## Place-Type Diversification

This volume presents chapters that go beyond home, assisted living and skilled care to discuss nascent and evolving place types such as adult foster care, rehabilitation clinics, and "last places," hospices. Each is discussed as a response to specific phenomenon of the aging experience and provides nuanced physical settings in response to them. This only begins to scratch at the surface of what is likely to emerge over the coming decades. The very premises in regard to both the opportunities of these

K. D. Moore
College of Architecture and Planning, School of Architecture, University of Utah, Salt Lake City, UT, USA

F. Ferdous, E. Roberts (eds.), *(Re)designing the Continuum of Care for Older Adults*, https://doi.org/10.1007/978-3-031-20970-3

various place types and their limitations will be questioned. The first two chapters raise the likelihood of the type of (dis)abilities likely to age successfully in the home to expand due to the "prosthesis" of evolving digital technology. What are the changes in both digital and human support that may enable the home environment to foster greater aging-in-place? With pandemic life, could we now possibly imagine a definition of aging-in-place that *does not* address digital technology as an essential component of what that term necessarily means?

Thus, home environments will be asked to afford a wider range of compensatory supports. The home will be considered as part of a care environment ecosystem or "environmental convoy" (c.f. Diaz Moore et.al., 2019) wherein the ability of the home's environmental convoy to provide social connectedness, meal assistance, medication delivery, and beyond will be essential. Social connectedness may be enhanced through more inclusively designed pathways but also through socially assistive robots (SARs). Meals and medications could be delivered by delivery robots at the command of a voice-activated assistive device. This would extend to more "care intensive" services such as the Acute Hospital at Home Program (AHHP) (Bishop et.al., this volume). As Bishop et al. (this volume) write, "the goal (is) to extend the time persons are able to age-in-place despite functional health impairment or physical disablement." Quite simply, over the next couple of decades, the expectations of home in the aging experience will continue to extend into the "assisted living" part of the continuum and thereby challenge the need for assisted living as a place type. How to provide the affordances necessary for such an extended expectation of aging-in-place, particularly through the renovation of existing housing stock, will prove an essential challenge. Concomitantly, what to do with existing assisted living facilities that may well become "white elephants" will be a pressing design question as well.

While skilled nursing facilities (SNFs) have often been viewed as the "bad guy" in the long-term care continuum, the intensive nature of care required by some older adults is quite real. But here, the challenge will be for SNFs to become smaller and more "assisted living-like" as found in smaller homes such as Green Houses. Equally so, SNFs will need to become more integrated into age-friendly communities to avoid the age segregation imposed by where such facilities are often zoned. This is not to say age-segregated communities will disappear, but they will become amenity communities that older adults actively seek out such segregation by choice such as in Sun City or the Villages. Age-integration will become the norm. The opportunity for creative adaptive re-use to meet the needs of an age-friendly society is not only real, but essential.

Lastly, Kader's (this volume) identification of hospice as "last places" and Greer and Diaz Moore's (this volume) mention of transitional housing for "housing precarious" older adults point to the likelihood of new place types emerging at the seams within our traditional continuum of long-term care. Greer and Diaz Moore cite Canham et al. (2021) who question the built in assumption that older adults will age-in-place at home, as some older adults do not have a home. Kader is at the other end of the continuum and finds intensive care environments anathema to dignified dying, raising the notion of the last place. Both challenge the closed system of places articulated by Oldenburg (1999) of first (home), second (work), and third places (social). Places will adopt new purposes and therefore emergent orientations. For instance, the acute hospital at home program moves acute care from a work-place to the home or from a second place to a first place. One could also imagine care settings, such as medical offices, becoming more hybrid. Why wait in a waiting room when you could be called in from the neighborhood café a level down? This begins to have implications for greater granularity and agility to land use zoning than is typically found. The opportunities for innovation in geriatric-capable set-tings are simply enormous.

## Placemaking as Process

As exciting as these new purposes and therefore new places will be, we must not overlook a powerful and essential second theme found in the volume: that our approach to placemaking for older adults needs radical reconsideration. There is an intrinsic critique of our current long-term continuum in that much of it deprives older adults of their personhood. Certainly the concept of "person-centered care" is replete throughout the collection, but interestingly so is the follow-on concept of co-design. Whether spoken of directly as co-design, as in chapters "Bridging the Digital Divide: Smart Aging-in-Place and the Future of Gerontology", "The Home as a Place for Rehabilitation After Stroke: Emerging Empirical Findings", or "Autonomy, Identity, and Design in the COVID-19 Era", addressing it in alternative terms such as participatory design as in chapters "Adult Family Care: A Homelike Environment for Community-Based Care" and "A Theory of Creating *At-Homeness* Across the Long-Term Care Continuum", or presenting such models as in chapters "Designing for Dementia: An Approach that Works for Everyone", "Adaptive Reuse of Closed Malls for Dementia Programs and Services: Community Focus Group Feedback", and "Creating a Tailored Approach: The Transformation of Jewish Senior Life", it is quite clear that the authors as a collective find traditional architec-tural practice as wanting in terms of providing places for older adults in which they may thrive.

There is a current zeitgeist to this in the architectural community that can find parallels in the evolution of accessibility toward inclusive design. Design for acces-sibility, or barrier-free design, is the provision of environmental elements that enable people of varying abilities to access the building—ramps and elevators being ubiq-uitous examples. This, unfortunately, results in a "two-class" system; one set of environmental experiences for those without disabilities that differs from a set of solutions for those with disabilities. Recently, Maisel et al. (2018) provided a useful advance by recognizing that truly inclusive design only occurs when it is central within and at the origin of the design process. In their words, they offer "a view of inclusive design *as a process*, rather than as an end product or feature….The aim of inclusive design, seen through this lens, then, is to identify and refine architectural ways of thinking and working that improve the self-efficacy and self-actualization of all building occupants" (Maisel et al., 2018: 4). As expressed in the various chapters identified above, co-design is characterized by wider participation of people with divergent life experiences, knowledge bases, and perspectives in the design process, beginning with problem identification. A careful reading of these chapters suggests a need to reconceptualize the process of architectural design in order to better further self-efficacy for all.

Finally, this collection, focused on the question of redesigning long-term care settings, provides a useful list of contemporary exemplars that all in the field should now view as the baseline and not the aspiration of design for older adults. Clear touchstones include Woodside Place, the Green House in Tupelo, Mississippi, the Hogeweyk Dementia Village in the Netherlands, Park Homes in Kansas, and perhaps now Jewish Senior Life in New York. As wonderful as these projects are, there is not a one that rises to all the opportunities outlined in this collection of thought-provoking chapters.

Still what these exemplars had suggested for long-term care settings for the past 30 years—smaller-scale, private rooms, more socially integrated into age-friendly neighborhoods, "dementia-capable"—all would have lessened the toll COVID-19 took on older adults in long-term care and their families and friends. While perhaps not suggested for those reasons, as is often the case, good design must simply not be compromised as the purposes inclusive design principles accomplish are not singular in nature but rather are multi-valent, "bundled hypotheses." The coming decades will provide ample opportunities for innovation to recast long-term care as not something to ostracize on the outskirts of town, but may well be the catalyst for creating inclusive, resilient, enabling places—ones that promote health, productivity, and social connectivity for all of us.

March 11, 2022

# References

Bishop, A. J., Sheng, W., Carlson, B. W., & Firdausya Jones, N. (this volume). The evolution and rise of robotic health assistants: The new human-machine frontier of geriatric home care. In F. Ferdous & E. Roberts (Eds.), *(Re)designing the continuum of care for older adults: The future of long-term care settings*. Springer.

Canham, S. L., Humphries, J., Moore, P., Burns, V., & Mahmood, A. (2021). Shelter/housing options, supports and interventions for older people experiencing homelessness. *Ageing and Society, 42*(11), 2615–2641. https://doi.org/10.1017/S0144686X21000234

Diaz Moore, K., Garcia, I., & Kim, J. Y. (2019). Healthy places and the social life of older adults. In L. Kane & C. Singer (Eds.), *Social isolation of older adults: Strategies to bolster health and well-being* (pp. 103–118). Springer.

Greer, V., & Diaz Moore, K. (this volume). Autonomy, identity and design in the COVID-19 era. In F. Ferdous & E. Roberts (Eds.), *(Re)designing the continuum of care for older adults: The future of long-term care settings*. Springer.

Kader, S. (this volume). Designing the post-pandemic hospice environment: "The Last Place". In F. Ferdous & E. Roberts (Eds.), *(Re)designing the continuum of care for older adults: The future of long-term care settings*. Springer.

Maisel, J., Steinfeld, E., Basnak, M., Smith, K., & Tauke, B. (2018). *Inclusive design: implementation and evaluation*. Routledge.

Oldenburg, R. (1999). *The great good place: cafés, coffee shops, bookstores, bars, hair salons, and other hangouts at the heart of a community*. Marlowe.

# Index